Mobile Phone and Internet Addiction: Risk Factors, Assessment and Treatment

Mobile Phone and Internet Addiction: Risk Factors, Assessment and Treatment

Editor: Henry Taylor

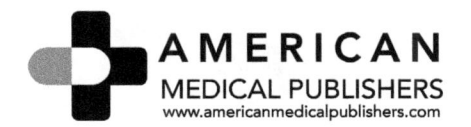

AMERICAN MEDICAL PUBLISHERS
www.americanmedicalpublishers.com

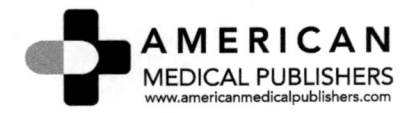

AMERICAN
MEDICAL PUBLISHERS
www.americanmedicalpublishers.com

Cataloging-in-Publication Data

Mobile phone and internet addiction : risk factors, assessment and treatment / edited by Henry Taylor.
   p. cm.
Includes bibliographical references and index.
ISBN 979-8-88740-271-0
1. Nomophobia. 2. Cell phones--Psychological aspects. 3. Internet addiction. 4. Digital media--Psychological aspects.
5. Compulsive behavior--Risk assessment. 6. Compulsive behavior--Diagnosis. 7. Compulsive behavior--Treatment.
8. Psychiatry. I. Taylor, Henry.
RC552.N66 M633 2023
616.858 4--dc23

American Medical Publishers,
41 Flatbush Avenue,
1st Floor, New York,
NY 11217, USA

ISBN 979-8-88740-271-0 (Hardback)

Contents

Preface

I am honored to present to you this unique book which encompasses the most up-to-date data in the field. I was extremely pleased to get this opportunity of editing the work of experts from across the globe. I have also written papers in this field and researched the various aspects revolving around the progress of the discipline. I have tried to unify my knowledge along with that of stalwarts from every corner of the world, to produce a text which not only benefits the readers but also facilitates the growth of the field.

Mobile phone addiction is the obsessive use of a mobile phone that negatively affects the physical and mental health of a person. The main cause of mobile phone addiction is internet addiction disorder in which the technology purposely keeps its users engaged through various applications and games. Emotional regulation and depression are the risk factors associated with the addiction of internet and smart phones. Chronic phone usage leads to conditions, such as GABA dysfunction, decrease in grey matter in the brain and depression. There are several methods of treating addiction to mobile phone and internet, which include counseling, group therapy, group support, cognitive-behavioral therapy, psychotherapy, motivational interviewing and medication-assisted treatment. This book examines the risk factors of mobile phone and internet addiction along with its assessment and treatment methods. Researchers and students actively engaged in this field will find it full of crucial and unexplored concepts.

Finally, I would like to thank all the contributing authors for their valuable time and contributions. This book would not have been possible without their efforts. I would also like to thank my friends and family for their constant support.

Editor

Long-Term Symptoms of Mobile Phone Use on Mobile Phone Addiction and Depression Among Korean Adolescents

So-Young Park [1]🄳, **Sonam Yang** [2], **Chang-Sik Shin** [3], **Hyunseok Jang** [2] **and So-Youn Park** [2,*]

[1] Ewha Institute for Age Integration Research, Ewha Womans University, 52, Ewhayeodae-gil, Seodaemun-gu, Seoul 03760, Korea; syp279@gmail.com

[2] Kyonggi University, San 94-6, Iui-dong, Yeongtong-gu, Suwon, Kyonggi-do 16227, Korea; snyang@kyonggi.ac.kr (S.Y.); hsjang@kyonggi.ac.kr (H.J.)

[3] Daejeon University, 62, Daehak-ro, Dong-gu, Daejeon 34520, Korea; csshin@dju.kr

* Correspondence: spark831@gmail.com

Abstract: This study aimed to compare the mean scores of mobile phone use, mobile phone addiction, and depressive symptoms at three-time points among Korean adolescents according to gender and to examine the differences in the long-term relationships among the three abovementioned variables between Korean boys and girls in a four-year period. Data for 1794 adolescents (897 boys and 897 girls) were obtained from three waves of the second panel of the Korean Children and Youth Panel Survey. Multigroup structural equation modeling was used for data analyses. The study findings showed that at each of the three-time points, Korean girls tended to use their mobile phones more frequently and were at a higher risk of mobile phone addiction and depressive symptoms than Korean boys. Significant changes were observed in the longitudinal relationships among phone use, mobile phone addiction, and depressive symptoms in Korean adolescents across time periods, but no gender differences were found in the strengths of these relationships. These findings contribute to expanding the knowledge base of mobile phone addiction and depressive symptoms among Korean adolescents.

Keywords: mobile phone use; mobile phone addiction; depression; Korean adolescents

1. Introduction

Today's adolescents are generally considered as the digital generation [1]. They have grown up using mobile phones, which have become an important part of their life and have reshaped their social life and behavior. Although mobile phones have many advantages such as the convenience of searching information, researchers have expressed concern regarding the potential negative effects of problematic mobile phone use, such as depression, anxiety, sleep disturbance, technostress, and poor academic performance [2,3]. In this regard, Korean adolescents have been found to be at considerable risk of mobile phone addiction. A recent national survey in South Korea in 2018 revealed that 29.3% of adolescents were dependent on mobile phones [4].

Various terms have been used to describe varying degrees of potential problems related to uncontrolled mobile phone use; the terms of problematic mobile phone use [5], mobile phone dependence [6], and mobile phone addiction [7] are used interchangeably. Although researchers have not reached a consensus regarding the definition of mobile phone addiction, potential indicators of mobile phone addiction include preoccupation with one's mobile phone, conflicts with one's family members resulting from the excessive use of the mobile phone, use of the mobile phone to handle changes in mood, and feeling of unease when mobile phone use is inhibited [7].

Researchers have identified gender differences in mobile phone use and mobile phone addiction [1,6,8]. Several studies have reported that female youth are likely to spend more time on their mobile phones than male youth [6,8], suggesting that females are potentially more vulnerable to mobile phone addiction than males [8]. In addition, gender differences have been found in the patterns of mobile phone usage. For example, female adolescents tend to use their mobile phones for text messaging, social media, for playing online games and for other forms of entertainment [6,8].

As regards the association between problematic mobile phone addiction and mental health issues, mobile phone addiction is consistently linked to depression [9]. Behavioral addiction such as internet addiction and mobile phone addiction during adolescence can be understood with a developmental psychopathology framework [10]. Adolescents go through the rapid development of emotional, social, and psychological changes, and, in particular, impulsive tendency is demonstrated during this time. Such impulsive behavior of the adolescent is intensified if the self-control is limited. This adolescent's limited ability for self-control may be more vulnerable and susceptible to addictive behavior [11].

Most cross-sectional studies on mobile phone addiction have yielded inconclusive findings, but a few longitudinal studies have shown a bidirectional association between mobile phone addiction and depression [12,13]. For instance, Jun [12] investigated reciprocal effects between mobile phone addiction and depression using autoregressive cross-lagged modeling and determined the bidirectional associations between mobile phone addiction and depression over time. Specifically, significant reciprocal relationships were found over a period of three years, and both mobile phone addiction and depression became severe with time. On the other hand, Coyne Stockdale, and Summers [14] tested a bidirectional longitudinal model representing the relationship between depression and problematic mobile phone use and did not find any bidirectional relationship between them.

Considering these mixed findings on the directional relationships between mobile phone addiction and depression, we aimed to fill the gaps found in previous studies in a number of ways. In particular, the present study expanded on the earlier study by Jun [12], which showed the reciprocal association between mobile phone addiction and depression using the same Korean Children and Youth Panel Survey (KCYPS) data. First, this study included mobile phone use data, which were not included in Jun's study [12], and examined the longitudinal associations among mobile phone use, mobile phone addiction, and depression. Several studies have found relationships between the frequency or duration of mobile phone use and mobile phone addiction [15,16], suggesting that an increase in mobile phone use causes mobile phone addiction. Second, the present study incorporated important factors related to family (i.e., parents' education and income) and school (i.e., academic activity and relationships with peers), which were not controlled in Jun's study [12]. Jun [12] mentioned that one of the limitations of his study was that it did not include relevant variables associated with mobile phone addiction and depressive symptoms. Third, considering that several studies found gender differences in various relationships, this study further investigated the role of gender in the longitudinal relationships among mobile phone use, mobile phone addiction, and depression in Korean youth.

Therefore, the purposes of this study were as follows: (1) to compare differences between Korean boys and girls regarding the mean scores of mobile phone use, mobile phone addiction, and depression across three time points, and (2) to investigate gender differences in the longitudinal relationships among mobile phone use, mobile phone addiction, and depression across different time periods.

2. Present Study

The structural model used in this study is displayed in Figure 1. The hypotheses are as follow:

Hypothesis 1 (H1). *The mean values of mobile phone use, mobile phone addiction, and depression for Korean girls will be higher than those for Korean boys in the second year of middle school (Time 1), first year of high school (Time 2), and third year of high school (Time 3).*

Hypothesis 2 (H2). *The longitudinal relationships among mobile phone use, mobile phone addiction, and depression will change from Time 1 to Time 3, and the strengths of these changes will differ between Korean boys and girls.*

H2a. There will be contemporaneous effects of mobile phone use on mobile phone addiction at each time point (Path a, Path b, and Path c).

H2b. There will be first-order autoregressive effects of mobile phone use (Paths d and e), mobile phone addiction (Path f and Path g), and depression (Path h and Path i) across time periods.

H2c. There will be second-order autoregressive effects of mobile phone use, mobile phone addiction, and depression (Path j, Path k, and Path l) from Time 1 to Time 3.

H2d. There will be cross-lagged effects between mobile phone use and mobile phone addiction (Path m, Path n, Path o, and Path p) and between mobile phone addiction and depression (Path q, Path r, Path s, and Path t) across time periods.

H2e. There will be bidirectional relationships between mobile phone addiction and depression at each time point (Path u, Path v, and Path w).

H2f. There will be gender differences in the hypotheses (H2a~H2e) stated previously.

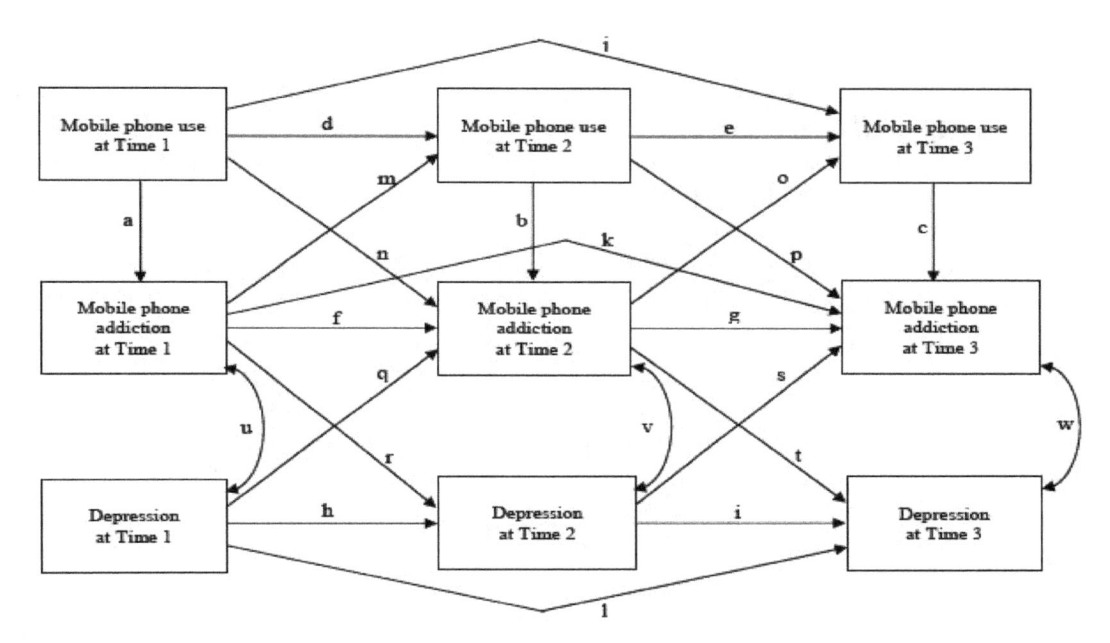

Figure 1. Structural model.

3. Materials and Methods

3.1. Data Source and Sample

This study used the second panel of the KCYPS data collected by the National Youth Policy Institute (www.nypi.re.kr/archive) from 2010 to 2016. The KCYPS is a nationally representative longitudinal panel survey that repeatedly collects data of three cohorts of Korean children and adolescents. The sampling frame of the KCYPS was based on stratified multistage cluster sampling. Specific data collection procedures used in the KCYPS have been described in the literature [17].

The present study used the middle school student cohort data from the second wave (the year of 2011, 2nd grade in middle school, 14-year-old, Time 1), fourth wave (the year of 2013, 16-year-old, 1st grade in high school, Time 2), and sixth wave (the year of 2015, 3rd grade in high school, 18-year-old, Time 3) of the KCYPS. The observed sample at Time 1 consisted of a total of 2280 adolescents (1152 boys and 1128 girls). We included only those adolescents who had owned mobile phones in each time period when the data were collected. A final sample was 1794 adolescents (897 boys and 897 girls) [17].

This study was exempt from the Institutional Review Board (IRB) for the protection of human subjects (IRB No: 1040647-201810-HR-006).

3.2. Measures

Mobile Phone Use. The KCYPS assessed mobile phone use using a set of nine items [17]. Items assessed the frequency of mobile phone use by asking the respondents how often they used their mobile phones, such as 'How often do you use your mobile phone to talk to your family?' 'How often do you use your mobile phone to text or message your friends?' 'How often do you use your phone to use game applications?' Items were rated on a four-point Likert scale ranging from 1 (not at all) to 4 (very frequently). All the items required reverse coding, higher scores indicated higher levels of mobile phone use. The alpha coefficients for this measure in this study were 0.690 (Time 1), 0.703 (Time 2), and 0.706 (Time 3).

Mobile Phone Dependence. Mobile phone addiction was assessed according to a seven-item version of the Inventory for Mobile Phone Dependency (IMPD) [18]. It examines how much the respondents were addicted to their mobile phones, for instance: 'I feel anxious without my mobile phone when I go out of the house,' 'I lose track of time when using my mobile phone,' and 'I cannot live without my mobile phone.' The responses were rated on a four-point Likert scale ranging from 1 (never true) to 4 (always true), and all the items required reverse coding. Higher scores indicated greater levels of mobile phone dependency. Cronbach's alpha coefficients in this study were 0.898 (Time 1), 0.884 (Time 2), and 0.867 (Time 3).

Depression. Depression was measured according to a shorter 10-item version of the Korean Manual of Symptom Checklist (KMSC) [19] such as 'I have little energy,' 'I feel unhappy and depressed,' 'I have many worries,' and 'Everything is overwhelming for me.' These items were rated on a four-point Likert scale ranging from 1 (never true) to 4 (always true), and all the items were reverse-scored. Higher scores indicated more severe depression. The alpha coefficients in this study were 0.901 (Time 1), 0.888 (Time 2), and 0.880 (Time 3).

Covariates. Covariates included factors related to family (i.e., two-income family, both parents living in the household, father's education, and mother's education, annual household income) and school (i.e., academic activity, compliance with school rules, and youth relationships with peers and teachers). Gender was used as a moderator.

The factor "two-income family" was dichotomized into two categories: both parents were working (1) and at least one parent was not working (0). The factor "both parents living in the household" was assessed by asking respondents whether or not they were living with both their parents, the responses were scored as either 1 (yes) or 0 (no). The annual household income was categorized into four categories as follow: 1 = less than $30,000, 2 = $30,000 to $40,000, 3 = $40,000 to $55,000, and 4 = greater than $55,000. The educational level of parents was scored as follows: 1 = less than high school, 2 = high school graduate, 3 = two-year college graduate, and 4 = four-year college graduate or above.

The School Adjustment Inventory was composed of 19 items with four subscales: academic activity, compliance with school rules, relationships with peers, and relationships with teachers [17]. The subscale "relationships with peers" consisted of four items, whereas the other three subscales included five items. The responses were rated on a four-point Likert scale ranging from 1 (never true) to 4 (always true). Higher scores indicated a greater level of school adjustment. Cronbach's alpha coefficients for the four abovementioned subscales in this study were 0.696, 0.783, 0.677, and 0.835, respectively.

3.3. Strategy for Data Analyses

The family and school factors were descriptively examined for Korean boys and girls and compared using *t*-tests and chi-square tests. The *t*-tests were used to compute group mean comparisons of mobile phone use, mobile phone addiction, and depression in boys and girls at each time point.

A measurement invariance model was tested to ensure the metric equivalence of the three factors between boys and girls. Then, a multiple group structural equation modeling (MGSEM) approach was performed to compare gender group differences in unstandardized coefficients for the paths in Figure 1 [20]. First, an unconstrained model without equality constraints was estimated across the entire set of boys and girls. Second, a constrained model with equality constraints was separately estimated across groups. Then, a nested chi-square difference test was performed to compare the constrained and unconstrained models. Model fit was estimated using the following indices: the overall chi-square test ($p > 0.05$), the comparative fit index (CFI > 0.95), the root mean square error of approximation (RMSEA < 0.05), and the standardized root mean residual (SRMR $\leq$ 0.08) [21]. Missing data were dealt with using a full-information maximum likelihood approach [22]. Mplus 8.1 [23] and SPSS version 24.0 [24] were used for data analyses.

4. Results

4.1. Descriptive Analyses

Table 1 presents the group comparisons of family and school factors between Korean boys and girls in the second year of middle school (Time 1). Some significant differences between boys and girls were found for the school factor but not for the family factor. Among the school factors, girls reported higher levels of compliance with school rules ($t = 2.94$, $p < 0.01$) and relationships with peers ($t = 3.80$, $p < 0.001$).

Table 1. Group comparisons of family and school factors between boys and girls at Time 1 ($N = 1794$).

Variable	Boys (n = 897)		Girls (n = 897)		t/χ^2
	Frequency (%)	$M \pm SD$	Frequency (%)	$M \pm SD$	
Family factor					
Two-income Family					
Yes	492 (54.8)		509 (56.7)		0.65
No	405 (45.2)		388 (43.3)		
Both parents in household					
Yes	766 (87.7)		772 (89.9)		1.97
No	107 (12.3)		87 (10.1)		
Annual household income ($)					
0–30,000	283 (33.4)		258 (30.7)		5.31
30,000–40,000	193 (22.8)		177 (21.1)		
40,000–55,000	168 (19.8)		204 (24.3)		
≥55,000	203 (24.0)		201 (23.9)		
Father's education					
Less than high school	28 (3.5)		29 (3.6)		1.06
High school graduate	356 (44.2)		338 (42.1)		
Two-year college graduate	76 (9.5)		85 (10.6)		
Four-year college graduate or Above	344 (42.8)		351 (43.7)		
Mother's education					
Less than high School	22 (2.7)		29 (3.5)		2.01
High school graduate	463 (57.7)		455 (55.3)		
Two-year college graduate	83 (10.3)		80 (9.7)		
Four-year college graduate or Above	235 (29.3)		259 (31.5)		
School factor					
Learning activity		13.64 ± 2.64		13.72 ± 2.46	0.68
Compliance with school rules		13.81 ± 2.87		14.18 ± 2.54	2.94 **
Youth relationships with peers		12.11 ± 2.04		12.45 ± 1.73	3.80 ***
Youth relationships with teachers		14.12 ± 3.34		13.95 ± 3.24	1.06

Note: *** $p < 0.001$, ** $p < 0.01$. M = mean, SD = standard deviation.

4.2. Group Comparisons

Table 2 lists the group mean comparisons of mobile phone use, mobile phone addiction, and depression between boys and girls. Statistically significant group differences were found in the means of mobile phone use, mobile phone addiction, and depression at Times 1, 2, and 3. Mobile phone use for girls was higher than that for boys across time periods (Time 1: $t = 7.25$, $p < 0.001$, Time 2: $t = 5.44$, $p < 0.001$, Time 3: $t = 4.94$, $p < 0.001$). Similarly, girls showed higher mobile phone addiction than boys at each time point (Time 1: $t = 8.20$, $p < 0.001$, Time 2: $t = 6.49$, $p < 0.001$, Time 3: $t = 5.80$, $p < 0.001$). The means of the depression for girls were also higher than those for boys over time (Time 1: $t = 6.12$, $p < 0.001$, Time 2: $t = 7.71$, $p < 0.001$, Time 3: $t = 7.50$, $p < 0.001$). Therefore, hypothesis H1 was supported.

Table 2. Group mean comparisons of major variables between boys and girls ($N = 1794$).

Variable	Boys (n = 897)	Girls (n = 897)	t
	$M \pm SD$	$M \pm SD$	
2nd Grade of middle school at Time 1 (14-year-old)			
Mobile phone use	27.68 ± 4.27	29.04 ± 3.63	7.25 ***
Mobile phone addiction	15.07 ± 4.97	17.06 ± 5.32	8.20 ***
Depression	18.36 ± 5.94	20.09 ± 6.02	6.12 ***
1st Grade of high school at Time 2 (16-year-old)			
Mobile phone use	29.43 ± 4.08	30.40 ± 3.50	5.44 ***
Mobile phone addiction	15.98 ± 4.53	17.42 ± 4.89	6.49 ***
Depression	17.79 ± 5.34	19.78 ± 5.60	7.71 ***
3rd Grade of high school at Time 3 (18-year-old)			
Mobile phone use	29.57 ± 4.01	30.47 ± 3.70	4.94 ***
Mobile phone addiction	15.68 ± 4.51	16.91 ± 4.46	5.80 ***
Depression	17.75 ± 5.41	19.65 ± 5.34	7.50 ***

Note: *** $p < 0.001$. M = mean, SD = standard deviation.

4.3. Structural Equation Model

Measurement invariance tests were performed for mobile phone use, mobile phone addiction, and depression among boys and girls using multiple-group confirmatory factor analyses. Among the 69 group comparisons, 15 paths linking from the unobserved variables to the observed indicators were statistically significant. These links represented 21.7% of all the group contrasts, which indicated that the path coefficients for the three factors largely measured the mobile phone use, mobile phone addiction, and depression in a similar manner between boys and girls. Thus, this study used latent composite variables to examine the structural model shown in Figure 1.

To test hypothesis 2, the structural model of mobile phone use, mobile phone addiction, and depression in boys and girls were tested using an MGSEM strategy with a Huber–White maximum likelihood estimator. The model fit was good (χ^2(df = 26) = 33.826, $p > 0.05$, CFI = 0.998, RMSEA = 0.018, SRMR = 0.008, 90% C.I. = (0.000, 0.034)). Focused fit tests revealed no theoretically meaningful significant points of ill fit. Figure 2 shows the unstandardized path coefficient comparisons between boys and girls. For each of the two groups, statistically significant path coefficients were found for the contemporaneous effects of mobile phone use on mobile phone addiction at Times 1, 2, and 3 for boys (path coefficients = 0.397, 0.314, and 0.245, respectively) and girls (path coefficients = 0.448, 0.353, and 0.318, respectively). Therefore, hypothesis H2a was supported.

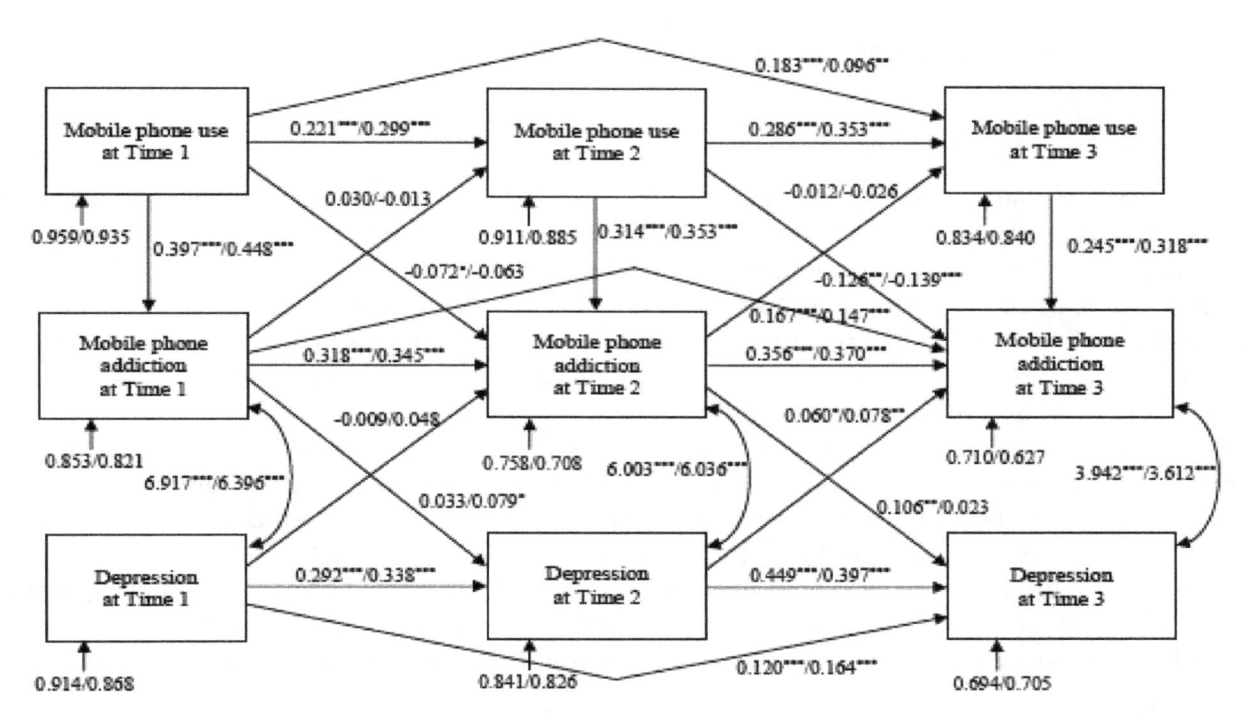

Figure 2. Autoregressive cross-lagged multiple-group structural equation model (Note: *** $p < 0.001$, ** $p < 0.01$, * $p < 0.05$. The first coefficient is the unstandardized path coefficient for boys, the second coe cient is the unstandardized path coefficient for girls. All coefficients are unstandardized path coefficients but disturbance values are standardized. Covariates include two-income family, both parents in the household, father's education, mother's education, annual household income, academic activity, compliance with school rules, and youth relationships with peers and teachers).

For the first-order autoregressive effects of mobile phone use, statistically significant effects were found for boys (Time 1 to Time 2: path coefficient = 0.221, Time 2 to Time 3: path coefficient = 0.286) and girls (Time 1 to Time 2: path coefficient = 0.299, Time 2 to Time 3: path coefficient = 0.353). Similarly, the first-order autoregressive effects of mobile phone addiction were observed for boys (Time 1 to Time 2: path coefficient = 0.318, Time 2 to Time 3: path coefficient = 0.356) and girls (Time 1 to Time 2: path coefficient = 0.345, Time 2 to Time 3: path coefficient = 0.370). For depression, the predicted first-order autoregressive effects from Time 1 to Time 2 and from Time 2 to Time 3 were observed for boys (path coefficients = 0.292 and 0.449) and Korean girls (path coefficients = 0.338 and 0.397). Additionally, the second-order autoregressive effects of mobile phone use, mobile phone addiction, and depression were found from Time 1 to Time 3 for boys (path coefficients = 0.183, 0.167, and 0.120) and girls (path coefficients = 0.096, 0.147, and 0.164). Therefore, hypotheses H2b and H2c were supported.

As for cross-lagged effects, statistically significant path coefficients were found between mobile phone use at Time 1 and mobile phone addiction at Time 2 for boys (path coefficient = 0.072) and between mobile phone use at Time 2 and mobile phone addiction at Time 3 for boys (path coefficient = −0.126) and girls (path coefficient = −0.139). However, no reciprocal causal relationships were found between mobile phone use and mobile phone addiction across time periods for both groups. Statistically significant path coefficients were found from mobile phone addiction at Time 1 to depression at Time 2 for girls (path coefficient = 0.079) and from mobile phone addiction at Time 2 to depression at Time 3 for boys (path coefficient = 0.106). Reciprocal causal relationships linking depression at Time 1 to mobile phone addiction at Time 2 were not observed, but reciprocal causal relationships linking depression at Time 2 to mobile phone addiction at Time 3 were found for boys (path coefficient = 0.060) and girls (path coefficient = 0.078). Therefore, hypothesis H2d was partially supported.

For bidirectional relationships, statistically significant path coefficients were found between mobile phone addiction and depression at each time point for boys (path coefficients = 6.917, 6.003, and 3.942) and girls (path coefficients = 6.396, 6.036, and 3.612). Therefore, hypothesis H2e was supported.

Finally, there were no gender differences for each path in the structural model. Thus, hypothesis H2f was not supported.

5. Discussion

This study aimed to investigate the gender differences in the mean scores of mobile phone use, mobile phone addiction, and depression among Korean youth and to compare differences in the longitudinal relationships of these three variables among boys and girls for a four-year period. The following four main points are discussed: (1) gender differences in the mean values of mobile phone use, mobile phone addiction, and depression, (2) longitudinal effects of mobile phone use, mobile phone addiction, and depression, (3) bidirectional relationships between mobile phone addiction and depression, and (4) gender differences in the structural model.

First, the mean values of mobile phone use, mobile phone addiction, and depression were differed by gender. Compared to boys, Korean girls were likely to use their mobile phones more and were at a higher risk of mobile phone addiction and depression during the second year of middle school (Time 1), the first year of high school (Time 2), and the third year of high school (Time3). These findings were consistent with those of a previous study by Sánchez-Martínez and Otero [6], which reported that female adolescents tended to use their mobile phones more often and were more likely to depend on mobile phone devices than their male counterparts. Similarly, girls were more likely to have depression than boys [25].

With regard to the autoregressive effects of mobile phone use, mobile phone addiction, and depression over time, the present study found that early mobile phone use, mobile phone addiction, and depression during middle school were associated with later mobile phone use, mobile phone addiction, and depression during high school. Frequent mobile phone users at middle school showed the tendency to use their mobile phones frequently even in high school. Similarly, Korean adolescents who showed higher levels of mobile phone addiction during the junior high school period were more likely to depend on their mobile phones during the high school period. This finding was consistent with previous studies [14,26], which indicated that mobile phone addiction tended to increase over time. As for depression, Korean adolescents with higher depression during the early adolescence period were at a higher risk of developing depression during the late adolescence period, which was consistent with the results of a previous study [25].

Regarding the cross-lagged effects of mobile phone use, mobile phone addiction, and depression, the present study found that the frequency of mobile phone use could not predict mobile phone addiction at a later time period. However, mobile phone addiction and depression concurrently predicted each other across time periods. First, frequent mobile phone users in middle school were less likely to addict to their mobile phones in high school. This finding was contrary to our hypothesis. The inconsistent finding might be attributable to the use of different measurement tools. Haug et al. [27] found that smartphone addiction was more strongly associated with the total time spent per day using smartphones than the frequency of smartphone use. In contrast, Lin et al. [28] reported that the frequency of mobile phone use was an indicator of smartphone addiction rather than the total time spent using mobile phones. These two studies [27,28] used both the frequency of mobile phone use and the total time spent using mobile phones and mainly carried out cross-sectional analysis. The present study did not include the variable of the total time spent using mobile phones but longitudinally analyzed the relationship between the frequency of mobile phone use and mobile phone addiction. Therefore, further longitudinal study is warranted to examine the relationships among the total time spent using mobile phones, the frequency of mobile phone use, and mobile phone addiction. Second, earlier depression in the first year of high school (Time 2) was associated with later mobile phone addiction in the third year of high school (Time 3). This finding supports that of a previous study, which indicated that depression was a predictor of mobile phone addiction [29]. Third, this present study found that earlier mobile phone addiction was associated with later depression. This finding, that supported the study by Coyne et al. [14], indicated that early problematic mobile phone use was a significant predictor of depression.

This study confirmed that the bidirectional relationship between mobile phone addiction and depression persisted even after the other variables were controlled. This finding is consistent with Jun's study [12]. There are some possible explanations for this causal pathway. Adolescents with depression are more likely to be addicted to their mobile phones because mobile phones may provide an environment where such adolescents can relate to others in a safer and less demanding environment [6]. Inversely, a possible explanation of why mobile phone addiction may lead to depression is that adolescents with higher levels of mobile phone addiction might be at an increased risk of interpersonal problems, resulting in depression later [30]. This finding highlights the importance of providing simultaneous intervention for reducing both depression and mobile phone addiction.

Finally, contrary to our expectation, the present study found no gender differences for each path in the structural model. A plausible explanation for this finding is that the sample considered in this study consisted of middle and high school Korean students. In particular, high school students have less time to use their mobile phones than young adults because high school students need to prepare for university entrance exams. This commonality of adolescent life in South Korea may result in there being no gender differences. Although the present study analyzed data longitudinally, four years of research might not be sufficient to investigate gender differences in the relationships among mobile phone use, mobile phone addiction, and depression. Prior literature reported that gender was an important predictor in the relationship between the internet or mobile phone use and mental health outcomes but these studies were cross-sectional [1,31]. Few studies have explored the causal effects of gender on this issue, thus, more studies are needed to conduct with longitudinal data.

This study has some limitations. First, considering the nature of the secondary analysis, the present study was limited by the measurement of mobile phone use. The KCYPS did not measure the actual time and frequency of mobile phone use, which may yield different results regarding the relationship between mobile phone use and mobile phone addiction. A further longitudinal study is warranted to examine the relationships among the total time spent using mobile phones, the frequency of mobile phone use, and mobile phone addiction. Second, our study did not distinguish between different types of mobile phone devices but treated them (from the most advanced smartphones to standard cell phones) as the same. Thus, the findings of this study should be interpreted with caution. Future research is warranted to investigate whether the types of mobile phone devices are related to adolescents' patterns of mobile phone use. Third, although we found significant associations among mobile phone use, mobile phone addiction, and depression over time in this study, causal inferences among these variables are limited due to the inconsistent results on this topic. Lastly, although this study included parents' socio-economic variables such as income and education, it did not include parents' psychological status such as mobile phone use of parents, which may affect their children's mobile phone use. Future research is needed to examine the effect of parents' psychological status on their children's mobile phone use and mobile phone addiction.

6. Conclusions

In summary, excessive mobile phone use and mobile phone addiction have been increasing concerns among Korean adolescents. Findings of this study revealed that Korean girls were more exposed to mobile phone use and they were at higher risk of mobile phone addiction and depressive symptoms. In addition, the longitudinal relationships among mobile phone use, mobile phone addiction, and depressive symptoms were observed in Korean adolescents. This study implies that it is necessary to acknowledge the negative effects of mobile phone use and to design adequate intervention strategies to prevent mobile phone addiction and depressive symptoms among adolescents.

Author Contributions: Conceptualization, S.-Y.P. (So-Young Park) and S.-Y.P. (So-Youn Park); methodology, S.-Y.P. (So-Young Park) and H.J.; software, S.-Y.P. (So-Young Park) and S.-Y.P. (So-Youn Park); validation, S.Y., H.J., and C.-S.S.; formal analysis, S.-Y.P. (So-Young Park) and S.-Y.P. (So-Youn Park); investigation, C.-S.S.; resources, S.-Y.P. (So-Young Park), S.Y., H.J., and S.-Y.P. (So-Youn Park); data curation, S.-Y.P. (So-Young Park) and S.-Y.P. (So-Youn Park); writing-original draft preparation, S.-Y.P. (So-Young Park), S.Y. and S.-Y.P. (So-Youn Park); writing-review and editing, C.-S.S., and H.J.; visualization, S.-Y.P. (So-Young Park); supervision, S.Y., C.-S.S., and S.-Y.P. (So-Youn Park); project administration, S.-Y.P. (So-Youn Park); funding acquisition, S.-Y.P. (So-Youn Park).

References

1.   Chen, B.; Liu, F.; Ding, S.; Ying, X.; Wang, L.; Wen, Y. Gender difference in factors associated with smartphone addiction: A cross-sectional study among medical college students. *BMC Psychiatry* **2017**, *17*, 341. [CrossRef]

2.   Lee, Y.; Chang, C.; Cheng, Z. The dark side of smartphone usage: Psychological traits, compulsive behavior and technostress. *Comput. Hum. Behav.* **2014**, *31*, 373–383. [CrossRef]

3.   Sanaha, M.; Hawi, N.S. Relationships among smartphone addiction, stress, academic performance, and satisfaction with life. *Comput. Hum. Behav.* **2016**, *57*, 321–325. [CrossRef]

4.   Ministry of Science and ICT and the National Information Society Agency. Results of Prevalence Study on Smartphone Overdependence in 2018. Available online: https://msit.go.kr (accessed on 5 June 2019).

5.   Billieux, J.; Maurage, P.; Lopez-Fernandez, O.L.; Kuss, D.J.; Griffiths, M.D. Can disorder mobile phone use be considered a behavioral addiction? An update on current evidence and a comprehensive model for future research. *Curr. Addict. Rep.* **2015**, *2*, 156–162. [CrossRef]

6.   Sánchez-Martínez, M.; Otero, A. Factors associated with cell phone use in adolescents in the community of Madrid (Spain). *Cyberpsychol. Behav.* **2009**, *12*, 131–137. [CrossRef]

7.   Csibi, S.; Griffiths, M.D.; Cook, B.; Demetrovics, Z.; Szabo, A. The psychometric properties of the Smartphone Application-Based Addiction Scale (SABAS). *Int. J. Mental Health Addict.* **2018**, *16*, 393–403. [CrossRef]

8.   Roberts, J.A.; Yaya, C.; Manolis, C. The invisible addiction: A cell-phone activities and addiction among male and female college students. *J. Behav. Addict.* **2014**, *3*, 254–265. [CrossRef]

9.   Elhai, J.D.; Dvorak, R.D.; Levine, J.C.; Hall, B.J. Problematic smartphone use: A conceptual overview and systematic review of relations with anxiety and depression psychopathology. *J. Affect. Disord.* **2017**, *207*, 251–259. [CrossRef]

10.   Ciccheti, D.; Rogosch, F.A. A developmental psychopathology perspective on adolescence. *J. Consult. Clin. Psychol.* **2002**, *70*, 6–20. [CrossRef]

11.   Cerniglia, L.; Zoratto, F.; Cimino, S.; Laviola, G.; Ammaniti, M.; Adriani, W. Internet addiction in adolescences: Neurobiological, psychosocial and clinical issues. *Neurosci. Biobehav. Rev.* **2017**, *76*, 174–184. [CrossRef]

12.   Jun, S. The reciprocal longitudinal relationships between mobile phone addiction and depressive symptoms among Korean adolescents. *Comput. Hum. Behav.* **2016**, *58*, 179–186. [CrossRef]

13.   Van den Eijnden, R.J.; Meerkerk, G.J.; Vermulst, A.A.; Spijkerman, R.; Engles, R.C. Online communication, compulsive internet use, and psychosocial well-being among adolescents: A longitudinal study. *Dev. Psychol.* **2008**, *44*, 655–665. [CrossRef] [PubMed]

14.   Coyne, S.M.; Stockdale, L.; Summers, K. Problematic cell phone use, depression, anxiety, and self-regulation: Evidence from a three year longitudinal study from adolescence to emerging adulthood. *Comput. Hum. Behav.* **2019**, *96*, 78–84. [CrossRef]

15.   Cha, S.S.; Seo, B.K. Smartphone use and smartphone addiction in middle school students in Korea: Prevalence, social networking service, and game use. *Health Psychol. Open* **2018**, *5*, 1–15. [CrossRef] [PubMed]

16.   Jeong, J.Y.; Kim, D.H. A study on the addicted use of mobile phone among the high school students. *Korean J. Epidemiol.* **2005**, *27*, 140–153.

17.   National Youth Policy Institute. *Korean Youth and Children Panel Survey 1–7th Wave User's Guide*; National Youth Policy Institute: Sejong, Korea, 2017.

18.   Lee, S.; Kim, H.; Na, E.; Lee, S.; Kim, S.; Bae, J. *A Study on the Effects of Mobile Phone Use of Adolescents*; Report No. 2002-1; Samsung Life Public Welfare Foundation: Seoul, Korea, 2002.

19.   Kim, K.; Kim, J.; Won, H. *Korean Manual of Symptom Checklist-90-Revision*; Choong-Ang Aptitude Laboratory: Seoul, Korea, 1984.

20.   Brown, T.A. *Confirmatory Factor Analysis for Applied Research*; Guilford Press: New York, NY, USA, 2006.

21. Schreiber, J.B.; Stage, F.K.; King, J.; Nora, A.; Barlow, E.A. Reporting structural equation modelling and confirmatory factor analysis results: A review. *J. Educ. Res.* **2006**, *99*, 323–337. [CrossRef]
22. Enders, C. *Applied Missing Data Analysis*; Guilford Press: New York, NY, USA, 2010.
23. Muthén, L.K.; Muthén, B.O. *Mplus User's Guide*, 8th ed.; Muthén & Muthén: Los Angeles, CA, USA, 2017.
24. IBM Corp. *IBM SPSS Statistics for Windows*, version 24.0; IBM Corp.: Armonk, NY, USA, 2016.
25. Galambos, N.L.; Leadbeater, B.J.; Barker, E.T. Gender differences in and risk factors for depression in adolescence: A 4-year longitudinal study. *Int. J. Behav. Dev.* **2004**, *28*, 16–25. [CrossRef]
26. Herreo, J.; Uruena, A.; Torres, A.; Hidalgo, A. Socially connected but still isolated: Smartphone addiction decreases social support over time. *Soc. Sci. Comput. Rev.* **2019**, *37*, 73–88. [CrossRef]
27. Haug, S.; Castro, R.; Kwon, M.; Filler, A.; Kowatsch, T.; Schaub, M.P. Smartphone use and smartphone addiction among young people in Switzerland. *J. Behav. Addict.* **2015**, *4*, 299–307. [CrossRef] [PubMed]
28. Lin, Y.H.; Chang, L.R.; Lee, Y.H.; Tseng, H.W.; Kuo, T.B.; Chen, S.H. Development and validation of the Smartphone Addiction Inventory (SPAI). *PLoS ONE* **2014**, *9*, e98312. [CrossRef] [PubMed]
29. Demirci, K.; Akgonul, M.; Akpinar, A. Relationship of smartphone use severity with sleep quality, depression, and anxiety in university students. *J. Behav. Addict.* **2015**, *4*, 85–92. [CrossRef] [PubMed]
30. Kim, Y.; Jang, H.M.; Lee, Y.; Lee, D.; Kim, D. Effects of internet and smartphone addictions on depression and anxiety based on propensity score matching analysis. *Int. J. Environ. Res. Public Health* **2018**, *15*, 859. [CrossRef] [PubMed]
31. Wang, J.; Sheng, J.; Wang, H. The association between mobile game addiction and depression, social anxiety, and loneliness. *Front Public Health* **2019**, *7*, 247. [CrossRef]

Generalised Versus Specific Internet Use-Related Addiction Problems: A Mixed Methods Study on Internet, Gaming and Social Networking Behaviours

Olatz Lopez-Fernandez [1,2,3]

1 Turning Point, Eastern Health Clinical School, Monash University, 110 Church Street, Richmond VIC 2131, Australia; olatz.lopez-fernandez@monash.edu or lopez.olatz@gmail.com

2 International Gaming Research Unit, Psychology Department, Nottingham Trent University, Nottingham NG1 4FQ, UK

3 Laboratory for Experimental Psychopathology, Psychological Sciences Research Institute, Catholic University of Louvain, 1348 Louvain-la-Neuve, Belgium

Abstract: The field of technological behavioural addictions is moving towards specific problems (i.e., gaming disorder). However, more evidence of generalised versus specific Internet use-related addiction problems (generalised pathological Internet use (GPIU) vs. specific pathological Internet use (SPIU)) is still needed. This mixed methods study aimed to disentangle GPIU from SPIU. A partially mixed sequential equal status study design (QUAN→QUAL) was undertaken. First, through an online survey, which adapted the compulsive Internet use scale (CIUS) for three types of problems (i.e., generalised Internet use, and specific online gaming and social networking). Second, potential problem users' perceptions of the evolution of these problems (aetiology, development, consequences, and factors) were ascertained, through semi-structured interviews, together with their opinion on present Internet gaming disorder (IGD) criteria adapted to each problem studied. Findings showed the CIUS remains valid and reliable for GPIU and SPIUs examined; a prevalence between 10.8% and 37.4% was estimated for potential at-risk problem gamers and Internet users, respectively, who reported their preference for maintaining their virtual lives. Half of the sample had a risk of a unique or mixed profile of these problems. Moreover, device patterns, gender, and age issues emerged, such as problem gamers being proportionally equal male and female young or middle-aged adults. GPIU was highly associated with problem social networking use, and weakly with problematic gaming, but both SPIUs were independent. Concerning addictive symptoms, salience, deception, and tolerance required redefinition, especially for SPIUs, while better-valued IGD criteria applied to GPIU and SPIUs were: Risk relationships or opportunities, give up other activities, withdrawal, and continue despite problems. Thus, although problems studied are present as risk behaviours, SPIUs seem to cover the addictive symptomatology in those categorised as potential problem users, online gaming being the most severe behavioural addiction problem.

Keywords: behavioural addictions; generalised versus specific problem Internet uses; Internet addiction; gaming disorder; social networking; mixed methods research

---

1. Introduction

The field of behavioural addictions related to technological uses (i.e., technological behavioural addictions) has been growing exponentially since 1995 [1–4] and not without scientific, clinical, and social debates. In mid-nineties, the phenomenon was recognised by the umbrella term of 'Internet addiction', a generalised addiction problem covering all online activities together. Almost automatically, this was conceptualised as a clinical disorder [5], initially closely aligned with 'impulse control disorder'. In 2013, it was proposed as a future 'addictive disorder' in the third appendix of the fifth Diagnostic and Statistical Manual of Mental Disorders (DSM-5) by the American Psychiatric Association (APA) [6], and at present it has been recognised as a health disease in the eleventh revision of the International Classification of Diseases (ICD-11) by the World Health Organization (WHO) [7]. However, this international recognition has come about solely for a specific technological addictive problem—problematic gaming—even though other technological use-related addiction problems coexist (e.g., cybersex addiction).

The terminology requires an update, as it covers the emergent health issues related to excessive online uses, which emerged together with the development of technologies at the end of last century, and it has been consolidated in the 21st Century. Thus, although it seems Internet use-related addiction problems were initially mainly studied as a generalised problem [8], there is a scientific and clinical production of other specific problems simultaneously studied, such as problematic video gaming [9] or social networking [10]. Both generalised and specific Internet use-related addiction problems seem to produce addictive symptomatology (i.e., the classic symptoms for substance use or gambling disorders) in a few users, together with functional physical or psychological impairments (i.e., when the online activity(-ies) negatively affects other areas of a user's organism or lives; e.g., sight or academic/work facets), and distress (i.e., when the online activity(-ies) may reflect a maladaptive behaviour, failure in coping or adaptation processes).

Concerning statistics records, the International Telecommunication Union (ITU) has published its Information and Communication Technologies (ICT) Facts and Figures 2017 [11], showing the continuous worldwide expansion of Internet use through fixed or mobile subscriptions. For instance, in 2017, 3578 million individuals were using the Internet (compared to 495 million in 2001), 830 million being young people (i.e., 15–24-year-olds), which represents 80 per cent of the youth population in the 104 countries studied (see Figure 1).

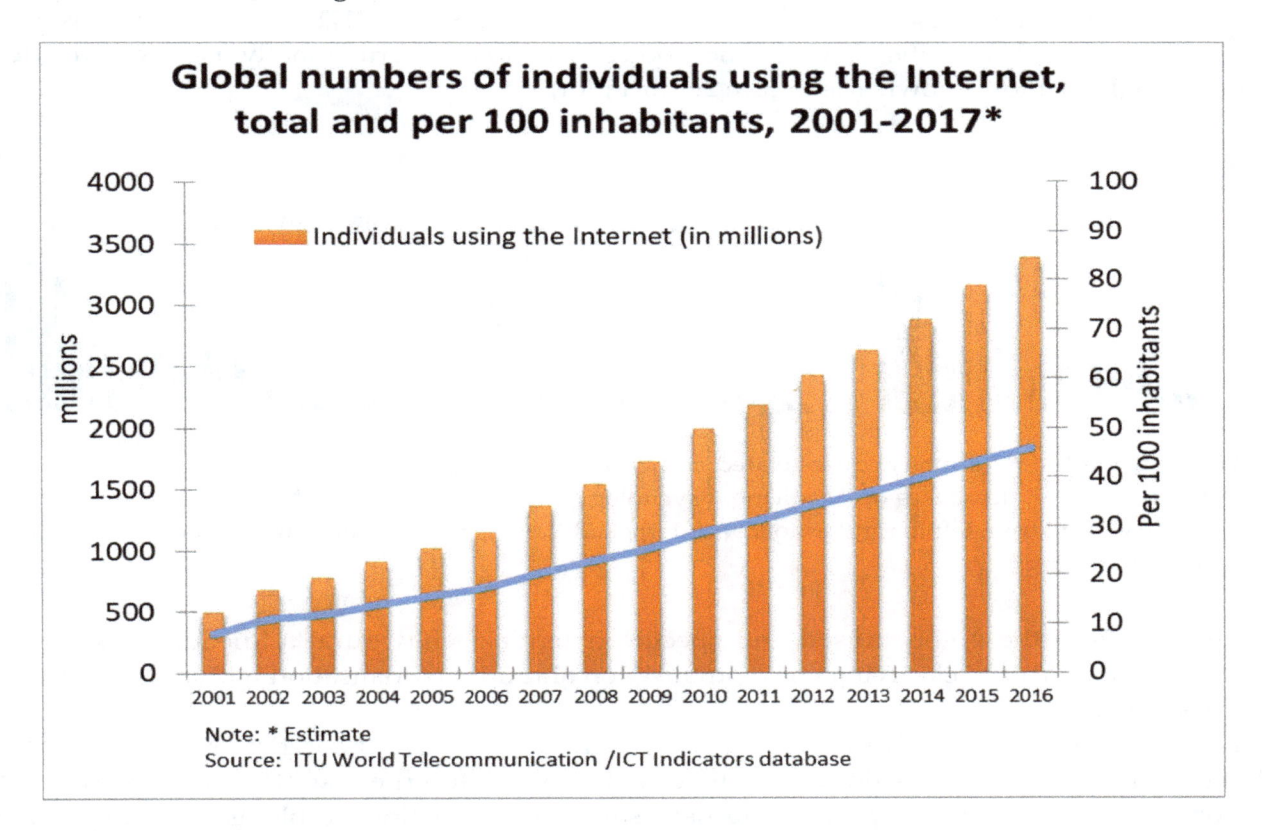

Figure 1. Evolution of global Information and Communication Technologies (ICT) from 2001 to 2017 (according to the International Telecommunication Union [ITU] World Telecommunications and its ICT indicators database).

Similarly, bibliometric evidence extracted from three ProQuest Central scientific databases (i.e., Health and Medical Collection, Psychology Database, and Public Health Database [12]) shows this impactful increase in research on Internet use-related addiction problems during the last two decades (1995–2017), which have especially risen from the beginning of the 21st century [13].

Indeed, an advanced search was conducted to observe the increase of production on these addiction problems. The procedure for the search of Internet addiction production was: It was introduced the terms 'Internet addiction' OR 'problem* Internet use' OR 'pathological Internet use' OR 'excessive Internet use' (to cover the main terminology used in Internet addiction). Simultaneously, the options to refine the search were: 'Peer reviewed' (i.e., to ensure the outputs were articles from official editorial processes), 'Exclude duplicate documents' (i.e., to avoid any article is detected more than once through the databases selected), 'Show additional terms included in the search' (to suggest and add alternative terminology used in relation to the terms selected), and a period from 1 January 1995 to 31 December 2017. A total of 116,455 outputs were obtained, showing a growing tendency in its bibliometric production, where each bar corresponded to the number of articles published in a year, going from 146 records in 1995 to 11,630 in 2017 (see Figure 2, first plot). The same procedure was used with the other two specific online behavioural addiction problems studied. Concerning problematic gaming (i.e., 'gaming addiction' OR 'problem* gaming use' OR 'pathological gaming use' OR 'excessive gaming use' OR 'gaming disorder' OR 'internet gaming disorder'), 7246 outputs were addressing problems within video gaming (e.g., computer gaming, digital or electronic game addiction). These ranged from 35 records in 1995 to 839 in 2017, with a progressive increment from 2010 and especially from 2014 (after the inclusion of 'Internet gaming disorder' (IGD) in the appendix of the DSM-5 by the APA [6]; see Figure 2, second plot). Similarly, problematic social networking obtained the most outputs in the search: A total of 202,045 (using as keywords: 'social network* addiction' OR 'problem* social network* use' OR 'pathological social network* use' OR 'excessive social network* use' OR 'social network* disorder'); from 1474 in 1995 to 18,595 in 2017; with a continuous growth accelerating since 2008 (i.e., the year that Facebook started to be internationally used with the design and functionalities most known; see Figure 2, third plot).

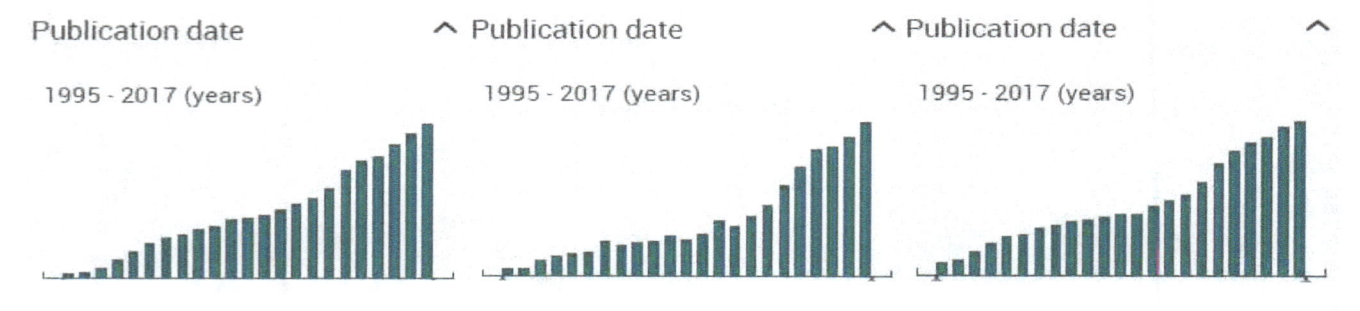

Figure 2. Evolution of Internet use-related addiction problems from 1995 to 2017 (according to the ProQuest Central databases on Medicine, Psychology, and Public Health). Note: The diagrams of bars are ordered from left to right as follow: Internet addiction, problematic gaming, and problematic social networking.

Research into these generalised and specific potential behavioural addictions has provided fundamental advances in clarifying conceptualisation and operationalisation within the spectrum of these problems.

Firstly, Davis in 2001 [14] introduced one of the few existing theoretical models on Internet addiction. His cognitive–behavioural model of pathological Internet use (PIU) proposed dividing the problem into two types: Specific Internet use-related addiction problems (SPIU, referring to the condition in which an individual pathologically uses the Internet for a purpose; e.g., online gaming) and generalised PIU (GPIU, referring to the global set of online behaviours). The basic idea was that cognitive distortions (e.g., thoughts such as 'the Internet is the only place where I am respected') were automatically and unintentionally enacted whenever a stimulus associated with the Internet was available, resulting in emotional or behavioural outputs (i.e., GPIU or SPIU symptoms). Thus, maladaptive cognitions impact SPIU or GPIU, but the latter type was found to be more complicated, as several external factors could be the cause (e.g., social isolation, lack of social support), with negative consequences, such as procrastination and other daily functioning problems (e.g., putting off responsibilities to be online without a directive purpose). To the authors' knowledge, no previous author has asked yet why the same external problems would not be present in generalised and specific Internet-use addition problems. This is a central question, as few works have addressed these factors in SPIUs, which are precisely the ones being treated, studied, and even recognised internationally in the case of gaming disorder.

Between 2002 and 2010, Caplan [15,16] tested and updated this model for GPIU, indicating some users had a preference for online social interactions and used the Internet for mood regulation, which predicted deficient online self-regulation (i.e., compulsive Internet use and a cognitive preoccupation regarding the Internet). Subsequently, Haagsma and colleagues in 2013 [17] tested the model for a SPIU (i.e., online gaming) into an adolescent population and obtained similar findings. However, although these studies showed a few readjustments in Davis' model (e.g., internal factors, such as a preference for online interaction, online mood regulation, and online deficient self-regulation could predict both GPIU or SPIU), there is still a need for more theoretical development on generalised and specific online problems, especially addressing external (i.e., environmental) factors and structural (i.e., video games) factors.

Secondly, Griffiths in 2005 [18] adapted Brown's [19] proposal for gambling and developed the component model of addiction to operationalise the common features among substance and behavioural addictions. The addictive problem is formed in a biopsychosocial framework (i.e., as a consequence of individual, situational, and structural factors) and could be defined by six components (i.e., symptoms; see Table 1). Recently, Griffiths [20] has clarified common components are essential keys to delineate behavioural and substance addictions, as although different addictions have idiosyncrasies, these also have similarities (i.e., components), which are critical to the behaviour being labelled as an addiction. Thus, the six components need to be endorsed to operationally define an addiction (e.g., independently if generalised or specific problems). However, in public and mental health organisations (e.g., APA), and in their respective health manuals (e.g., the DSM), the components are usually articulated as criteria. Thus, to diagnose a disease or a mental health illness, the patient has to endorse a number of criteria (e.g., in the IGD proposed by the DSM-5, it is five out of nine). This quantitative approach has generated concern to estimate the prevalence of potential problematic users, as it has been dependent on several factors (e.g., the criteria, psychometric tools). Moreover, some criteria are more prominent and relevant than others, which have been tackled by few authors.

Thirdly, concerning Internet addiction, Tao and colleagues [21] proposed renowned diagnostic criteria for Internet addiction (see Table 1). This had an operationalisation which introduced specifications: First, the relevance of symptoms (i.e., some being more important than others); second, the timing for the problem course (i.e., the addictive problem requires a period over which to be developed); third, exclusion tactics to diagnose the problem (i.e., the addictive problem should be differentiated from other disorders); fourth, the importance of the functional impairment (i.e., the addictive problem affects users' real-life, impeding at least a facet of a user's functioning). In concrete terms, they stated preoccupation and withdrawal should always be present, as these are the most important symptoms. Subsequently, at least one of the other symptoms should also be present (i.e., tolerance, persistent desire and difficulty to control it, continued use disregarding harmful consequences, loss of interests, or alleviation of negative emotions). The exclusion criteria were psychotic or bipolar I disorders, together with the need for a clinical impairment criterion (in other duties or relationships), and course the criterion of using the Internet excessively for at least three months for six hours per day as entertainment. Tao and colleagues' proposal [21] together with substance use disorder (SUD) and gambling disorder criteria were taken as a source by the APA to propose the IGD criteria [22], which slightly differ in the symptoms, time of development (i.e., a year), and exclusion criteria (other excessive Internet uses). The IGD criteria are: (1) Preoccupation, (2) withdrawal, (3) tolerance, (4) reduction/stop, (5) giving up other activities, (6) continuing despite problems, (7) deceit/cover-up, (8) escaping adverse moods, (9) risk/loss of relationships/opportunities (the wording proposed for these criteria has been introduced in Table 1). Nevertheless, the field has recently been characterised by intense debate on whether and how IGD or Internet addiction (among other addiction problems) should become official disorders. These debates are central to the question of how general versus specific behavioural addiction forms.

Thus, critiques of the component model, Internet addiction (i.e., as GPIU), or IGD (i.e., as SPIU) have emerged [23,24]. For instance, Griffiths' and Tao's proposals were criticised by Van Rooij and Prause [23], as they considered that the evidence base was not enough to support the diagnostic of the generalised Internet addiction as a behavioural addiction. They suggested studying common unpaired dimensions with the support of neuroimaging proofs, and identifying the changes in the rewarding element of using the Internet (e.g., if users are responding to the hedonic reward indistinctly if it is sex, drugs, or online behaviours, and how this response changes their usage pattern) [23]. Similarly, Kardefelt-Winther [24] criticised the IGD criteria for being too adhered to other previous addictive disorders included in the fourth DSM (DSM-IV), rather than capturing the phenomenology of online gaming; he argued some criteria were weak to diagnose SPIU (e.g., preoccupation, withdrawal, loss of interests, and tolerance; especially the later one, which belongs to SUDs). Moreover, it is worth noting how a relevant component, such as salience, which originally covered person's thinking, feelings, and behaviours [18,19] has been reduced to a sole cognitive facet in this century's research and clinical works; even the Davis model was only based on the cognitive approach of the maladaptive behaviour of Internet addiction.

Fourthly, Charlton and Danforth in 2007 [25] stated the distinction between Internet use-related addiction problems and high online engagements through specific components (i.e., criteria). They established the difference between core and peripheral criteria for behavioural addictions, initially performed for the GPIU, and subsequently applied to an SPIU: Online gaming (i.e., massively multiplayer online game playing [MMORPG]; e.g., Asheron's call; see Table 1). The core criteria which defined an addictive problem were: Conflict (with other personal activities or other persons), withdrawal, relapse and reinstatement, and behavioural salience; while peripheral criteria were present in nonproblem online users (i.e., high-engagement users): Cognitive salience (e.g., preoccupation), tolerance, and euphoria. Moreover, time spent on online gaming was positively associated with those who highly scored on the core criteria. A study recently carried out by Lehenbauer and Fohringer [26] has found similar results regarding online gaming. They adapted the version of a previous MMORPG (i.e., World of Warcraft), and found differences between highly-engaged and addicted gamers to the same core versus peripheral criteria, together with more time spent on the core criteria (i.e., addicted gamers were gaming 30 h per week, while highly-engaged players played around 20 h). Furthermore, this study also showed the quality of life for addict gamers was significantly lower than highly-engaged players, especially in physical and psychological health indicators.

For problem Internet and gaming addictions, other research has been undertaken this decade and provided evidence about other potential behavioural addictions which could be classed into this spectrum of online addiction problems [27]. However, the existing theoretical studies (e.g., critiques, reviews) have scarce theoretical development, and only a few of the classic studies have developed attempts of theoretical models (e.g., Davis' model [14]). Studies are usually empirical and use a quantitative approach (e.g., surveys), while qualitative or mixed methods approaches are still scarce, as in other complementary fields, such as behavioural or educational sciences [28,29]. At present, there is a need for knowledge on the phenomenology (i.e., nature) of these problems and more theoretical development. Young developed the latest published study addressing the phenomenon of Internet addiction in 2004 [30], eight years after she coined the term [2,5]. She provided awareness about the nature of Internet use and its potential abuse, as a decade ago this phenomenon had not been identified and defined yet [31,32]. Similarly, recent research has been published, tackling the phenomenology of traditional gaming versus gaming addiction through insights from the gamers' perspective [33], especially in younger generations. Thus, GPIU and SPIU (gaming) might become emerging public health problems as, according to Grant, Schreiber, and Odlaug [34], behavioural addictions are characterised by the inability to resist a drive, resulting in actions that are harmful to oneself and others.

There is a need to cover the gap to start ascertaining the addictive nature of these Internet use-related addiction problems; especially when a public health organisation, such as the WHO, has included 'gaming disorder' as a behavioural addiction into the category for 'Disorders due to substance use or addictive behaviours', subcategory 'Disorders due to addictive behaviours', together with gambling (WHO, 2018 [7]). Furthermore, it seems that while other potential addictive problems connected to technological uses are still under investigation by academic and clinical professionals, there is limited evidence to consider their official recognition yet. This is the case of social media or social networking addiction, where a small number of controversial studies have reported these problems related to the maladaptive use of these media as entertainment and communication tools [35,36]. However, although a few psychometric instruments have been developed to measure this new phenomenon (based on previous addictive criteria, such as SUDs or IGD [37,38]), the evidence is limited and concentrated on adolescents and young adults.

On the other hand, it seems to be established that the existing scales which have been developed in the field of technological (behavioural) addictions have usually been developed through other current addiction criteria and validated using student community samples. An outstanding scale is the compulsive Internet use scale (CIUS [39]), which has been recognised as one of the most psychometrically stable tools (e.g., similar factorial structure among several language adaptations) to measure both generalised and specific (i.e., cybersex) use-related addiction problems. In this study, this scale has been selected to quantitatively measure the phenomena of GPIU (i.e., Internet) and SPIUs (i.e., gaming and social networking), respectively (see Table 1). Indeed, psychometrically, the CIUS has excellent reliability, a unique factor structure demonstrated by exploratory and confirmatory approaches, and has shown measurement invariance [39]. However, as the purpose of this paper is to go further in depth and observe the commonalities and differences among GPIU versus SPIUs, a qualitative measure was performed by interviewing participants potentially classed as problem Internet, gaming, and/or social network users. This strategy required a mixed methods approach of a community sample, accomplishing the following methodological requirements provided below.

Thus, the principal aim is to understand adults' online uses in their personal sphere (i.e., non-academic or professional) to ascertain if these behaviours could be classed as GPIU and/or SPIU and to know about the problems from those who could be categorised as potential problem users. This is articulated in a four-fold specific aim: (i) To validate the CIUS adapted to these three Internet use-related addiction problems (i.e., Internet, gaming, and social networking) to compare them; (ii) to estimate the prevalence of potential problem Internet, gaming, and social networkers users to explore them by sociodemographic variables and addictive symptomatology; (iii) to examine potential problem users' knowledge, experiences, and perceptions with regard to the nature and development of these problems; and (iv) to know their opinion on IGD criteria adapted to the GPIU and SPIUs studied.

Table 1. Comparison of components, criteria, criterions in GPIUs and SPIUs proposals.

Components/Criteria	Subcomponents/Criterions	GPIU (Addiction; Griffiths, 2005 [18])	GPIU (Internet addiction; Tao et al., 2010 [21])	SPIU (IGD; APA, 2013 [22])	SPIU (online gaming; Charlton & Danforth, 2007 [25])	GPIU (CIUS; Meerkerk, Van Den Eijnden, Vermulst, & Garretsen, 2009 [39])
Salience [18,39], Preoccupation [21,22,25]	Cognitive salience [25,39]	When the activity becomes the most important thing and dominates person's thinking, feelings, and behaviours	A strong thinking ongoing online	Do you spend a lot of time thinking about games even when you are not playing, or planning when you can play next?	I rarely think about playing when I am not using a computer	6. Do you think about the Internet, even when not online? 7. Do you look forward to your next Internet session?
	Behavioural salience [25,39]				I often fail to get enough sleep/miss meals because of playing	4. Do you prefer to use the Internet instead of spending time with others (e.g., partner, children, parents)?
Mood modification [18,25], alleviation of negative emotions [21,39], deceit or cover up [22] or escaping adverse moods [22,39]	Manage tension	Subjective experience as a consequence of engaging in the activity to increase or decrease tension to escape, or disconnect		Do you lie to family, friends or others about how much you game, or try to keep your family or friends from knowing how much you game?	I often experience a buzz of excitement while playing	12. Do you go on the Internet when you are feeling down?
	To escape or relieve		Being online to escape or being relieved	Do you game to escape from or forget about personal problems, or to relieve uncomfortable feelings, such as guilt, anxiety, helplessness or depression?		13. Do you use the Internet to escape from your sorrows or get relief from negative feelings?
Tolerance [18,21,22,25]		The need to increase amounts of the activity to achieve the preceding pleasant effects	Marked increase in online use to achieve satisfaction	Do you feel the need to play for increasing amounts of time, play more exciting games, or use more powerful equipment to get the same amount of excitement you used to get?	I tend to want to spend increasing amounts of time playing	
Withdrawal [18,21,25,39]		Unpleasant feeling states or physical effects when the activity is reduced or stopped	Dysphoric mood, anxiety, or boredom after days without online activity	Do you feel restless, irritable, moody, angry, anxious or sad when attempting to cut down or stop gaming, or when you are unable to play?	When I am not playing, I often feel agitated	14. Do you feel restless, frustrated, or irritated when you cannot use the Internet?

Table 1. *Cont.*

Components/Criteria	Subcomponents/Criterions	GPIU (Addiction; Griffiths, 2005 [18])	GPIU (Internet addiction; Tao et al., 2010 [21])	SPIU (IGD; APA, 2013 [22])	SPIU (online gaming; Charlton & Danforth, 2007 [25])	GPIU (CIUS; Meerkerk, Van Den Eijnden, Vermulst, & Garretsen, 2009 [39])
Conflict [18,25,39], loss of interests [21], give up other activities [22]	Intrapersonal [18,25,39], clinical impairment [21]	Conflicts from within the individual themselves		Do you lose interest in or reduce participation in other recreational activities (hobbies, meetings with friends) due to gaming? Do you risk or lose significant relationships, or job, educational or career opportunities because of gaming?	My social life/work has sometimes suffered because of my playing	8. Do you think you should use the Internet less often? 10. Do you rush through your (home) work in order to go on the Internet?
	Interpersonal [18,39], loss of interests and clinical impairment [21]	Conflicts between the addict and those around them	Online use substitutes (e.g., hobbies)		Arguments have sometimes arisen at home because of the time I spend playing	3. Do others (e.g., partner, children, parents) say you should use the Internet less? 11. Do you neglect your daily obligations (work, school, or family life) because you prefer to go on the Internet?
Relapse [18] and relapse reinstatement [25]		Tendency for repeated reversions to earlier patterns of the activity to be quickly restored after time of abstinence or control			I have made unsuccessful attempts to reduce the time I spend playing	
Persistent desire and difficulty to control it [21,39], reduction/stop [22,39]			Not being able to maintain a regular online usage pattern	Do you feel that you should play less, but are unable to cut back on the amount of time you spend playing games?		1. Do you find it difficult to stop using the Internet when you are online? 2. Do you continue to use the Internet despite your intention to stop? 5. Are you short of sleep because of the Internet? 9. Have you unsuccessfully tried to spend less time on the Internet?
Continued use disregarding harmful consequences [21,22]			Being online even causing psychological or physical harm to oneself	Do you continue to play games even though you are aware of negative consequences, such as not getting enough sleep, being late to school/work, spending too much money, having arguments with others, or neglecting important duties?		

Note: GPIU = Generalised Problematic Internet Use; SPIU = Specific Problematic Internet Use; IGD = Internet Gaming Disorder; APA = American Psychiatric Association; CIUS = Compulsive Internet Use Scale.

2. Materials and Methods

Permission to conduct this study was obtained from the ethics committee of the Psychological Science Research Institute (IPSY) at the Catholic University of Louvain (UcL; Belgium) in 2014. Respondents participated in leading research, which builds upon the Tech Use Disorders (TUD; [40]) project, carried out between 2014 and 2016. The qualitative part was undertaken at UcL, which is the main reason only Belgian results have been included in this paper. None of the data analysed in this paper have been used in any other article from this Marie Curie Intra-European Fellowship (FP7-PEOPLE-2013-IEF; ID 627999 [40–44]).

2.1. Design

Following the notation proposed by Morse [45] for the mixed methods designs, and according to the combination of data collection strategy (i.e., sequential implementation/time orientation) and priority (i.e., equal weight/emphasis) [46], a partially mixed sequential equal status ('QUAN→QUAL') design was used. The purpose of this design was to integrate in the discussion of the present study two different types of data [47–49] to clarify and illustrate the results obtained with the quantitative method by applying the qualitative one (i.e., whereby the interviews may help to evaluate and interpret the psychometric results obtained, estimating potential problem users who excessively perform a general or a specific online use(s)). A few of the previous studies on problematic online gaming have recently requested and undertaken this strategy [33] or the qualitative approach [50], but more should be done to cover the methodological gaps of finding what is behind the phenomena usually extracted from a sole psychometric measure. Another complementary purpose was to enable expansion (i.e., seeking to analyse and explore different facets of the GPIU and SPIU phenomena studied; e.g., to know if they seem independent or are interconnected, and in what sense). The mixed methods research in this study attempts to look for the way both methods complement each other to obtain a more productive, realistic, and detailed understanding of Internet addiction (as GPIU), online gaming disorder (as $SPIU_1$), and maladaptive use of social networks (as $SPIU_2$).

2.2. Participants and Procedure

2.2.1. Quantitative

The study online surveyed a convenience sample from Belgian higher education environments with 581 adult participants (85% originally francophone; 25.5% male; age range 18–79 years, mean (M) age 26.9 years, standard deviation (SD) = 12 years), with student and staff members who voluntarily agreed to participate. Participants had an information sheet and consent form on the first page of the survey and they provided informed consent and voluntarily participated following assurance of confidentiality and anonymity. The invitation to join the online survey used three recruitment strategies: Undergraduates' lectures, master or doctoral supervisions; via electronic requests or pools in online academic environments; and web sites or quick response code advertisements.

2.2.2. Qualitative

Participants who scored equal or over 21 in each CIUS [51] were invited to interviews, as they could potentially be classed as problem users. They were usually university students (except one who was an employee), all speaking fluent French. The invitation to participate in the qualitative part of the study was included at the end of the survey. The author contacted all participants who achieved the inclusion criteria reported and eight (1.4% of the overall sample) agreed to engage in the interview with an economic compensation (20 euros). They received an information sheet, provided informed consent by signing an agreement, and voluntarily participated following assurance of confidentiality and anonymity using pseudonyms. Interviews had a duration between 45 min and an hour, which took place at the IPSY (UcL). Permission was received for audio-recording.

2.3. Instrument and Analytical Strategy

2.3.1. Quantitative

The quantitative method was an online survey developed using Qualtrics which comprised: (i) Sociodemographics (gender, age, civil status, occupation status); (ii) online usage time (i.e., usual minutes per week day, and usual minutes per weekend day); (iii) technologies (i.e., fixed/desktop computer, laptop/notebook, tablet, smartphone, fixed game console or nonportable console, portable game console, television, other devices); (iv) main online activity used (i.e., emails (e.g., Google Mail, Oulook.com), messaging and chat (e.g., Skype, Hangouts), maintaining a blog (e.g., WordPress, Tumblr), online videos or streaming (e.g., YouTube, Netflix), downloads (e.g., music, movies), reading (e.g., newspapers, e-books), search for specific information (e.g., weather forecasts, city maps), casual games (e.g., Candy Crush, Farmville), solo video games (e.g., Dragon age, Assassin's Creed), vehicle simulation games (e.g., Euro Truck Simulator, Flight Simulator), strategy and management games (e.g., Age of Empire, StarCraft, Civilization), sport games (e.g., Pro Evolution Soccer, Virtua Tennis), shooting games online or first-person shooter (FPS; e.g., Call of duty, Planet side 2), multiplayer online battle arena (MOBA; e.g., League of Legends, Dota 2), MMORPG (e.g., World of Warcraft, Guild Wars 2), online gambling (e.g., PlayHugeLottos.com, OnlineBingo.eu), sport bets (e.g., PMU, horseracing, football), poker online (e.g., PokerStars.com), online casino (e.g., Casino Online, Blackjack), online slot machines, dating sites (e.g., Match, Meetic), erotic sites (e.g., Erotica), pornographic sites (e.g., Youporn), online shopping (e.g., eBay, Amazon), social networks (e.g., Facebook, Twitter)); and (v) the psychometric scales assessing generalised and specific Internet use-related addiction problems reported. Other studies have used and analysed other sections of this survey (e.g., other questionnaires in other samples from different countries or group ages), usually related to problematic mobile phone use and gaming [41–44].

Sociodemographics examined gender, age, relationship status (i.e., single, in a relationship, legally cohabitating, married, separated, divorced, or other), profession (i.e., student, employed, unemployed, retired, housewife/husband, self-employed, or other). The CIUS [39] measures general problem or compulsive Internet use (i.e., Internet addiction). It is based on the fourth DSM criterion for SUDs and pathological gambling. It contains 14 items rated from 0 "never" to 4 "very often". Scores ranged from 0–56, with the higher scores meaning to the more top potential generalised compulsive online use. The original scale in Dutch showed factorial, content, and concurrent validity and excellent reliability (Cronbach α between 0.89 and 0.90), as did the French adaptation used [52], which obtained similar outstanding psychometric properties (i.e., Cronbach α = 91). In this study, the original item had three options to be answered: General Internet use, online gaming, and social networking. For instance, item 1 (in French: 'A quelle fréquence, trouvez-vous difficile d'arrêter d'utiliser Internet pendant que vous êtes en ligne (c'est à dire s'arrêter, stopper l'activité)'; in English: How often do you find it difficult to stop using the Internet when you are online?) had three responses: (a) For Internet in general (CIUS), (b) for online gaming (CIUS-G), and (c) for social networking (CIUS-SNS). Thus, participants completed each item with these online uses. This innovation allows to assume more than one online use could be present simultaneously for any participant.

All statistical analyses were performed using IBM SPSS (version 23) software (IBM Corp. Released, Armonk, NY, USA) and a significance level of $p < 0.05$. Concerning the psychometric properties, the factor validity of each scale adaptation was assessed by exploratory factor analysis (EFA) using the principal components technique, with the Kaiser–Mayer–Olkin index (KMO) and Bartlett's test of sphericity to confirm the adequacy of the sample and procedure, respectively. The rationale for using the EFA is no study has adapted the CIUS to measure other specific Internet use-related addiction problems until the present, as far as the author is aware. The analysis yielded one factor, which is consistent with the theory and previous research using the CIUS [39]; with eigenvalues above 1 (factor loading > 0.4) to obtain an acceptable factor based on its explained variance. Internal consistency was estimated through the Cronbach's alpha coefficient, and an item analysis was performed to compare all

CIUS forms. Construct and content validity were obtained through associations of the total score with several indicators (i.e., time spent online using the Internet in general, or spent mainly gaming or mainly on social networks; or activities usually used by each of the CIUS studied). Comparisons between CIUS total scores and sociodemographic variables (i.e., gender and age groups) were performed through t and U Mann–Whitney tests. The proposed cut-off score reported by Guertler and colleagues [51] was chosen (i.e., score of 21 out of 56) to estimate the prevalence of potential problem users. However, caution should be considered, as present cut-offs still do not represent a threshold for clinical relevance and impairment. The sum of all potential problem users was computed to know how many participants could have one (or more) of the problems studied, together with the items and symptoms endorsed. Finally, to compare core versus peripheral symptoms [25,26] in those classed as potential problem users, the three CIUS were divided in two subgroups, according to Meerkerk and colleagues' [39] and Charlton and Danforth's [25] proposals (core symptoms: Items 3, 4, 5, 8, 10, 11, 14; peripheral symptoms: Items 1, 2, 6, 7, 9, 12, 13). Only an item (5) was modified from Meerkerk's proposal (i.e., from 'loss of control' was moved to 'intrapersonal conflict').

2.3.2. Qualitative

The interviews were undertaken and transcribed. The methods selected for the qualitative data analysis were two [53]: First, thematic analysis [54,55] with an etic coding strategy (i.e., coding from the perspective of the observer based on the literature) was used for examining perceptions and attitudes about potential Internet use-related addiction problems (causes, development, consequences, factors). Second, content analysis [56,57] to focus at a more micro level to provide both counts and opinions on IGD criteria proposed by the APA applied to the three problems studied. Both methods belong to qualitative descriptive phenomenological approaches [53], with a lower level of interpretation, but higher detail on the description of the meanings (i.e., focused on the knowledge that can originate and establish new definitions and substantial findings). At this stage of the development of the field, detail is needed on the nature of these problems. Synthetically, thematic analysis constitutes a purely qualitative approach used for identifying, analysing (codes), reporting patterns (themes) within textual data (i.e., involving the search for and identification of common threads), and interpreting aspects of the research question [56]. On the other hand, content analysis is a systematic coding and categorising approach used to explore text in detail to find patterns of words used, their frequencies (counts), their relationships, and their structures, which will allow answering the research questions [58].

3. Results

3.1. Quantitative

3.1.1. Participants Characteristics: Sociodemographic, Technologies Usage Patterns, and Online Activities

The majority of the sample (71.8%) were students (only 17.3% were employees, and the rest were 2.9% self-employed, 2% retired, 1.1% unemployed, 0.05% housewives or househusbands, among other). Half of the sample (58.2%) were single (36.5% were couples/in legal cohabitation/married, 4.9% separated/divorced, among other), without children (only 15.3% had progeny); their maximum education level was above all between secondary (59.8%) and higher education (38.8%). The participants (99.8%) had an Internet connection where they lived, had at least a computer (desktop or laptop; 97.5%) and a mobile phone (99.3%: without Internet access (25.1%) or a smartphone (74.2%)), and a third had (34.7%) a Tablet (e.g., iPad, Samsung galaxy tab). In all technologies, they usually had monthly contracts (i.e., Internet at home 95.5% of the sample, in the mobile phone 75.1%, and for the Tablet 35.3%).

3.1.2. Psychometric Properties of the French Generalised and Specific CIUS in Belgium

The CIUS as a GPIU psychometric tool was previously validated [39,52], but not the CIUS as SPIUs scales in gaming and social networking. In this study, the three measures showed factorial validity (i.e., CIUS: KMO = 0.91, $\chi^2_{(91)}$ = 2673.09, $p < 0.001$; CIUS–G: KMO = 0.93, $\chi^2_{(91)}$ = 5223.13, $p < 0.001$; CIUS–SNS: KMO = 0.93, $\chi^2_{(91)}$ = 3519.31, $p < 0.001$) and excellent internal consistency (see Table 2; where the descriptive, Cronbach alpha coefficients, and correlations between the three CIUS are reported). It is worth noting the high positive association between CIUS and CIUS–SNS, and the low positive association between CIUS and CIUS–G; however, between the two specific uses (CIUS–G and CIUS–SNS), there is no correlation.

Table 2. Descriptive, reliability, and correlation matrix across all adaptations for the CIUS.

			CIUS Adaptations		
Scale Adaptations	Descriptive *M(SD)*; Range	Cronbach alpha	CIUS	CIUS–G	CIUS–SNS
CIUS	14.63(10.10); 0–56	0.90	-		
CIUS–G	4.78(8.97); 0–51	0.95	0.22 **	-	
CIUS–SNS	11.63(10.79); 0–56	0.93	0.59 **	−0.02	-

Note: CIUS: Compulsive Internet use scale; CIUS–G: CIUS for gaming; CIUS–SNS: CIUS for social networking sites; *M*: Mean; *SD*: Standard deviation; ** $p < 0.01$.

The CIUS yielded one factor (i.e., generalised problematic Internet use), which explained 48.86% of the total variance with loads to this sole factor between 0.85 (item 14) to 0.72 (item 10); such as the CIUS–G (i.e., specific problematic (video) gaming) that explained 60.12% with loads to between 0.69 (item 9) to 0.84 (item 7), and the CIUS–SNS (i.e., specific problematic social networking) that explained 50.50% with loads to between 0.58 (item 4) to 0.79 (item 2). The scree plots of the three versions show the one-factor of these adaptations (see Figure 3), which allows to compare items by descriptive, correlations, and factors loadings (see Table 3).

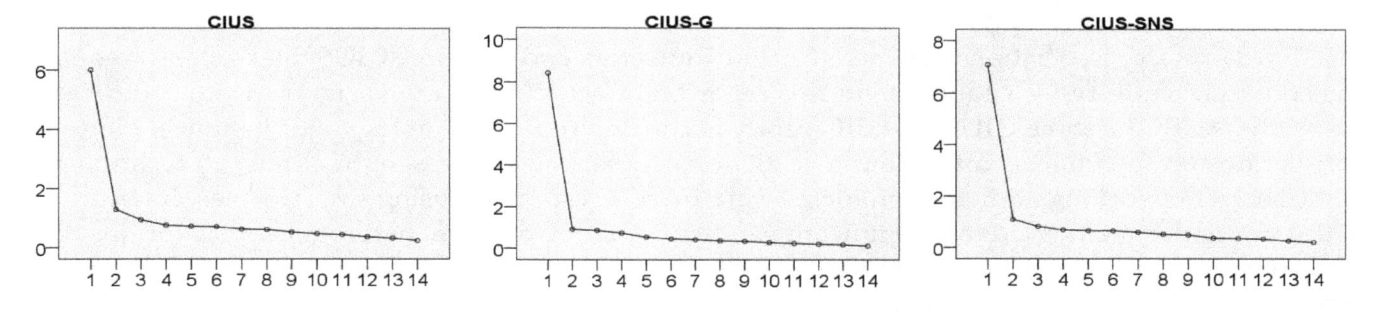

Figure 3. Scree plots from the original CIUS (GPIU), the adaptation for gaming (CIUS–G; SPIU$_1$), and the adaptation for social networking (CIUS–SNS; SPIU$_2$); in the y axis the eigenvalues, and in the x axis the component numbers.

Table 3. Item analysis: descriptive, correlation item per total correlation, and factor loadings across all adaptations for the CIUS.

Items	Descriptive *M(SD)*			Correlation Item-Total Correlation Per CIUS Adaptations			Factor Loading Per CIUS Adaptations		
	CIUS	CIUS–G	CIUS–SNS	CIUS	CIUS–G	CIUS–SNS	CIUS	CIUS–G	CIUS–SNS
1	1.98(1.267)	0.66(1.159)	1.84(1.372)	0.60	0.79	0.71	0.67	0.82	0.76
2	1.84(1.354)	0.52(1045)	1.73(1.468)	0.65	0.76	0.74	0.71	0.79	0.79
3	0.80(1.089)	0.27(0.765)	0.78(1.131)	0.46	0.63	0.61	0.53	0.69	0.67
4	0.90(1.003)	0.31(0.768)	0.63(0.945)	0.56	0.75	0.52	0.63	0.78	0.58
5	1.07(1.147)	0.28(0.750)	0.79(1.094)	0.57	0.68	0.64	0.64	0.73	0.69

Table 3. *Cont.*

Items	Descriptive *M*(SD)			Correlation Item-Total Correlation Per CIUS Adaptations			Factor Loading Per CIUS Adaptations		
	CIUS	CIUS–G	CIUS–SNS	CIUS	CIUS–G	CIUS–SNS	CIUS	CIUS–G	CIUS–SNS
6	0.99(1.045)	0.29(0.716)	1.06(1.087)	0.56	0.74	0.67	0.63	0.79	0.72
7	1.16(1.107)	0.39(0.863)	1.00(1.103)	0.56	0.80	0.64	0.64	0.84	0.70
8	1.33(1.187)	0.39(0.872)	1.39(1.321)	0.59	0.75	0.65	0.66	0.79	0.71
9	0.78(1.017)	0.22(0.615)	0.82(1.094)	0.63	0.64	0.62	0.70	0.69	0.68
10	1.01(1.090)	0.29(0.739)	0.84(1.107)	0.66	0.78	0.69	0.72	0.83	0.75
11	1.07(1.175)	0.28(0.718)	0.89(1.137)	0.63	0.74	0.64	0.70	0.79	0.69
12	2.05(1.240)	0.57(1.095)	1.69(1.419)	0.60	0.79	0.71	0.67	0.82	0.75
13	1.54(1.304)	0.41(0.943)	1.18(1.318)	0.59	0.72	0.65	0.66	0.76	0.71
14	1.20(1.172)	0.23(0.657)	0.91(1.132)	0.51	0.69	0.67	0.85	0.74	0.73

Note: CIUS: Compulsive Internet use scale; CIUS–G: CIUS for gaming; CIUS–SNS: CIUS for social networking sites; *M*: Mean; *SD*: Standard deviation.

Regarding descriptive results per item in each version, CIUS and CIUS–SNS have higher scores than CIUS–G. The higher punctuations in all of them being for items 1, 2, and 12 (which were associated with loss of control and mood modification symptoms [39]). However, differences between adaptations emerged in the lowest scores: Item 9 on Internet and gaming (loss of control [39]), and item 4 in social networking (preoccupation [39]). Concerning the correlation of each item with the total correlation of each adaptation, all CIUS presented high positive correlations between each item and the total score, especially the gaming version (r between 0.63 and 0.80). Concerning factor loading, all were greater than 0.5; by order from higher to lower scores: Gaming (minimum 0.69), social networking (minimum 0.58), and Internet (minimum 0.53). Consequently, when dividing the CIUS scores by core and peripheral symptoms, descriptive results were higher for peripheral ones (i.e., Internet use in general ($M = 10.34$, $SD = 5.87$), social networking ($M = 9.32$, $SD = 6.77$), and gaming ($M = 3.06$, $SD = 5.25$)) than the core symptoms (i.e., Internet ($M = 7.38$, $SD = 5.32$), social networking ($M = 6.23$, $SD = 5.70$), and gaming ($M = 2.04$, $SD = 4.12$)).

Furthermore, associations between the time indicators and the three CIUS total scores strengthen the construct validity (see Table 4). In this regard, almost all the time variables were significantly associated with the three CIUS, but differently according to the technology. For instance, moderate correlations on the Internet and gaming addiction problems were present in almost all technologies, while social networking addiction problems were present, especially using smartphones. Interestingly, a device pattern emerged as significant associations were quite heterogeneous; for instance, all technologies were associated with time per days (weekday or weekend day) when using Internet in general, but when gaming, only computers and tablets were correlated with time per days, and when social networking, only computers and smartphones were associated with time spent on a day. However, the maximum time spent as leisure was usually on computers.

Similarly, content validity was also established through associations to CIUS total scores and across all the online activities as follows: Firstly, the CIUS (GPIU) with 'messages and chats' ($r = 0.19$, $p < 0.001$), 'online videos and streaming' ($r = 0.17$, $p < 0.001$), 'Twitter' ($r = 0.16$, $p < 0.001$), 'Facebook' ($r = 0.14$, $p < 0.001$), 'Instagram' ($r = 0.12$, $p < 0.05$), 'Hi5' ($r = 0.11$, $p < 0.05$), 'blogs' ($r = 0.10$, $p < 0.05$), and 'porn sites' ($r = 0.09$, $p < 0.05$). Secondly, the CIUS–G (SPIU$_1$) was associated to the following games: 'MOBA' ($r = 0.45$, $p < 0.001$), 'MMORPG' ($r = 0.43$, $p < 0.001$), 'Solo games' ($r = 0.42$, $p < 0.001$),

'FPS' ($r = 0.39$, $p < 0.001$), 'games strategy' ($r = 0.33$, $p < 0.001$), 'casual games' ($r = 0.23$, $p < 0.001$), and 'simulation games' ($r = 0.22$, $p < 0.001$), together with porn sites ($r = 0.24$, $p < 0.001$), and reading ($r = 0.1$, $p < 0.05$). Lastly, the CIUS–SNS (SPIU$_2$) was related to the following social networks: 'Facebook' ($r = 0.36$, $p < 0.001$), 'Instagram' ($r = 0.18$, $p < 0.05$), and 'Twitter' ($r = 0.14$, $p < 0.001$), including messages and chats ($r = 0.23$, $p < 0.01$), downloading ($r = 0.2$, $p < 0.001$), streaming ($r = 0.18$, $p < 0.001$), and blogging ($r = 0.1$, $p < 0.05$).

3.1.3. Prevalence of the French Generalised and Specific CIUS in Belgium

In this study, no statistical difference was found between the original CIUS total score per gender ($t_{(469)} = -0.08$, $p = 0.94$; male: $M = 17.65$, $SD = 11.05$; female: $M = 17.75$, $SD = 10.48$), but differences between gender were found in the specific CIUS: CIUS–G ($U = 13{,}420$, $p < 0.001$; male: $M = 10.05$, $SD = 12.30$; female: $M = 3.68$, $SD = 7.42$), CIUS–SNS ($U = 13{,}945$, $p < 0.001$; male: $M = 11.25$, $SD = 10.55$; female: $M = 16.78$, $SD = 12.03$). With respect to the age groups, young adults (i.e., 18–39 years old) compared to middle-aged adults (i.e., 40–65 years old) presented significant differences in all measures: CIUS ($t_{(459)} = -5.54$, $p < 0.001$; young: $M = 18.58$, $SD = 10.35$; middle-aged: $M = 10.41$, $SD = 8.85$), CIUS–G ($U = 9160$, $p < 0.05$; young: $M = 5.34$, $SD = 9.37$; middle-aged: $M = 2.81$, $SD = 6.42$), and CIUS–SNS ($U = 4493.5$, $p < 0.001$; young: $M = 17.05$, $SD = 11.70$; middle-aged: $M = 5.89$, $SD = 7.66$).

Concerning GPIU, taking into account the overall 471 participants as potential problem users, there were 176 potential Internet addicts (37.4%: 8.1% males and 29.3% females, $\chi^2_{(1)} = 23.58$, $p < 0.001$; 39.8% young and 13% middle-aged, $\chi^2_{(1)} = 14.79$, $p < 0.001$), 51 potential problematic online gamers (10.8%: 5.3% males and 5.5% females, $\chi^2_{(1)} = 0.08$, $p = 0.78$; 11.3% young and 3.7% middle-aged, $\chi^2_{(1)} = 2.95$, $p = 0.09$), and 153 problematic social networkers (32.5%: 3.4% males and 29.1% females, $\chi^2_{(1)} = 18.09$, $p < 0.001$; 32.4% young and 7.4% middle-aged, $\chi^2_{(1)} = 23.58$, $p < 0.001$). Finally, when computing the potential problem users, 49.7% of the sample has not classed in any user problem category, 23.6% had only one problematic online use, 23.1% had two potential online problems, and 3.6% had all the problems.

From these three groups of problem users, descriptive and endorsements to each item (i.e., on the basis of answering 'often' or 'very often' should be considered) were computed (see Table 5). Interestingly, the highest scores and endorsement in all GPIU and SPIUs were in items 1 and 2 for the loss of control symptom, and item 12 for the mood modification symptom; while the lower scores and endorsements were more heterogeneous. For instance, item 3 (conflict) being lower in the problematic Internet (CIUS), but the less endorsed were items 4 (preoccupation) and 9 (loss of control); while in gaming (CIUS–G) item 9 (loss of control) was the one with lower score and the less endorsed by none potential problem gamer; lastly, item 4 (preoccupation) obtained the lower score and endorsement in problematic social networking.

Table 4. Descriptive and correlation across all validated adaptations for the CIUS in relation to time.

Scales and Descriptive	Days Per Week (Weekly Frequency) r			Minutes Per Day in a Weekly Day r			Minutes Per Day in a Weekend Day r		
	Computers	Tablets	Phones	Computers	Tablets	Phones	Computers	Tablets	Phones
CIUS	0.18**	0.08	0.09	0.37**	0.25**	0.24**	0.39**	0.28**	0.21**
CIUS-G	0.14**	0.27**	0.07	0.27**	0.26**	0.05	0.22**	0.21**	0.02
CIUS-SNS	0.09	-0.02	0.21**	0.11*	0.08	0.35**	0.22**	0.13	0.37*
M(SD)	6.17(1.62)	3.87(2.80)	4.62(2.98)	118.71(93.45)	46.10(64.99)	82.70(116.08)	183.91(200.53)	68.16(100.13)	90.99(124.45)

Note: Weekly Day: from Monday to Friday; Weekend Day: from Saturday to Sunday; CIUS: Compulsive Internet use scale; CIUS-G: CIUS for gaming; CIUS-SNS: CIUS for social networking sites; r: r Pearson (correlation); M: Mean; SD: Standard deviation; * p < 0.05; ** p < 0.01.

Table 5. Item and symptoms from potential problem users: descriptive, and frequency of endorsement across all adaptations for the CIUS.

Item Number, Symptom According to Meerkerk et al., 2009 [39] and Charlton & Danforth, 2007 [25]	Descriptive M(SD)			Endorsement f i (%)		
	CIUS	CIUS-G	CIUS-SNS	CIUS (n = 176)	CIUS-G (n = 51)	CIUS-SNS (n = 153)
1—Loss of control–Peripheral	2.86(0.942)	2.86(1.02)	3.08(0.924)	114(64.8)	34(66.7)	112(73.2)
2—Loss of control–Peripheral	2.91(0.987)	2.59(1.134)	3.07(0.926)	124(70.5)	28(54.9)	113(73.9)
3—Conflict–Core	1.48(1.214)	1.55(1.301)	1.73(1.262)	31(17.6)	12(23.5)	38(24.8)
4—Preoccupation–Core	1.53(1.008)	1.82(0.974)	1.25(1.079)	26(14.8)	11(21.6)	18(11.8)
5—Loss of control–Core	1.85(1.162)	1.59(1.236)	1.67(1.261)	43(24.4)	13(25.5)	41(26.8)
6—Preoccupation–Peripheral	1.70(1.039)	1.71(1.082)	2.04(0.973)	39(22.2)	9(17.6)	46(30.1)
7—Preoccupation–Peripheral	1.9(1.057)	2.18(1.072)	1.94(1.04)	52(29.5)	19(37.3)	41(26.8)
8—Conflict–Core	2.19(1.082)	2.02(0.99)	2.46(1.088)	68(38.6)	14(27.5)	77(50.3)
9—Loss of control–Peripheral	1.56(1.057)	1.20(1.077)	1.70(1.181)	29(16.5)	7(13.7)	37(24.2)
10—Conflict–Core	1.86(1.073)	1.80(1.114)	1.85(1.146)	52(29.5)	13(25.5)	43(28.1)
11—Conflict–Core	1.97(1.146)	1.67(1.089)	1.82(1.227)	53(30.1)	12(23.5)	40(26.1)
12—Mood modification–Peripheral	2.92(0.977)	2.59(1.268)	2.95(1.022)	124(70.5)	30(58.8)	113(73.9)
13—Mood modification–Peripheral	2.48(1.181)	2.12(1.291)	2.30(1.22)	97(55.1)	20(39.2)	67(43.8)
14—Withdrawal–Core	1.89(1.175)	1.43(1.171)	1.90(1.134)	55(31.3)	11(21.6)	47(30.7)

Note: CIUS: Compulsive Internet use scale; CIUS-G: CIUS for gaming; CIUS-SNS: CIUS for social networking sites; M: Mean; SD: Standard deviation; f i: frequency; % is valid percentage; n: Subsample size; and item 5 was moved from 'Loss of control' [39] to Conflict by the author, for this reason has been classed as Core symptom [25].

Finally, when comparing core and peripheral symptoms in each CIUS peripheral ones used to have higher punctuation than core ones in the potential problem users in GPIU and SPIUs (see Table 5). Furthermore, for those categorised as problem Internet users, moderate associations between time variables and core or peripheral items were significant in the time spent using Internet on a weekday (core: $r = 0.19$, $p < 0.05$; peripheral: $r = 0.21$, $p < 0.05$) or a weekend day (core: $r = 0.23$, $p < 0.01$; peripheral: $r = 0.22$, $p < 0.05$); while in problem social networkers there existed only an association between the core symptoms and weekend days ($r = 0.25$, $p < 0.01$), and none association existed in problem gamers (e.g., core: Time spent gaming in a weekday ($r = 0.21$, $p = 0.19$)).

3.2. Qualitative

3.2.1. Participants Characteristics: Sociodemographic, Technologies Usage Patterns, and Online Activities

A total of 165 (out of 581) provided their contact details to participate in the qualitative part of this study; eight of them (4.85% of those who left this information) accepted the invitation to participate in an individual interview. Participants' characteristics are reported in Table 6.

Table 6. Participant sociodemographic characteristics and potential problem online uses.

Pseudonyms	Variables					
	Gender	Age	Civil Status	CIUS	CIUS–G	CIUS–SNS
Leia	Female	31	Partner	**24**	**29**	17
Moira	Female	20	Single	**26**	5	**28**
Aneka	Female	20	Partner	**37**	14	**37**
Victor	Male	20	Single	**36**	**31**	**37**
Elektra	Female	35	Divorced	23	5	8
Carol	Female	21	Partner	13	**25**	19
Scarlet	Female	18	Single	8	0	**21**
Martin	Male	19	Partner	9	**22**	4

Note: CIUS: Compulsive Internet use scale; CIUS–G: CIUS for Gaming; CIUS–SNS: CIUS for Social networking sites; numbers in bold are the scores above the cut-off in each CIUS adaptation as potential problems.

Almost all participants were female Belgian young adults who scored as potential problem users of Internet in general ($n = 5$), gaming ($n = 4$), and/or social networking ($n = 4$). Therefore, half of them had mixed problem profiles, usually as excessive Internet in general and social network users, except one presenting all problems studied (i.e., GPIU, SPIU$_1$, and SPIU$_2$), who was a young male.

3.2.2. Themes Related to Generalised Internet Problem, and Specific Gaming and Social Networking Problems

Themes Related to Its Evolution: Causes, Development, and Consequences

Individuals' experiences and reflections mapped into the central themes which are presented in Tables 7–10 below by types of GPIU vs. SPIU.

The causes of excessively using specific online activities were diverse (see Table 7), and they could be summarised in three types of aetiological facets: the individual, the social, and the contextual ones. First, the individual aspect relates to avoiding boredom and to escaping reality (as a daily routine or because of a trauma). In the case of gamers, it seems there is a profile: they tend to be tech-savvy (i.e., study or work in informatics or the technologies sector) or really enjoy technologies (to be daily connected, multitasking, and managing studies/work and leisure), together with being a homebody person with an introvert personality, and to have a specific desire or mood to only play video games. By contrast, social networkers would like to have consistent updates in all areas and use SNS obsessively to scrutinise others' lives and compare them with their own life. Second, the social facet seems to be related to sharing a hobby with others who have similar interests in technologies and online activities (e.g., relatives, boyfriend/girlfriend, friends from real life, virtual colleagues); gamers usually are highly committed to their guild and tend to supply (or complement) their social life through virtual social friendships developed (or maintained) through the game. It seems online users tend to build (or strengthen) bonds with those who share the same online activities and they are constantly connected through games and networks sharing information (e.g., about competitions, gossips). Third, the contextual facet is usually linked to having plenty of free time (e.g., because they are studying at secondary school or university, unemployed, in convalescence, or they are housewives/househusbands); a perceived 'poor' or 'hostile' external context (e.g., difficult relationships (or not fulfilling ones) with family, partner, colleagues), an environment where everybody is connected to the Internet (e.g., gamer guilds, Facebook profiles), being in a post-traumatic recovery (e.g., having lost a loved one(s), having lost a job), or feeling the need to consume technology when something new and appealing appears in the market (e.g., new video game, new social network, latest version). Interestingly, no quote was extracted from GPIU, and almost all were obtained from gaming.

Table 7. Superordinate and subordinate themes about the aetiology of the SPIUs studied, together with a few quotations (adapted from French to English) as illustration.

Theme	Subthemes		
		CIUS–G	CIUS–SNS
Causes	Individual facet	'I started to be a gamer at the same time I started at the university. It is quite usual in people who like technologies to have online hobbies, as we have difficulties communicating with other people; games could be an escape' (Leia) 'I think the pathology in gaming appears when you cannot avoid craving; when the negative feelings emerge from not being able to play, it is the lack of something in you' (Victor)	'In the game, when you win you feel you are valorised; on Facebook, you only see positive things and this makes people feel positive, as it is easier to see someone through Facebook than call him or her' (Elektra)
	Social facet	'What makes me play more and more is playing online with those I know, to compete among us' (Victor) 'I play League of Legends, a MMORPG, not a MOBA, as it needs an objective and it is a network; you play with friends, and this is what I really like' (Martin)	'It is the wish to share; as sharing your emotions. Above all when there is good news you share it through Facebook' (Moira)
	Contextual facet	'Gaming can increase if there is a lot of free time, studying at university or being unemployed. Also because external relations are difficult, at school, friendships and above all in the family' (Leia)	'With all technologies around us, you feel the obligation to be connected all the time, to know what is happening' (Moira)

Note: CIUS–G: Compulsive Internet use scale for gaming; CIUS–SNS: CIUS for social networking sites; MMORPG: massively multiplayer online role-playing games; MOBA: multiplayer online battle arena.

The development of these Internet problems is described as a process, which starts during adolescence with an acquired enjoyable habit that slowly and unconsciously takes progressively more and more from the user (i.e., not only more time; by coming above all other life aspects of the user, such as feelings, emotions, cognitions, behaviours, relationships, activities). This gradual mining of the problematic online uses could be observed through the addictive symptomatology described by excessive users (see Table 8).

Regarding salience, it is usually described covering emotional and cognitive facets (i.e., craving or preoccupation respectively; e.g., as a personal drive or desire to be connected or worrying, even being obsessive about personal or social online duties, such as updating your profile, tending to notifications in the SNS, or accomplishing guild expectations in a role-play game). Sometimes, it is associated with an unconscious need to be connected even when not possible, or an alleviation of negative emotions, such as wanting to escape or being 'anesthetised'. It seems to be quite a usual symptom in the three problems studied.

With regard to mood modification, salience is present in the GPIU and SPIUs studied, but it seems more prevalent in gaming. Gamers report using various kinds of games to produce different types of moods, such as MMORPG or FPS to induce tension, and casual games to relax; they state they balance their spirit in each moment through the games they choose to play. Similarly, social networkers, for instance, use Facebook to channel emotions (e.g., to share good news vs. to look for someone to cheer up). Networkers state they use SNS to share positive things (e.g., positive messages, images, videos). SNS contents seem to be positively biased, but networkers are aware and happy with it. However, sometimes, images or other information observed through the SNS could affect a user's humour negatively (e.g., as the user could compare his or her life with others; especially in adolescence), and feel upset caused by negative feelings (e.g., jealousy, sadness). This could also happen with the online series that people watch in streaming too, usually used to relax (e.g., users could compare their lives, and this could affect them, especially when being an adolescent).

Tolerance is a symptom which only emerged in both SPIUs studied. In gaming, it seems to be linked to all types of continuous increments: Time, expertise, the sensation of progress, achievement, and advancement in the game to produce similar satisfaction or rewards. Therefore, the 'dose' is not only a quantity of time playing, it is also an increment of intensity and development of the gamer's skills in the game, as well as the level of personal achievement in the game (e.g., score, level) or the level of social recognition by other gamers (e.g., status in the guild). Similarly, in social networking, the tolerance symptom could be understood for the continuous need and increment of publishing information (e.g., posts, pictures) about one's own (or another's) life, to observe social reactions (e.g., how many likes and/or comments the post received). This reinforces specific online behaviours, as the user self-perceives his or her life as a gamer or networker good enough to be valued by those who share the same online activity (e.g., through score comparisons, others' life achievements).

The other classic addictive symptom studied was withdrawal, which has usually been associated with negative feelings (i.e., frustration, irritability) when not being connected for gaming. This sense is directly linked to the need of connection after interruption or a forced stop. It seems being disconnected is being in severe discomfort, above all when the user is younger (e.g., an adolescent), alone at home (i.e., with plenty of time to play games), and a gamer (i.e., playing 'big video games', which usually are MMORPG, FPS, or MOBA). Thus, in the GPIU and SPIU related to SNS, withdrawal has not emerged as a subtheme.

Concerning conflicts, intrapersonal and interpersonal facets have emerged for all Internet use-related addiction problems. Gamers are the users who appeal more often to intrapersonal conflicts, as they play everywhere when a computer is available to them (e.g., university, work, or home), and when they supposedly should do other activities (e.g., attending a session in university, working in a workplace, or sleeping during night). However, social networkers have reported similar problems with depression, anxiety, and stress, as well as sleep or meal deprivation, which could affect their duties or relationships. Subsequently, there are problems with family, friends, or partners because of excessive online behaviours, which cause disputes, possible loss of contacts (e.g., boyfriend, girlfriend) or less of other relevant activities (e.g., studies, job).

Concerning relapse, this only appeared once in a gamer interview, who expressed how rigid rules created by the guild could constrain the gamer and obligate him or her to play. If the player leaves the game, social pressure appears by the guild, as well as the loss of the feelings of being in a 'virtual world' created by the gamers during an extended period. Thus, the gamer continually returns to the game.

The persistent desire and difficulty to control, reduce, or stop online behaviour is a common difficulty for all excessive Internet users. For instance, gaming is an extended hobby with an industry which supports periodic updates to play better and differently (e.g., characters, collections, the system of dropping). Moreover, the fact that some games reproduce 'persistent worlds' facilitates continuous playing (e.g., to compete). Similarly, the continued use with disregard of harmful consequences (e.g., physical problems or unhealthy attitudes or behaviours) is usually due to the habit already created to manage the user's mood, user's time, social relationships, etc. It seems essential to be continuously connected to the Internet, games, or SNS to maintain users' personal and social life actively.

Lastly, deceit or cover-up has only appeared in problematic gaming, as gamers usually report they live a 'secret double life', the one in the 'real world' and the one in the 'virtual world' (i.e., the game(s)). Gamers are quite aware they invert time and effort in the games; contrary to other established addictive behaviours, gamers work hard and actively to maintain their gaming behaviour. One reason is other gamers (e.g., the guild) when playing in the 'big games' share their own online spaces and codes to constantly communicate (even if they know themselves or not in 'real life', as sometimes gamers are from other countries or cultures). Thus, deception is not only hiding what is consumed through technology to others (e.g., hiding playing games at night to their parents), it is a more complex issue (i.e., managing languages, identities, relationships, and duties in different 'worlds'). In this sense, they express that those who do not play games usually cannot understand them; they directly maintain this 'other (online) life' in secret for many reasons: To avoid conflicts, to be judged, along with other reasons.

Concerning the consequences (see Table 9), the positive outcomes are usually associated with enriching users' social lives, as they could experience other 'virtual (online) worlds' and relationships that they consider improving their lives. For instance, they can connect differently with others who are more related to them (i.e., transmitting the online 'virtual self' through SNS or through an avatar in a game, creating and maintaining friendships or affective relationships through private online spaces in SNS or through games (e.g., 'feeling together'), dating and finding partners). They have other types of connections parallel to their 'real life' ones (i.e., relatives, partner, peers, colleagues, friends, or other persons with whom they interact face-to-face). Furthermore, gamers report an improvement in their cognitive processes (e.g., memory, attention, and learning).

However, the adverse self-perceived outcomes by heavy users are mainly those problems which have been unconscious developed until they became aware of the addiction problem, as something (or someone) alerted them. This discovery usually requires them to start behaving differently to naturally recover from a maladaptive to an adaptive pattern of usage. Only in gamers has natural recovery emerged as a process of maturity (i.e., need to develop other life challenges), such as to enter the workplace (which requires responsibility, time, effort, energy, among other skills before invested above all in the game); although, sometimes, they cannot do it by themselves. For instance, it has been reported heavy gamers are living in 'another world' which is alternative to real life, and not all of them know how to manage both or do not see the benefit in renouncing 'virtual life'. A few of them have lost studies/jobs, friends/partners, even some aspects of their health; a few have experienced chronic sleeping and eating problems, and discomfort in some bones, muscles, and organs, probably due to the maintained tension during extended periods (e.g., cervical, hands, or eyes, respectively). Those who mix gaming with drug consumption (e.g., cannabis) experience other problems (e.g., see images of the game when the player was not gaming).

With regard to neutral consequences, users appeal to curiosity and relationships reinforced by the virtual connections. It is observed that female gamers seem to have boyfriend gamers, as they have met them and/or matched with them better as a couple because of sharing this hobby or passion for games, which ensures their common understanding as gamers and lets them share their virtual lives. Similarly, social networkers report the relevance of being intellectually fed by being updated continuously. Thus, related to these consequences, detail has been provided only for SPIUs.

Finally, few risk factors were reported and directly connected with the symptomatology in all Internet use-related addiction problems (see Table 10), where developmental and contextual factors seem the most impactful ones. For instance, some of them are: Parent styles, such as authoritarian, partner already 'addicted' to gaming, drug consumption together with gaming, the tendency to be indoors with online hobbies, lost someone(s) loved, adolescent crisis, games substituting 'virtual' prices with money. Only a few protective factors have also emerged (i.e., family limits, activities outdoors, and transforming the online activity to a healthy activity or profession: 'eSport').

Table 8. Superordinate and subordinate themes about the development (i.e., addictive symptomatology) of the GPIU and SPIUs studied, together with a few quotations (adapted from French to English) as illustration.

Theme	Subthemes	Quotes		
		CIUS	CIUS-G	CIUS-SNS
Development (addictive symptoms)	Salience	'If you have a need, such as looking for a job, and you always have your smartphone with you, you could get obsessive about checking the Internet continuously. You are in your own world. If I am not checking it, I think I am losing opportunities' (Aneka)	'Gaming is excessive when it is a priority. Years ago, I felt I needed to play when I was going out with others, and I realised I had a problem. It is not a question of time playing. It is about when you cannot be without gaming, and there is no Internet. For instance, a gamer will take public transport for hours until finding a place with Internet to play video games. The gamer substitutes going out with friends for video gaming, and gamers are always connected even through a smartphone' (Carol) 'There are guild obligations, as we agree to be there to do something, and if you do not do it, you put people in trouble' (Leia) 'The "vagaries" of life, there are periods when I wish to play; I do not think craving is in myself or my brain; I think it is outside' (Carol)	'In the SNS we think of other things, to free our minds of negative feelings' (Moira)
	Mood modification	'If I am sad, I watch an online series or films to cheer up, which sometimes is better than gaming' (Carol)	'I integrate myself in the story and into a character of an MMORPG to disconnect with reality. When you have had a stressed day, your reward is gaming. As I made an effort, I have the right to escape; it is very relaxing' (Carol) 'When gaming (RPG or FPS) we can quickly become annoyed or nervous, but sometimes it's the contrary, playing casual games helps you to relax. I have all types of different games I play depending on my mood, and how I want to balance my emotions' (Leia) 'When I am alone and upset, I play to calm myself, but I do not regulate myself as I feel tense or nervous after stopping' (Martin)	'You go to Facebook to look for something to cheer you up' (Moira)
	Tolerance		'The feelings of success and gratification could be a stimulus that makes us think of the game and makes us feel well, and produces the wish to play' (Carol) 'I need to have my little dose every day to feel like I'm advancing in the game. Before I could play for 15 hours daily, but now only 2 h. For example, if you stop for a day everything is reset, so sometimes we have to play to keep the game and the gamers together, and when you win you are happy' (Leia)	'It is the need to look into other's lives. It is about being jealous, to posting pictures, messages, and to observing reactions through the numbers of likes and comments we receive, as these reinforce you' (Elektra)
	Withdrawal		'Ten years ago, I had to play games on my computer. If I couldn't, I was frustrated; it was emotionally automatic. I had only one desire: to enter the game and play' (Leia) 'Once we were on vacation for weeks and I could not access the Internet, I felt the craving. I was thinking all the time about it. I learnt I could not put gaming as a priority, and I started to control the periods of gaming or not gaming' (Carol)	
	Conflict (intrapersonal and interpersonal)	'Problematic use is when the use of the Internet is affecting the family or the couple. Or if it is affecting sleep, work, or social life' (Elektra)	'I was gaming in class sessions, when I came back home I spent whole nights on my computer gaming. I could play 15 or 16 hours per day, but other people left or hindered their studies or jobs, or had conflicts with their partners' (Leia) 'You neglect other activities, your course, your family, other social contacts, even your health. Gamers have a lack of vitamin D because they do not go out, they eat poorly and quickly, so they can return to the game' (Carol) 'Excessive gaming is evident as lack of sleep shows in your eyes; hygiene, as you are not taking showers for gaming; the body, as you skip meals. These have consequences for your family, life, and work. It is the same problem during adolescence or adulthood, but the consequences are worst in adulthood. It causes tiredness. It is a loop' (Martin) 'I think the more you play, the more it affects your vision; as you start to seeing images from your thoughts; and these are engaged with the game' (Martin)	'When I am online too much, without sleeping and with troubles in my daily life, I have observed others like me have real problems with their studies, with both games and SNS' (Moira)
	Relapse		'If you want to leave a game such as a FPS, the group require you to return to maintain the same number of gamers in the teams as before. If not, they need to look for other gamers who are not so good. It is like a team sport, we have microphones, it is not simply a game, and it is another dimension. It is about speaking, planning strategies, indeed it is a world that we develop for a long time. Thus, when dates are fixed it is too restrictive' (Victor)	
	Difficulty to control it	'When I come home, I connect myself to Facebook from 5 to 10 or 11 pm, and if I cannot sleep, I use the Internet' (Aneka)	'Each new version of an RPG causes an increment of gamers and game play again. These are persistent worlds and being in one country or another does not change anything' (Leia) 'You make a false plan; it's almost a fake virtual plan' (Victor) 'One of my relatives was online gaming in an RPG with a guild, and we told him he needed to do something else, but he did not stop' (Victor)	'When I play with my partner, he cannot stop gaming if he is not winning. It is a fact of being successful, to have a goal. When a gamer develops an addiction, I think it is because they are attached to a world which is not real life. This is different from SNS users who are overly connected with real life. Gaming and SNS are really different' (Moira)
	Continued use disregard		'I passed hours gaming even when my eyes hurt' (Martin)	
	Deceive		'I had an alternative life; it is like private groups in Facebook, but in the game, and we are constantly in communication through software. We have the impression of living a double life, we do not speak about our real lives in the game, because people ask questions and judge us. It is a secret double life, it is a habit, like a drug' (Leia)	

Note: CIUS: Compulsive Internet use scale; CIUS-G: CIUS for gaming; CIUS-SNS: CIUS for social networking sites; MMORPG: massively multiplayer online role-playing games; RPG: role-playing games; FPS: first-person shooter.

Table 9. Superordinate and subordinate themes about the consequences of the GPIU and SPIUs studied, together with a few quotations (adapted from French to English) as illustration.

Theme	Subthemes	CIUS–G	CIUS–SNS
Consequences	Positive	'I play for the strategy, the research, the challenge, the learning through connections of things. We get into to a story and this promotes your memory, intelligence, and the capacity to maintain attention and quickly answer, to plan and foresee consequences, to adapt yourself. We are less confined in a virtual world and we could see and live more and differently than in real life' (Leia)	'Facebook could be a place to meet with my partner, to communicate or play games. I need to maintain this bond daily to maintain our news' (Moira)
	Negative	'Gaming is addictive without knowing exactly why. The people around you or your financial situation will not stop you, only the circumstances such as the professional world, physical problems, and a partner if he or she is not a gamer. Gamers can be confined and isolated; some of them have lost courses, jobs, partners; it can be dramatic' (Leia) 'Online games sometimes cause negative consequences at a social level, because these are simultaneously promoting isolation of the gamer; maybe there were previous social problems which promoted this isolation through online games. In any case, there is a progressive reclusion, I have observed this in a close friend' (Victor)	'Playing games excessively is a step out of reality; they should go outdoors more, as SNS users usually do' (Moira)
	Neutral	'Gaming is for curiosity, for enjoyment; gaming makes you happy; it does not always affect your real life' (Carol)	'I am also very curious about newsfeeds' (Moira)

Note: CIUS–G: Compulsive Internet use scale for gaming; CIUS–SNS: CIUS for social networking sites.

Table 10. Superordinate and subordinate themes about the prevention of the GPIU and SPIUs studied, together with a few quotations (adapted from French to English) as illustration.

Theme	Subthemes	Quotes		
		CIUS	CIUS–G	CIUS–SNS
Prevention	Risk factors	'A close friend lost a relative, and he was gaming between 5-6 hours per day, plus watching online series, which affected his studies. It was to compensate for the loss. Now he has reduced his gaming and we do other things' (Carol)	'I had a growing crisis in my adolescence; I had to detach from my family, and I could not do it physically, only through the games. I discovered another world and friends' (Carol) 'When I was an adolescent, I spent a lot of time at home alone gaming. In University you live alone, and you do what you want' (Martin) 'I had a friend who had difficulties with his father, then he played games to prove his value, as he needed to valorise himself, to obtain recognition' (Carol) 'I had a boyfriend who introduced me to gaming; it became a vicious circle. There were a lot of external thoughts that made us think about the game, remembering our wellbeing when gaming or the feeling to do something which challenged us was hard; but I started to look for real accomplishments' (Carol) 'I know someone who was an extreme gamer, and he smoked cannabis and played video games simultaneously which became a habit. The cannabis was only reinforcing the habit. The cause was that he was living alone with a parent who worked a lot. He only stopped to help his parent, but he spent the money to buy things for the MMORPG, or to buy cannabis' (Martin) 'There is a system that makes you play more, as you win and you are repaid receiving points. These points let you buy characters without real money; although you could buy things for the game with real money. It is a vicious cycle. The virtual money is the points you accumulate, and there is a ranking; then reputation also makes you play more' (Martin)	'A trauma could encourage you to stay behind the computer' (Moira) 'I had a close friend who was using the SNS all day until she found a partner. Problematic use could appear in a period of solitude to replace the lack of relationships with others' (Elektra) 'I was on Facebook a lot when I broke up with my partner; to avoid thinking' (Scarlet)
	Protective factors		'I had a friend who could not control his time online. I recommended dancing to him, as I had other hobbies apart of the Internet, like dancing 4 hours per week which diminished the hours of my gaming' (Carol) 'There is eSport at a global level, which is a way to win money, where you have to have real teams to compete. They are famous, and win a lot of money with sponsors. I think these gamers are not addicts, as their rewards are real, they are professional gamers; this is a career' (Martin)	'My parents were against the technologies. We did not receive education about them, and we were too connected at home. Thus, they started to switch off the Wi-Fi in the evening, encouraged us to go out, to start doing other activities: dance, music' (Moira)

Note: CIUS: Compulsive Internet use scale; CIUS–G: CIUS for gaming; CIUS–SNS: CIUS for social networking sites; MMORPG: massively multiplayer online role-playing games.

3.2.3. Themes Related to IGD Criteria Adapted for the Three Problems

The nine IGD criteria adapted (to excessive general Internet use, video game use (original IGD), or social networks use) were first quantitatively analysed by codes: by frequency (i.e., 2 = essential criterion without a problem detected in its wording; 1 = good criterion with a problem detected; 0 = not an adequate criterion with problems detected; thus, the minimum score was 0, and maximum was 18); with some quotes as illustrations presented in Table 11 below.

The criteria were ranked by order (i.e., from higher to lower frequency of agreement) and the most positively valued and important ones were: Risk or loss of relationships or opportunities, giving up other activities, withdrawal, and continuing despite problems. Following the first set of crucial symptoms which emerged, a second rank order appeared: Escape adverse moods, deceit or cover-up, preoccupation, and being unable to reduce or stop. Moreover, users stated that some of these criteria should not be stated like they are proposed in the criteria set, and in the scales, as usually users are not aware of them and probably select that they do not fulfil these criteria when they do, but are unaware of it (i.e., false negatives). This was usually happening in the following criteria: Preoccupation, reduction or stop, continuing despite problems, deceit or cover-up, and risk or loss of relationships or opportunities. Thus, clinical external evaluation is needed to explore if criteria are met or not by the user. Almost all criteria were well valued except tolerance, as users requested that it be reworded or that it cover not only quantitative time online, but also frequency, money spent on the game, accumulating points/accomplishments/likes, along with other similar elements.

Table 11. Internet, gaming, and social networking criteria encoded through the frequency of agreement and a few quotations (adapted from French to English) as illustration.

Criteria	Frequency of Agreement	Quotes
1: Preoccupation	$\Sigma = 8$	'This is a good criterion, if we are only thinking about what is happening through Facebook, it's as if we are addicted to it' (Moira, as a social networker) 'It remains in your head, we are permanently thinking, but it is also constantly in your feelings. Thus, I think this criterion should include feelings, and the cause of the suffering' (Victor, as a gamer) 'I would eliminate the phrase 'a lot of time', as it requires reflection' (Elektra, as a social networker) 'The problem is when you recognise your strange behaviour when not gaming: the gamer is thinking of the game outside the game, such as reflecting on strategies for playing. I have also observed this in girls who excessively shop online' (Carol, as a gamer)
2: Withdrawal	$\Sigma = 10$	'This is a good criterion, it is difficult to stop using Facebook. I am a bit addicted as I am on it 3-4 hours a day. I have started to tell myself I should do another thing in these hours, but I have not stopped. It is a need, but it is different from other online activities because it's about being in touch' (Moira, as a social networker) 'This is the most important criterion because the diagnostic includes suffering, what the user feels' (Victor, as a gamer) 'I think it should be divided into two criterions as there are two different verbs which refer to two different things' (Elektra, as a social networker) 'These excessive gamers can be with you to a degree, but they are so nervous and anxious to return to the games' (Martin, as a gamer)
3: Tolerance	$\Sigma = 1$	'Only if the game is not on computers. I think it is not that relevant, as I did not have this need as stated, but I was addicted to games' (Leia, as a gamer) 'To have a hobby which you would like to do more or improve is not a problem, as long as there are no financial problems. Everybody is online' (Victor, as a gamer) 'I would eliminate the words 'excitation' and 'pleasure' as these are intimate words, the word 'satisfaction' is better. Should add the notion of frequency, as in the SNS we are not spending much time but a lot of times' (Elektra, as a social networker) 'When one is addicted to a game there is no need to play more for the same state of excitement; the problem is that we do not want to leave the game. This behaviour is not like drugs; we do not need to increment the dose, above all for MMORPG. For those who have problems, to invest money in improving their materials to play could be a sign. If the gamer has this problem is because he or she has trouble with the excitement. Gaming addicts want to acquire more and more, as the feeling is not to wait, because the game continues without the gamer. I only accumulate accomplishments for avoiding the fear of losing, for not losing events' (Carol, as a gamer) 'To have new materials improves your quality of playing games, then more time and more things, the question is complex' (Martin, as a gamer)

Table 11. *Cont.*

Criteria	Frequency of Agreement	Quotes
4: Reduce or stop	$\sum = 7$	'Some gamers are not aware of their problem, but when they realise, they have already achieved a step towards recovery' (Leia, as a gamer) 'I think this criterion is above all for those who spend too much time alone' (Moira, as a social networker) 'I think it is for users who are aware of their excessive use, but there are periods in life you are not aware of it; it is a global unhappiness' (Elektra, as a social networker) 'You never take the pauses even when thinking of them' (Martin, as a gamer)
5: Give up other activities	$\sum = 10$	'This is a good criterion, but it is important to be aware this affects real life' (Leia, as a gamer) 'This is a fundamental criterion. Others stop their activities to be in the SNS' (Moira, as a social networker) 'The problem is users could consider their online activity as a sole hobby' (Elektra, as a social networker) 'I know I had an excessive gaming behaviour, playing a lot with craving, but nobody knew about it, as I was doing 'normal' life in school, and with other activities. You could be an addict and not accomplish this criterion' (Carol, as a gamer) 'This is a discriminative criterion, the impact on your life, when will everything be affected. I have lived it. It lacks the notion of time, the frequency when gaming' (Martin, as a gamer)
6: Continue despite problems	$\sum = 10$	'It is a good criterion if SNS are affecting our relationships negatively; as when you are going out to dinner, and everybody is always on their smartphones chatting by the SNS instead of with those who are at the dinner' (Moira, as a social networker) 'It is important, but maybe the user is not aware and continues gaming' (Victor, as a gamer) 'As the previous one, you could be an addict gamer and not accomplish this criterion, as others will not observe it' (Carol, as a gamer) 'This is only useful if the person is conscious' (Martin, as a gamer)
7: Deceive or cover-up	$\sum = 9$	'This is a good criterion. Gamers are a bit ashamed as we live in persistent worlds and we communicate with friends who are gamers' (Leia, as a gamer) 'This is a good criterion, if the user is conscious he or she is addicted to SNS' (Moira, as a social networker) 'This depends on the context, such as a strict family which puts pressure on you, maybe you will secretly game '(Victor, as a gamer) 'In the moment the gamer lies he or she is conscious' (Martin, as a gamer)
8: Escape adverse moods	$\sum = 9$	'This is a good criterion, as there are users who use the games as a shelter' (Leia, as a gamer) 'This is a criterion for those who play video games, but it should differentiate those who play for coping with a traumatic experience and those who play without any excuse' (Moira, as a social networker) 'Some gamers play to compensate, but others for the adrenaline, some to be alone, some to be happy' (Carol, as a gamer) 'It is needs to include the notion of frequency to achieve the concept of habit' (Martin, as a gamer)
9: Risk or loss of relationships or opportunities	$\sum = 13$	'This is a good criterion too, as it is influencing real-life' (Leia, as a gamer) 'This is a good criterion, it is too extreme but exists' (Moira, as a social networker) 'It is a subjective criterion because maybe the gamer treats this activity as work and he is fine like this, but if he is not aware and it affects him negatively, it is a problem (Victor, as a gamer) 'If you say yes, you could be an addict gamer; but if you say no, maybe you are accomplishing the criterion without being aware of it, and you could pass as healthy when you are not' (Carol, as a gamer) 'This is the most discriminative, as we lost something for playing and the addiction takes something from you' (Martin, as a gamer)

Note: $\sum$ means to sum all quantitative values (codes). SNS: social networking sites; MMORPG: massively multiplayer online role-playing games.

4. Discussion

This mixed methods study had as a primary aim to understand potential technological behavioural addictions in young adults based on their self-reported online uses (i.e., Internet, gaming, and social networking) to compare generalised versus specific addiction problems and verify if these could be classed as public health outcomes. This approach has added an innovative research study type into the literature of this field, as the individuals were targeted based on unique trends of Internet use, gaming, and social networking simultaneously in a mixed methods study. The specific aims were: To validate the generalised and specific CIUS to compare these problems, to estimate their prevalence, and to examine problem users' perceptions regarding the phenomenology of these problems, and their opinion about the IGD criteria for the GPIU and SPIUs studied.

Concerning the first specific aim, the main psychometric properties were outstanding, showing the commonalities of the three CIUS adaptations tested. Findings showed excellent reliability in all versions (Cronbach alpha coefficients: From $\alpha_{CIUS} = 0.90$ to $\alpha_{CIUS-G} = 0.95$), which were even higher than the previous French version [52]. The scales' factor validity was consistent with its unidimensional model [39], achieving greater explained variance than the original version (from CIUS: 49% to CIUS–G: 60%), and with factor loadings being high enough (from CIUS with a minimum of 0.53 to CIUS–SNS with 0.58).

Regarding the construct validity, positive associations between the overall scores of each problem and time variables supported the degree to which the adaptations measure what they claim. Nevertheless, differences among the three problems started to appear. For instance, a device profile emerged for the different problems: The GPIU is mainly associated with computer use, although it was also moderately related to time spent per day with other devices (e.g., tablets and smartphones). Gaming only was modestly associated with daily time in computers and tablets, and social networks above all in smartphones (a part of computers on a weak basis). Thus, gaming is not a usual problem when playing on the mobile phone [44,59], as probably modern smartphones and mobile game apps are not yet developed enough for gamers, at least in Europe. However, computers seem to act as an object of these addiction problems and the Internet can provide a vehicle for facilitating some of the addictive symptomatology, as reported in other behavioural addictions (e.g., gambling [60]).

Concerning content validity, the three forms measured different facets of the 'Internet addiction' umbrella construct. For instance, general use was weakly associated with a set of common online behaviours, with messaging, viewing, social networking, and sex consumption standing out. An issue which emerged is the taste for online TV shows/series and film consumption, a recent research line developed in the field [61–63], which is usually linked to Internet addiction and gaming as a sedentary behaviour affecting mental health [64,65]. Regarding gaming, game genres with a strong association to this problematic use included by order: MOBA [66,67], MMORPG [50,68–71], FPS [70,72,73], and solo games [71] (i.e., almost all big games). It is unusual that MOBA and especially 'solo games' have emerged, as the literature around problem gaming tends to include only role-playing games. The 'solo games' genre makes sense based on the qualitative findings associated with the aetiology about excessively play to avoid or prevent loneliness and boredom, reported in problematic gaming research [71,74–77]. On the other hand, regarding problem SNS usage, only Facebook emerged as the leading network with which users present addiction symptoms similar to Internet addiction, as previous studies reported [10,78]. As far as the author knows, it has scarcely been clarified what activities are really under the labels of GPIU and these SPIUs, such as gaming [79,80].

Interestingly, another set of differences was found between the three problems at a psychometric level. The general Internet and social networking overall scores were strongly positively correlated, which probably means that their constructs are very close, as current SNS have plenty of resources (e.g., Facebook have options to communicate, to share files, to play games, to consume information, even online gambling) that are starting to emulate a generalised online use [10,78,81]. Moreover, the findings of the content validity supported why the general purpose of the Internet and the specific use of social networks were so close in their interpretation. This could explain why when analysing the scales by items, the CIUS and CIUS–SNS have a similar pattern with moderate scores (i.e., CIUS: a M from 0.78 in item 9 to 2.05 in item 12 out of 4; CIUS–SNS: An M from 0.63 in item 4 to 1.84 in item 1) compared to the CIUS–G (i.e., an M from 0.22 in item 9 to 0.66 in item 1). However, the association between general Internet use and gaming was weak, and it did not exist between gaming and social networking, meaning both SPIUs were independent between them. Moreover, qualitative findings support this different phenomenology of both constructs, as users state many differences between problem gaming and problem networking (e.g., the first being detached from real life, while the second overly attached to real life). This independence observed could be interpreted as those who mainly use

SNS are not heavy gamers, and inversely [82]. This is a crucial finding as, from a phenomenological perspective, this indicates gaming could not be classed as a social networking problem and vice versa. These findings also suggest that while from an adult's perspective, their potential addictive symptomatology is higher when using the Internet in general or when networking, only a few users play games in an excessive and problematic form, and these are all types of adults (i.e., males and females, young and middle-aged ones). In a recent study testing the spectrum hypothesis using the network approach, the umbrella construct of Internet addiction was also highlighted; this study recommended the focus on the specific Internet- and technology-mediated addictive behaviours: Gaming, smartphone, and cybersex [83]. Present quantitative and qualitative findings support the specificity of the SPIU of gaming. Regarding gender issues, the differences were detected on SPIUs at a descriptive level, as while descriptively males tend to be gamers and view online porn, females tend to use social networks, as Andreassen and colleagues also reported [82]. However, when analysing only those classed as problem users, findings change.

Concerning the second specific aim, the estimated prevalence of potential at-risk addiction problem users, findings were (in descending order): 37.4% Internet addicts (generally women and young adults), 32.5% problematic social networkers (usually women and young adults too), and 10.8% problematic online gamers (both genders equally, as well as all group ages in adulthood). Thus, this suggests women are starting to be problem users, especially in addictive gaming, which traditionally was a problem in males [84]. Moreover, while young adulthood has a higher prevalence in general Internet and social networking uses, in the case of gaming, all adults have a similar level of addiction problems, as previously reported [85]. These findings provide evidence for IGD proposal and gaming disorder [6,7], as the problem is extended to both genders and adult group ages. The prevalence estimated was higher than usual for a European study, as reported previously by Laconi and colleagues [80,86]. This overestimation is probably due to a set of methodological factors, the different scales selected in similar studies (e.g., the Internet addiction test; IAT [5] vs. the CIUS [39]), the different interpretation of the symptoms measured as addiction criteria (e.g., see Table 1), and the cut-off score applied to the CIUS, which could be considered a threshold for risk instead of an addiction problem (i.e., as the theoretical median of the CIUS is 28, and 21 was used based on Guertler and colleagues' study [47], which it was found in the sole self-reported measures from German problem and pathological gamblers, but without clinical support as it is usual in the field). Furthermore, the cut-off was not performed by gender and by type of problem use, and the present sample was mainly composed of women, as it was based on Belgian academic environments of social sciences in higher education. However, almost no research has provided validated cut-off scores using the CIUS, except for the short CIUS [87], which implies a future research line. For this reason, prevalence should be taken with caution as a proposed proportion of users in risk of potential GPIU or SPIU.

Moreover, as a usual practice in the field, potential problem users were chosen by a psychometric measure, without explicit attention to the symptoms accomplished and their relevance [18,21,22,28] or clinical supervision. Other problems were the results obtained by endorsement per items, as there is no agreement on how to operationalise it (e.g., only extracting those who state 'often' and 'very often' or only 'very often' [88]). Interestingly, a clear difference between core and peripheral symptoms has not clearly emerged by the GPIU and SPIUs studied, contrary to other studies [89], as even the core ones were not related to time spent playing, unlike in previous research [25,26]. It is probably because the quantitative sample contained fewer gamers and problem gamers (the lower prevalence), and usually only players of the 'big games' seem to be the ones with more addictive problems [25,26,66–70,72]. Nevertheless, in the qualitative findings, the main addiction problem was gaming through 'big games', covering all symptomatology and causing more harm compared to the other two problems studied.

Thus, only half of the sample could be classed as potential or at risk of being a problem user, a quarter as having a potential Internet use-related addiction problem, and another quarter more than one problem (i.e., mixed profile: Usually by problem general Internet and networking uses), such as in another European study [80], which was closer in its phenomenology, as reported. It is worth noting that most prevalent symptoms in the quantitative evidence on GPIU and SPIUs studied were not those classed as core criteria according to Charlton and Danforth [25] (e.g., conflict, withdrawal) and Tao and colleagues [21] (i.e., preoccupation, withdrawal). Indeed, the commonality between the GPIU and SPIUs studied at a symptomatologic level was with items addressing loss of control and mood modification. This could highlight the fact that potential problematic users are being classed by criteria which are not the core ones, at least in problem gaming; in other words, the overestimation of these potential problem users could be due to a proportion of them being high enthusiasts of using the Internet in general, gaming and/or social networking. In this study, quantitative evidence has highlighted the loss of control was the symptom with high scores, and according to Griffiths, this is not central to addiction [90] (i.e., it is not a necessary component or a consequence of addictive behaviour). However, a few studies reported a difference in the conceptual and nosological entities of these problems using quantitative approaches, especially between GPIU versus SPIU (i.e., Internet addiction vs. problem online gaming [80]), although the distinction was mainly based on gender, which it seems to be changing based on present findings. Furthermore, the female gender seems at risk of these potential behavioural addictions, even gaming, which is a novel finding against the current literature [91]; this highlights that more research in female gamer in behavioural addictions is needed.

Regarding the third specific aim, the aetiology observed through the qualitative evidence shows more causes have emerged than in previous qualitative studies (e.g., usually only focused on boredom, mood feeling, stress, and escapism [58]); for instance, being an indoors person, with an introvert personality, real and virtual friendship with the guild, and being tech-savvy, feeling the need to be updated, connected, and obsessively informed by others in the case of social networkers. Curiously, environmental factors, such as weak or perceived difficult interpersonal context, have emerged as facilitating problematic gaming, but not other PIUs. Thus, maybe not all external factors facilitate same GPIU or SPIU. Similarly, Griffiths' component model was effective only for problem gaming [18], as a phenomenon caused by a biopsychosocial perspective; followed by problematic social networking; and finally, GPIU with less symptoms, which do not facilitate covering the need for more evidence to promote theoretical development on GPIUs [14] (e.g., only relapse was present as a symptom in problematic gaming).

According to addiction symptoms, salience seems not to only be a cognitive component, as its emotional facet has emerged, as it was stated by Griffiths [18], and it appears to include craving; however, it was not involved in other Internet addiction criteria or IGD [21,22]. Moreover, this addictive symptom is usually used to diagnose SUDs and gambling disorder, but not included in, for example, IGD [6,92]). Davis' model [15] did not cover this affective aspect of the nature of GPIU or SPIUs. Indeed, Caplan statements about the preference for online interaction, mood regulation, and deficient self-regulation [15,16] were supported by all interviewees. However, tolerance is more complicated than stated in the most contemporary proposals to diagnose behavioural addictions [21,22], especially in gaming [33]; as it is the increment of not only time (i.e., intensity, expertise, or advancement in the game), and not only for excitement or desire (wording usually used in IGD [22], which has been highly criticised in the interviews). Concerning deception or cover-up, like tolerance, it is more complicated than initially described in addictive symptomatology [18–21,28,33], as well as in the existing scales (e.g., the IAT [87]). It seems gamers usually maintain a 'secret double life' in the game, as they have explained, and as it has scanty been reported as a shared virtual environment among MMORPG players [93,94]. They have 'game friends' (the partner, guild or other teams) and their codes to communicate (own language), dedicating daily time to set goals and enjoy within the virtual world of the games; this essential element of gaming behaviour has not been studied in-depth yet [95]. If quantitative and qualitative findings are observed simultaneously, according to Tao and colleagues [21], preoccupation and withdrawal are weakly and moderately present, respectively, in the main sample. However, they are only present in the problematic gamers subsample, and persistent desire and difficult to control are strongly present in the sample for all (GPIU and SPIUs) studied, as well as in all problem users studied. Thus, based on Tao's criteria, problems studied could be classed as Internet use-related addiction problems with caution; only gaming seems to fit in their proposal. Nevertheless, for IGD [6,22] criteria, only gaming could also be categorised as SPIU based on all findings. Remarkably, the core components [25] could just be checked on the qualitative findings extracted from potential problem users, which concurrently stated conflict was the main addiction symptom (i.e., the one with a higher frequency of agreement), followed by withdrawal, giving up other activities, and continuing despite problems, as probable indicators of behavioural salience. In other words, matching all Charlton and Danforth core criteria for addictive gaming [25,26], qualitative findings support the health problem, together with IGD opinions, which are considered.

Regarding the consequences of excessive online uses, it should be highlighted not all of them are negative. Almost all of the users agreed they have experienced (or observed in others close to them) the risk of being addicted to the Internet or an online activity (usually gaming). They reported developmental and contextual factors as those supporting how a habit such as gaming could slowly and unconsciously develop into an addictive behaviour. For instance, to be a gamer and play video games during adolescence indoors during a long time, avoiding loneliness, establishing an identity in the game, and virtual social life may relate to real life (e.g., real friends are also gamers of the same role-playing games). The risk factors highlighted compared to the symptomatology reported [18–25], which were connected to both developmental and contextual factors (e.g., adolescent crises, parent styles) were found to be more important than individual factors (e.g., personality traits). This assertion goes against our current research in the field (i.e., focused on personality traits [73,96]), while few contextual or structural risk factors [97] or protective factors have been reported. Nevertheless, it should be argued that maybe these participants are not so aware of their characteristics that may help to develop extreme online behaviours, as in other addictive problems (e.g., SUDs). However, none of the interviewees recognised they might be a problem user at present, which questions the cut-off score selected in the adapted CIUS or supports that they probably had (or have had) an addiction problem (i.e., only one gamer recognised to have had this problem in the past, and another gamer described the game transfer phenomena [98]).

Finally, with respect to the fourth specific aim about IGD criteria opinions for diagnosing these problems, qualitative findings highlighted as the most critical addiction symptoms: Risk or loss of relationships or opportunities (conflict), giving up other activities, withdrawal, and continuing despite problems, which coin the core components previously pointed out [25] and match research findings [33]. Moreover, users clearly state 'intrapersonal or interpersonal conflict' [18] is equally important, sometimes associated with a 'functional impairment' [21]. The qualitative evidence seems to agree with critiques considering GPIU with not enough entity to be as a behavioural addiction [23,80], as a few subthemes did not provide evidence (e.g., not emerging in all addiction symptomatology analysed). In this sense, other excessive online behaviours, such as watching series online, have emerged and caused public health concerns with sedentary lifestyle and time in front of the screens [61–63]. Other criteria, such as escaping adverse moods, deceit or cover-up, preoccupation or not being able to reduce or stop online behaviour, are quite ordinary and excessive users agreed with them, the only criterion where users disagree being tolerance, one of which Kardefelt-Winther [24] criticised in the current IGD [22], and about which other authors have found similar evidence [33]. Tolerance, giving up other activities, or escaping adverse moods require a part of rewording them and covering their complexity, an indicator of frequency, as Ko [99] also stated when IGD was published in the DSM-5 appendix [6], as the need for using the intensity and frequency criteria to distinguish subjects with IGD from casual online gamers.

Some limitations of this cross-sectional and self-report study have been already discussed, but it could be added that it was performed with a non-random community and academic sample, with an online survey and interviewing only those who accepted the invitation to participate in the second part of this study (e.g., economic motivation). However, similar quantitative studies have been performed with smaller samples than the quantitative [80] and qualitative [50] parts of the study. The study's strengths include a survey with psychometric and epidemiological validated techniques, with a considerable and sufficient sample size based on Nunnally's recommendations for psychometrics [100], and Smith and Osborn's assertion [101] for the qualitative part of the study. The provision of a Belgian French adaptation of the CIUS and IGD for specific Internet use-related addiction problems was supported by previously validated adaptations [22,52]. The qualitative participants were psychometrically and theoretically selected after validating the CIUS scales to have the potential problem online users from all profiles studied to shed light on the phenomenology of these new addiction problems from adults.

In summary, technology uses are growing within contemporary societies and bibliographic productivity is attending these phenomena quantitatively. However, confirmatory approaches could have been chosen as a method for factor validity, which is a future research study under development. Finally, although this is not the first mixed methods study done in the field [33,92], it is one of the few that have been undertaken covering mixed user profiles of these problems. Therefore, it is an original contribution looking for mixed evidence on what seems to constitute the phenomenology of these problems through potential or at-risk adult problem users, although no functional impairment or other possible mental disorders were measured to disentangle the problem users with a clinical approach.

5. Conclusions

The present study is one of the first to ascertain what seems to be behind current psychometric measures and to start to disentangle generalised and specific Internet addiction problems, addressing their phenomenology with quantitative and qualitative evidence.

The findings show that around half of Belgian (European) adults seem to present at least a risk of Internet use-related addiction problems. However, a lower proportion could have a mixed profile, covering the risk of more than one problem. The CIUS for generalised problematic internet use and specific problematic gaming and social networking has been validated, and the potential prevalence in at-risk users have been estimated. Young or middle-aged adults in both genders have been shown to be equally vulnerable to problematic gaming. Furthermore, the addiction symptoms are present in the problems studied, but not with the same weight or level of importance. The higher scores are in general Internet addiction and problem social networking, which seem to have a common phenomenology, while problem gaming seems different. However, all of them have loss of control and mood modification as main prevalent symptoms. Nevertheless, when problem gaming is analysed in-depth, it is difficult to confirm all addictive components, symptoms, and criteria, in quantitative and qualitative findings. Furthermore, the classic core components have been tested but were only ratified in the qualitative results, where the relevant symptoms were conflicting, giving up other activities, withdrawal, and continuing despite problems.

An in-depth theoretical and empirical review of the public health approach usually used in behavioural addictions literature applied to generalised and specific addiction problems has been provided. This strategy together with analysing quantitative and qualitative evidence of these problems has shown what seems to be behind each addictive criterion usually used to screen users and classify them as a potential problem user (i.e., through DSM criteria, component addiction symptoms, and core vs. peripheral symptoms). Moreover, it has been documented that at-risk users' perceptions about the phenomenology of these problems, which start in adolescence and remain during adulthood, with a potential of increased harm. The aetiology is more diverse than previously described, and its development is supported by psychosocial, environmental, and technological factors, leading to a few cases of extreme problems. Potential at-risk problem users' opinions about IGD criteria have highlighted that some criteria (e.g., risk or loss of relationships or opportunities) are more important and better developed than others (e.g., tolerance), but the need to apply them with clinical resources is essential in the evaluation and diagnosis of these mental health problems. Nevertheless, natural recovery has emerged as a finding for some potential problem users, although mental health systems to support those users who have developed the problem(s) and cannot naturally recover are required.

Other preventive actions in education, social, and family relationships could promote the maintenance of users' health and wellbeing.

Thus, it seems these problems exist, but probably in a lower proportion than reported. However, when they do appear they present addictive symptomatology, especially in problem online gaming. These findings seem to provide evidence for the IGD proposed by the APA (with the restrictions and improvements suggested) and the recent recognition of gaming disorder by the WHO (especially for specific online gaming behaviours).

Acknowledgments: The author would like to thank Joel Billieux for supervising the project, to Jory Deleuze, Gaetan Devos, Aline Wery, and William De Brueger for supporting the survey design in French, and to Aurelien Cornil and Ophelie Devrient for supporting the interviews in French. Furthermore, the author would like to thank the ITU and the Proquest for their permission to publish the figures.

References

1. OReilly, M. Internet addiction: A new disorder enters the medical lexicon. *Can. Med. Assoc. J.* **1996**, *154*, 1882–1883.

2. Young, K.S. Psychology of computer use: XL. Addictive use of the Internet: A case that breaks the stereotype. *Psychol. Rep.* **1996**, *79*, 899–902. [CrossRef] [PubMed]

3. Stein, D.J. Internet addiction, Internet psychotherapy letter; comment. *J. Am. J. Psychiatry* **1997**, *154*, 890. [PubMed]

4. Griffiths, M. Internet addiction: Fact or fiction? *Psychologist* **1999**, *12*, 246–250. [CrossRef]

5. Young, K.S. Internet addiction: The emergence of a new clinical disorder. *CyberPsychol. Behav.* **1998**, *1*, 237–244. [CrossRef]

6. American Psychiatric Association (APA). *Diagnostic and Statistical Manual of Mental Disorders*, 5th ed.; American Psychiatric Association: Arlington, VA, USA, 2013.

7. World Health Organization (WHO). Gaming Disorder. WHO, 2018. Available online: https://icd.who.int/browse11/l-m/en#/http%3a%2f%2fid.who.int%2ficd%2fentity%2f1448597234 (accessed on 4 December 2018).

8. Shaw, M.; Black, D.W. Internet addiction: Definition, assessment, epidemiology and clinical management. *CNS Drugs* **2008**, *22*, 353–365. [CrossRef] [PubMed]

9. Ng, B.D.; Wiemer-Hastings, P. Addiction to the Internet and Online Gaming. *Cyberpsychol. Behav.* **2005**, *8*, 110–113. [CrossRef]

10. Kuss, D.J.; Griffiths, M.D. Social Networking Sites and Addiction: Ten Lessons Learned. *Int. J. Environ. Res. Public Health* **2017**, *14*, 311. [CrossRef]

11. International Telecommunication Union (ITU). ITU Committed to Connecting the World: ICT Facts and Figures 2017—Global ICT Developments. Available online: https://www.itu.int/en/ITU-D/Statistics/Pages/stat/default.aspx (accessed on 27 June 2018).

12. ProQuest. Search—All Databases. Available online: https://search.proquest.com/results/3E9BFDEC5154401PQ/1?accountid=14693 (accessed on 26 January 2018).

13. Becoña, E. Conductas adictivas: El problema del siglo XXI? *Psicol. Contemp.* **1998**, *5*, 4–15.

14. Davis, R.A. A cognitive–behavioral model of pathological Internet use. *Comput. Hum. Behav.* **2001**, *17*, 187–195. [CrossRef]

15. Caplan, S.E. Theory and measurement of generalized problematic internet use: A two-step approach. *Comput. Hum. Behav.* **2010**, *26*, 1089–1097. [CrossRef]

16. Caplan, S.E. Problematic Internet use and psychosocial well-being: Development of a theory-based cognitive-behavioral measurement instrument. *Comput. Hum. Behav.* **2002**, *18*, 553–575. [CrossRef]

17. Haagsma, M.C.; Caplan, S.E.; Peters, O.; Pieterse, M.E. A cognitive-behavioral model of problematic online gaming in adolescents aged 12–22 years. *Comput. Hum. Behav.* **2013**, *29*, 202–209. [CrossRef]

18. Griffiths, M.D. A "components" model of addiction within a biopsychosocial framework. *J. Subst. Use* **2005**, *10*, 191–197. [CrossRef]

19. Brown, R.I.F. Some contributions of the study of gambling to the study of other addictions. In *Gambling Behavior and Problem Gambling*; Eadington, W.R., Cornelius, J., Eds.; University of Nevada Press: Reno, NV, USA, 1993.

20. Griffiths, M.D. Behavioural addiction and substance addiction should be defined by their similarities not their dissimilarities. *Addiction* **2017**, *112*, 1718–1720. [CrossRef]

21. Tao, R.; Huang, X.; Wang, J.; Zhang, H.; Zhang, Y.; Li, M. Proposed diagnostic criteria for internet addiction. *Addiction* **2010**, *105*, 556–564. [CrossRef]

22. Petry, N.M.; Rehbein, F.; Gentile, D.A.; Lemmens, J.S.; Rumpf, H.; Mößle, T.; Bischof, G.; Tao, R.; Fung, D.S.; Borges, G.; et al. An international consensus for assessing internet gaming disorder using the new DSM-5 approach. *Addiction* **2014**, *109*, 1399–1406. [CrossRef]

23. van Rooij, A.J.; Prause, N. A critical review of "Internet addiction" criteria with suggestions for the future. *J. Behav. Addict.* **2014**, *3*, 203–213. [CrossRef]

24. Kardefelt-Winther, D. A critical account of DSM-5 criteria for Internet gaming disorder. *Addict. Res. Theory* **2015**, *23*, 93–98. [CrossRef]

25. Charlton, J.P.; Danforth, I.D.W. Distinguishing addiction and high engagement in the context of online game playing. *Comput. Hum. Behav.* **2007**, *23*, 1531–1548. [CrossRef]

26. Lehenbauer-Baum, M.; Fohringer, M. Towards classification criteria for internet gaming disorder: Debunking differences between addiction and high engagement in a German sample of World of Warcraft players. *Comput. Hum. Behav.* **2015**, *45*, 345–351. [CrossRef]

27. Lopez-Fernandez, O. How has internet addiction research evolved since the advent of internet gaming disorder? An overview of cyberaddictions from a psychological perspective. *Curr. Addict. Rep.* **2015**, *2*, 263–271. [CrossRef]

28. Lopez-Fernandez, O.; Molina-Azorin, J. The use of mixed methods research in the field of behavioural sciences. *Qual. Quant. Int. J. Methodol.* **2011**, *45*, 1459–1472. [CrossRef]

29. Lopez-Fernandez, O.; Molina-Azorin, J. The use of mixed methods research in interdisciplinary educational journals. *Int. J. Mult. Res. Approaches* **2011**, *5*, 269–283. [CrossRef]

30. Young, KS. Internet Addiction: A New Clinical Phenomenon and Its Consequences. *Am. Behav. Sci.* **2004**, *48*, 402–415. [CrossRef]

31. Stepien, K. Internet Addiction. The Phenomenon of Pathological Internet Use—Problems of Interpretation in the Definition and Diagnosis. *Intern. Secur.* **2014**, *6*, 79–90. [CrossRef]

32. Liu, T.C. Phenomenology and epidemiology of problematic Internet use. In *The Oxford Handbook of Impulse Control Disorders*; Grant, J.E., Potenza, M.N., Eds.; The Oxford Handbook of Impulse Control Disorders; Oxford University Press: New York, NY, USA, 2012; pp. 176–185, Chapter xvii.

33. Colder Carras, M.; Porter, A.M.; Van Rooij, A.J.; King, D.; Lange, A.; Carras, M.; Labrique, A. Gamers' insights into the phenomenology of normal gaming and game "addiction": A mixed methods study. *Comput. Hum. Behav.* **2018**, *79*, 238–246. [CrossRef]

34. Grant, J.E.; Schreiber, L.R.; Odlaug, B.L. Phenomenology and Treatment of Behavioural Addictions. *Can. J. Psychiatry* **2013**, *58*, 252–259. [CrossRef]

35. Andreassen, C.S. Online social network site addiction: A comprehensive review. *Curr. Addict. Rep.* **2015**, *2*, 175–184. [CrossRef]

36. Lee, E.W.J.; Ho, S.S.; Lwin, M.O. Explicating problematic social network sites use: A review of concepts, theoretical frameworks, and future directions for communication theorizing. *New Media Soc.* **2017**, *19*, 308–326. [CrossRef]

37. van den Eijnden, R.J.J.M.; Lemmens, J.S.; Valkenburg, P.M. The Social Media Disorder Scale. *Comput. Hum. Behav.* **2016**, *61*, 478–487. [CrossRef]

38. Hormes, J.M.; Kearns, B.; Timko, C.A. Craving Facebook? Behavioral addiction to online social networking and its association with emotion regulation deficits. *Addiction* **2014**, *109*, 2079–2088. [CrossRef] [PubMed]

39. Meerkerk, G.J.; van Den Eijnden, R.J.; Vermulst, A.A.; Garretsen, H.F. The compulsive internet use scale (CIUS): Some psychometric properties. *Cyberpsychol. Behav.* **2009**, *12*, 1–6. [CrossRef]

40. Tech Use Disorders. Technological Use Disorders: European Cross-Cultural Longitudinal and Experimental Studies for Internet and Smartphone Problem Uses. 12 July 2017. Available online: http://cordis.europa.eu/project/rcn/189961_en.html (accessed on 14 July 2017).

41. Lopez-Fernandez, O. Short version of the Smartphone Addiction Scale adapted to Spanish and French: Towards a cross-cultural research in problematic mobile phone use. *Addict. Behav.* **2017**, *64*, 275–280. [CrossRef] [PubMed]

42. Lopez-Fernandez, O.; Kuss, D.J.; Romo, L.; Morvan, Y.; Kern, L.; Graziani, P.; Rousseau, A.; Rumpf, H.-J.; Bischof, A.; Gässler, A.-K.; et al. Self-reported dependence on mobile phones in young adults: A European cross-cultural empirical survey. *J. Behav. Addict.* **2017**, *6*, 168–177. [CrossRef] [PubMed]

43. Lopez-Fernandez, O.; Männikkö, N.; Kääriäinen, M.; Griffiths, M.D.; Kuss, D.J. Mobile gaming and problematic smartphone use: A comparative study between Belgium and Finland. *J. Behav. Addict.* **2018**, *9*, 1–12. [CrossRef]

44. Lopez-Fernandez, O.; Kuss, D.J.; Pontes, H.M.; Griffiths, M.D.; Dawes, C.; Justice, L.V.; Männikkö, N.; Kääriäinen, M.; Rumpf, H.-J.; Bischof, A.; et al. Measurement Invariance of the Short Version of the Problematic Mobile Phone Use Questionnaire (PMPUQ-SV) across Eight Languages. *Int. J. Environ. Res. Public Health* **2018**, *15*, 1213. [CrossRef]

45. Morse, J. Approaches to qualitative-quantitative methodological triangulation. *Nurs. Res.* **1991**, *40*, 120–123. [CrossRef]

46. Johnson, B.; Onwuegbuzie, A. Mixed methods research: A research paradigm whose time has come. *Educ. Res.* **2004**, *33*, 14–26. [CrossRef]

47. Greene, J.; Caracelli, V.; Graham, W. Toward a conceptual framework for mixed-method evaluation designs. *Educ. Eval. Policy Anal.* **1989**, *11*, 255–274. [CrossRef]

48. Creswell, J. *Research Design: Qualitative, Quantitative and Mixed Methods Approaches*, 2nd ed.; Sage: Thousand Oaks, CA, USA, 2003.

49. Leech, N.; Onwuegbuzie, A. A typology of mixed methods research designs. *Qual. Quant. Int. J. Methodol.* **2009**, *43*, 265–275. [CrossRef]

50. Beranuy, M.; Carbonell, X.; Griffiths, M.D. A Qualitative Analysis of Online Gaming Addicts in Treatment. *Int. J. Ment. Health Addict.* **2013**, *11*, 149–161. [CrossRef]

51. Guertler, D.; Rumpf, H.; Bischof, A.; Kastirke, N.; Petersen, K.U.; John, U.; Meyer, C. Assessment of problematic internet use by the Compulsive Internet Use Scale and the Internet Addiction Test: A sample of problematic and pathological gamblers. *Eur. Addict. Res.* **2014**, *20*, 75–81. [CrossRef] [PubMed]

52. Khazaal, Y.; Chatton, A.; Horn, A.; Achab, S.; Thorens, G.; Zullino, D.; Billieux, J. French Validation of the Compulsive Internet Use Scale (CIUS). *Psychiatr. Q.* **2012**, *83*, 397–405. [CrossRef] [PubMed]

53. Vaismoradi, M.; Turunen, H.; Bondas, T. Content analysis and thematic analysis: Implications for conducting a qualitative descriptive study. *Nurs. Health Sci.* **2013**, *15*, 398–405. [CrossRef] [PubMed]

54. Braun, V.; Clarke, V. Using thematic analysis in psychology. *Qual. Res. Psychol.* **2006**, *3*, 77–101. [CrossRef]

55. Braun, V.; Clarke, V.; Terry, G. Thematic analysis. *Qual. Res. Clin. Health Psychol.* **2014**, *24*, 95–114.

56. Wilkinson, S. Women with Breast Cancer Talking Causes: Comparing Content, Biographical and Discursive Analyses. *Fem. Psychol.* **2000**, *10*, 431–460. [CrossRef]

57. Krippendorff, K. *Content Analysis: An Introduction to Its Methodology*, 2nd ed.; Sage Publications: London, UK, 2004.

58. Li, W.; O'Brien, J.E.; Snyder, SM.; Howard, M.O. Characteristics of internet addiction/pathological internet use in US university students: A qualitative-method investigation. *PLoS ONE* **2015**, *10*, e0117372. [CrossRef]

59. Roberts, J.A.; Petnji Yaya, L.H.; Manolis, C. The invisible addiction: Cell-phone activities and addiction among male and female college students. *J. Behav. Addict.* **2014**, *3*, 254–265. [CrossRef]

60. Shaffer, H.J. Understanding the means and objects of addiction: Technology, the internet and gambling. *J. Gambl. Stud.* **1996**, *12*, 461–469. [CrossRef] [PubMed]

61. Sussman, S.; Moran, MB. Hidden addiction: Television. *J. Behav. Addict.* **2013**, *2*, 125–132. [CrossRef] [PubMed]

62. Lopez-Fernandez, O. Chapter One: Online TV shows and series addiction: An exploratory francophone cross-country comparison. In *Combining Aesthetic and Psychological Approaches to TV Series Addiction*; Camart, N., Lefait, S., Paquet-Deyris, A.-M., Romo, L., Eds.; Cambridge Scholars Publishing: Newcastle upon Tyne, UK, 2018; pp. 1–16, ISBN 978-1-5275-0914-6.

63. Flayelle, M.; Maurage, P.; Billieux, J. Toward a qualitative understanding of binge-watching behaviors: A focus group approach. *J. Behav. Addict.* **2017**, *6*, 457–471. [CrossRef] [PubMed]

64. Hoare, E.; Milton, K.; Foster, C.; Allender, S. The associations between sedentary behaviour and mental health among adolescents: A systematic review. *Int. J. Behav. Nutr. Phys. Act.* **2016**, *13*. [CrossRef]

65. Gentile, D.A.; Berch, O.N.; Choo, H.; Khoo, A.; Walsh, D.A. Bedroom media: One risk factor for development. *Dev. Psychol.* **2017**, *12*, 2340–2355. [CrossRef]

66. Nuyens, F.; Deleuze, J.; Maurage, P.; Griffiths, M.D.; Kuss, D.J.; Billieux, J. Impulsivity in Multiplayer Online Battle Arena gamers: Preliminary results on experimental and self-report measures. *J. Behav. Addict.* **2016**, *5*, 351–356. [CrossRef]

67. Bertran, E.; Chamarro, A. Videojugadores del League of Legends: El papel de la pasión en el uso abusivo y en el rendimiento. *Adicciones* **2016**, *28*, 28–34. [CrossRef]

68. Achab, S.; Nicolier, M.; Mauny, F.; Monnin, J.; Trojak, B.; Vandel, P.; Sechter, D.; Gorwood, P.; Haffen, E. Massively multiplayer online role-playing games: Comparing characteristics of addict vs non-addict online recruited gamers in a French adult population. *BMC Psychiatry* **2011**, *11*, 12. [CrossRef]

69. Bergmark, K.H.; Bergmark, A. The diffusion of addiction to the field of MMORPGs. *Nordic Stud. Alcohol Drugs* **2009**, *26*, 415–426. [CrossRef]

70. Metcalf, O.; Pammer, K. Physiological arousal deficits in addicted gamers differ based on preferred game genre. *Eur. Addict. Res.* **2013**, *12*, 23–32. [CrossRef]

71. Männikkö, N.; Ruotsalainen, H.; Demetrovics, Z.; Lopez-Fernandez, O.; Myllymäki, L.; Miettunen, J.; Kääriäinen, M. Problematic gaming behavior among Finnish junior high school students: Relation to socio-demographics and gaming behavior characteristics. *Behav. Med.* **2018**, *44*, 324–334. [CrossRef] [PubMed]

72. Na, E.; Choi, I.; Lee, T.; Lee, H.; Rho, M.J.; Cho, H.; Jung, D.J.; Kim, D.J. The influence of game genre on Internet gaming disorder. *J. Behav. Addict.* **2017**, *6*, 248–255. [CrossRef] [PubMed]

73. Metcalf, O.; Pammer, K. Impulsivity and related neuropsychological features in regular and addictive first person shooter gaming. *Cyberpsychol. Behav. Soc. Netw.* **2014**, *17*, 147–152. [CrossRef] [PubMed]

74. Bergmark, K.H.; Bergmark, A.; Findahl, O. Extensive Internet Involvement-Addiction or Emerging Lifestyle? *Int. J. Environ. Res. Public Health* **2011**, *8*, 4488–4501. [CrossRef]

75. Myrseth, H.; Olsen, O.K.; Strand, L.Å.; Borud, E.K. Gaming behavior among conscripts: The role of lower psychosocial well-being factors in explaining gaming addiction. *Mil. Psychol.* **2017**, *29*, 128–142. [CrossRef]

76. Carras, M.C.; Van Rooij, A.J.; Van de Mheen, D.; Musci, R.; Xue, Q.; Mendelson, T. Video gaming in a hyperconnected world: A cross-sectional study of heavy gaming, problematic gaming symptoms, and online socializing in adolescents. *Comput. Hum. Behav.* **2017**, *68*, 472–479. [CrossRef] [PubMed]

77. Lemmens, J.S.; Valkenburg, P.M.; Gentile, D.A. The Internet Gaming Disorder Scale. *Psychol. Assess* **2015**, *27*, 567–582. [CrossRef] [PubMed]

78. Enrique, E.; De Corral, P. Addiction to new technologies and to online social networking in young people: A new challenge. *Adicciones* **2010**, *22*, 91–96. [CrossRef]

79. Király, O.; Griffiths, M.D.; Urbán, R.; Farkas, J.; Kökönyei, G.; Elekes, Z.; Tamás, D.; Demetrovics, Z. Problematic Internet use and problematic online gaming are not the same: Findings from a large nationally representative adolescent sample. *Cyberpsychol. Behav. Soc. Netw.* **2014**, *17*, 749–754. [CrossRef] [PubMed]

80. Laconi, S.; Tricard, N.; Chabrol, H. Differences between specific and generalized problematic internet uses according to gender, age, time spent online and psychopathological symptoms. *Comput. Hum. Behav.* **2015**, *48*, 236–244. [CrossRef]

81. Griffiths, M.D. Facebook addiction: Concerns, criticism, and recommendations—A response to Andreassen and colleagues. *Psychol. Rep.* **2012**, *110*, 518–520. [CrossRef] [PubMed]

82. Andreassen, C.S.; Billieux, J.; Griffiths, M.D.; Kuss, D.J.; Demetrovics, Z.; Mazzoni, E.; Pallesen, S. The relationship between addictive use of social media and video games and symptoms of psychiatric disorders: A large-scale cross-sectional study. *Psychol. Addict. Behav.* **2016**, *30*, 252–262. [CrossRef] [PubMed]

83. Baggio, S.; Starcevic, V.; Studer, J.; Simon, O.; Gainsbury, S.M.; Gmel, G.; Billieux, J. Technology-mediated addictive behaviors constitute a spectrum of related yet distinct conditions: A network perspective. *Psychol. Addict. Behav.* **2018**, *32*, 564–572. [CrossRef] [PubMed]

84. Ko, C.; Yen, J.; Chen, C.; Chen, S.; Yen, C. Gender Differences and Related Factors Affecting Online Gaming Addiction among Taiwanese Adolescents. *J. Nerv. Ment. Dis.* **2005**, *193*, 273–277. [CrossRef] [PubMed]

85. Scharkow, M.; Festl, R.; Quandt, T. Longitudinal patterns of problematic computer game use among adolescents and adults—A 2-year panel study. *Addiction* **2014**, *109*, 1910–1917. [CrossRef]

86. Laconi, S.; Kaliszewska-Czeremska, K.; Gnisci, A.; Sergi, I.; Barke, A.; Jeromin, F.; Groth, J.; Gamez-Guadix, M.; Ozcan, N.K.; Demetrovics, Z.; et al. Cross-cultural study of Problematic Internet Use in nine European countries. *Comput. Hum. Behav.* **2018**, *84*, 430–440. [CrossRef]

87. Besser, B.; Rumpf, H.; Bischof, A.; Meerkerk, G.; Higuchi, S.; Bischof, G. Internet-related disorders: Development of the Short Compulsive Internet Use Scale. *Cyberpsychol. Behav. Soc. Netw.* **2017**, *20*, 709–717. [CrossRef]

88. Stavropoulos, V.; Beard, C.; Griffiths, M.D.; Buleigh, T.; Gomez, R.; Pontes, H.M. Measurement invariance of the internet gaming disorder scale–short-form (igds9-sf) between Australia, the USA, and the UK. *Int. J. Ment. Health Addict.* **2018**, *16*, 377–392. [CrossRef]

89. Charlton, J.P.; Danforth, I.D. Validating the distinction between computer addiction and engagement: Online game playing and personality. *Behav. Inf. Technol.* **2010**, *29*, 601–613. [CrossRef]

90. Griffiths, M.D. Is "loss of control" always a consequence of addiction? *Front. Psychiatry* **2013**, *4*, 36. [CrossRef]

91. Paaßen, B.; Morgenroth, T.; Stratemeyer, M. What is a True Gamer? The Male Gamer Stereotype and the Marginalization of Women in Video Game Culture. *Sex Roles* **2017**, *76*, 421–435. [CrossRef]

92. Cornil, A.; Lopez-Fernandez, O.; Devos, G.; de Timary, P.; Goudriaan, A.E.; Billieux, J. Exploring gambling craving through the elaborated intrusion theory of desire: A mixed methods approach. *Int. Gambl. Stud.* **2018**, *18*, 1–21. [CrossRef]

93. Ramirez, F.A. From good associates to true friends: An exploration of friendship practices in massively multiplayer online games. In *Social Interactions in Virtual Worlds: An Interdisciplinary Perspective*; Lakkaraju, K., Sukthankar, G., Wigand, R.T., Eds.; Cambridge University Press: New York, NY, USA, 2018; pp. 62–79, Chapter xii; ISBN 9781107128828 (Hardcover).

94. Yee, N. The Psychology of Massively Multi-User Online Role-Playing Games: Motivations, Emotional Investment, Relationships and Problematic Usage. In *Avatars at Work and Play. Computer Supported Cooperative Work*; Schroeder, R., Axelsson, A.S., Eds.; Springer: Dordrecht, The Netherlands, 2006; Volume 34, Chapter 9, pp. 187–207, ISBN 978-1-4020-3883-9 (Printed). [CrossRef]

95. Farrow, R.; Iacovides, I. Gaming and the limits of digital embodiment. *Philos. Technol.* **2014**, *27*, 221–233. [CrossRef]

96. Ko, C.H.; Yen, J.Y.; Cheng-Chung, C.; Chen, S.; Wu, K.; Yen, C.F. Tridimensional Personality of Adolescents With Internet Addiction and Substance Use Experience. *Can. J. Psychiatry* **2006**, *51*, 887–894. [CrossRef] [PubMed]

97. Hull, D.C.; Williams, G.A.; Griffiths, M.D. Video game characteristics, happiness and flow as predictors of addiction among video game players: A pilot study. *J. Behav. Addict.* **2013**, *2*, 145–152. [CrossRef] [PubMed]

98. Ortiz de Gortari, A.B.; Aronsson, K.; Griffiths, M. Game Transfer Phenomena in video game playing: A qualitative interview study. *Int. J. Cyber Behav. Psychol. Learn. (IJCBPL)* **2011**, *1*, 15–33. [CrossRef]

99. Ko, C.H. Internet Gaming Disorder. *Curr. Addict. Rep.* **2014**, *1*, 177–185. [CrossRef]

100. Nunnally, J.C. *Psychometric Theory*, 2nd ed.; McGraw-Hill: New York, NY, USA, 1978.

101. Smith, J.A.; Osborn, M. Interpretive Phenomenological Analysis. In *Qualitative Psychology: A Practical Guide to Research Methods*; Smith, J.A., Ed.; SAGE Publications Ltd.: London, UK; Thousand Oaks, CA, USA; New Delhi, India; Singapore, 2007; pp. 53–81, ISBN 978-1-4129-3083-3.

Problematic Internet Use, Non-Medical Use of Prescription Drugs and Depressive Symptoms among Adolescents: A Large-Scale Study in China

Beifang Fan [1,†], Wanxing Wang [2,3,†], Tian Wang [2,3], Bo Xie [1], Huimin Zhang [1], Yuhua Liao [1], Ciyong Lu [2,3] and Lan Guo [2,3,*]

[1]   Department of Psychiatry, Shenzhen Nanshan Center for Chronic Disease Control, Shenzhen 518000, China; fanbf@foxmail.com (B.F.); sznsxb@163.com (B.X.); zhangzhanghuimin@163.com (H.Z.); liaoyuhua0011@163.com (Y.L.)

[2]   Department of Medical Statistics and Epidemiology, School of Public Health, Sun Yat-sen University, Guangzhou 510080, China; wgg0808@163.com (W.W.); wangt97@mail2.sysu.edu.cn (T.W.); luciyong@mail.sysu.edu.cn (C.L.)

[3]   Guangdong Engineering Technology Research Center of Nutrition Translation, Guangzhou, 510080, China

*   Correspondence: guolan3@mail.sysu.edu.cn

†   These authors contributed equally to this work.

Abstract: This large-scale study aimed to test, among Chinese adolescents, the association between problematic Internet use (PIU), non-medical use of prescription drugs (NMUPD), and depressive symptoms, as well as the mediating effects of NMUPD on the associations above. This study used the data from the 2017 National School-based Chinese Adolescents Health Survey, and 24,345 students' questionnaires qualified for the analyses. Generalized linear mixed models and path models were performed. In the models without mediation, PIU was associated with depressive symptoms (unstandardized β estimate = 0.26, 95% CI = 0.25–0.27); frequent use of opioid or sedative was also related to depressive symptoms (unstandardized β estimate for opioid = 2.77, 95% CI = 1.90–3.63; unstandardized β estimate for sedative = 4.45, 95% CI = 3.02–5.88). Additionally, the results of the path models indicated that opioid misuse partially mediated the association between PIU and depressive symptoms. PIU and opioid/sedative misuse were related to the increased risk of depressive symptoms, respectively. The association above might be complicated, and PIU may elevate the risk of opioid or sedative misuse and depressive symptoms, which in turn could worsen the situation of PIU and vice versa. Multidisciplinary health intervention programs to prevent adolescents involving in PIU, as well as NMPUD, are recommended to be provided.

Keywords: problematic Internet use; non-medical use of prescription drugs; depressive symptoms; adolescents

1. Introduction

Internet use has proliferated dramatically over the last decades and has become an internal part of contemporary life [1]. Excessive or maladaptive use of the Internet has been termed as "problematic Internet use (PIU)" or "Internet addiction", which has been reported to be related to a series of psychosocial impairments and substance-use problems (e.g., depression and drug use) [2,3]. Recently, Internet gaming disorder has been included in the section on addictive disorders in the 11th Revision of the International Classification of Diseases (ICD-11) as a pattern of behavior characterized by impaired control over gaming, indicating that PIU may develop into a severe social problem [4]. Adolescence represents a vulnerable developmental stage between childhood to adulthood, which is characterized by increased levels of novelty seeking and exploration along with a wide range of risk-taking behaviors or mental health problems [5]. The report of the World Health Organization (WHO) showed that adolescent PIU had been a public health concern worldwide, and China is no exception [6]. Considering the brain undergoes rapid development during adolescence, adolescents involved in PIU may be more vulnerable to psychological disorders, such as depressive symptoms.

Depressive symptoms are one of the most common mental disorders among adolescents. Evidence suggests that adolescent depressive symptoms can not only have long-lasting influences on the development of cognitive abilities and social skills into adulthood, but also may lead to clinical depression, placing a heavy financial burden on individuals, families, and society [7]. Previous studies in Western countries reported that approximately 20–50% of adolescents had suffered from long-term depressive symptoms [8], and our prior study in China also showed that about 6.4% of high school students reported having depressive symptoms with suicidal ideation [9]. Although the association between PIU and depressive symptoms has been documented in prior studies [10,11], the influence path of PIU on depressive symptoms is still unclear.

Over the last two decades, the rapid growth of non-medical use of prescription drugs (NMUPD) among adolescents has drawn increased attention [12]. According to the report of the 2014 National Survey on Drug Use and Health (NSDUH) in the United States, prescription drugs were the second most popular type of drugs among adolescents [13]. A recent study also demonstrated that 2.0% of Chinese high school students reported frequent use of opioids, and 1.8% admitted frequent use of sedatives [14]. Previous studies demonstrated that PIU was reported to be associated with substance use, and PIU and substance use may share similar biological characteristics (e.g., similar vulnerable brain regions) [3,15]. Moreover, substance use may affect an individual's brain function, as well as their ability to self-regulate, leading to the development of depressive symptoms [16,17]. Therefore, NMUPD may play a mediator role between PIU and depressive symptoms. First, Caplan's theory proposed that a preference for online social interaction and the use of the Internet for mood regulation can predict deficient self-regulation of Internet use (i.e., PIU), which was a significant predictor of depressive symptoms [18]. Besides, based on the cognitive–behavioral theory of generalized PIU introduced by Davis, depressive symptoms might predispose individuals to develop maladaptive Internet-related cognitions and behaviors that ultimately result in adverse outcomes (e.g., substance use or PIU) [19,20]. Then, there might be two mediation models (incorporating NMUPD as the mediators) in the association between PIU and depressive symptoms from two orders: (1) PIU—NMUPD—depressive symptoms; and (2) depressive symptoms—NMUPD—PIU.

With the modernization of society, Chinese adolescents are more easily exposed to PIU, NMUPD, and depressive symptoms. However, there is a lack of studies in China considering the effects of NMUPD on the association between PIU and depressive symptoms. Therefore, we conducted this large-scale study aimed to test, among Chinese adolescents, the association between PIU, NMUPD, and depressive symptoms, as well as the mediating effects of NMUPD on the association between PIU and depressive symptoms.

2. Materials and Methods

2.1. Study Design and Participants

This study adopted the data from the 2017 National School-based Chinese Adolescents Health Survey (SCAHS), which is an ongoing study about the health risk behaviors and mental health problems among Chinese adolescents (7th–12th grade) conducted by our group. SCAHS performed a series of large-scale cross-sectional surveys every two years since 2007. The 2017 SCAHS utilized a multi-stage stratified cluster random sampling method to recruit a representative sample of adolescents in Guangdong province, and the procedures for data collection have been described in detail in previous publications [21]. Briefly, Guangdong province was firstly categorized into three stratifications according to geographic locations (Yue Dong, Yue Xi, Yue Bei, and Pearl River Delta) and gross domestic product (GDP) per capita (high-level, middle-level, and low-level). Then, we randomly selected two representative cities from each stratification. Considering adolescence is often described as occurring between 13 and 18 years of age (roughly the period of high school for much of the world) [22], in the present study, four vocational high schools and four general high schools were selected from each chosen city. Finally, two classes were randomly selected from each grade within the chosen schools. All available students were invited to participate in this study voluntarily, and 24,345 students' questionnaires were completed and qualified for analyses, resulting in a response rate of 92.1%. The anonymity of the questionnaires was guaranteed to elevate the validity of self-reports of stigmatized behaviors [23], and our research assistants administered these questionnaires during a regular class period without the presence of teachers (to avoid any potential information bias). Of the total sample, 51.5% (12,526) were boys, and the mean age of the students was 15.2 ± 1.8 years. The study procedures were carried out in accordance with the Declaration of Helsinki. The School of Public Health Institutional Review Board of the Sun Yat-sen University approved the study (the ethic code: L201720). All participants were informed about the study, and all provided written informed consents. If the participant was under 18 years of age, a written informed consent letter was obtained from one of the student's parents (or legal guardian).

2.2. Measures

Depressive symptoms were estimated by the Center for Epidemiologic Studies Depression (CES-D) Scale proposed by Radloff (1977), which has been validated and widely used among Chinese adolescents with satisfactory psychometric properties [24], and the Cronbach's alpha for this CES-D scale was 0.88 in the present study (the Cronbach's alpha ranging from 0.85 to 0.90 in Radloff's study). The total CES-D score ranges from 0 to 60, where higher scores indicate more significant depressive symptoms [25]. A cutoff score of 28 points was utilized to identify students at risk for clinical depression, also calling having depressive symptoms. This cutoff score has been used in previous studies in Chinese adolescents [26,27].

PIU was measured by Young's Internet Addiction Test (IAT) proposed by Young (1998), which has been validated and utilized among Chinese adolescents with satisfactory psychometric properties [28,29], and the Cronbach's alpha for IAT was 0.91 in this study. The IAT includes 20 items rated on a five-point Likert scale (from 1 = not at all to 5 = always) [30], where the total IAT score ranges from 20 to 100 and a higher score representing a greater level of inclination to PIU.

In the present study, NMUPD consists of non-medical use of opioids and sedatives. This list of opioids and sedatives was developed according to the report of the Guangdong Food and Drug Administration, with a focus on the prescription medications that have been widely used by adolescent drug abusers in rehabilitation centers of China. Opioids consist of compounded cough syrup with codeine (codeine), compounded licorice tablets (opium), tramadol hydrochloride, and diphenoxylate. Sedatives included diazepam or triazolam (benzodiazepines), compounded aminopyrine phenacetine tablets (barbiturates), and scopolamine hydrobromide tablets (barbiturates). Non-medical use of opioids or sedatives was measured by asking students how many times have you used the prescription medications as mentioned above for a non-medical purpose in the past year, and response options included "never", "once or twice", and "at least 3 times". Students who selected "never" were considered as abstainers, those who answered "once or twice" were thought as experimenters, and those who selected "at least three times" were treated as frequent users [30].

Information on sociodemographic variables were also collected, including gender (1 = boy, 2 = girl), age, living arrangement (responses were coded as "living in a two-parent family" = 1, "living in a single-parent family" = 2, and "living with others" = 3), household socioeconomic status (HSS, available responses were "above average" = 1, "average" = 2, and "below average" = 3), academic performance (responses were also coded as "above average" = 1, "average" = 2, and "below average" = 3). Family relationships, classmate relations, and relationships with teachers were assessed by asking how students perceived their relationships with family members, classmates, and teachers (available responses included "good" = 1, "average" = 2, and "poor" = 3).

2.3. Statistical Analysis

First, descriptive analyses were used to describe sample characteristics, and the t-tests and one-way ANOVA tests were performed to compare the differences in the CES-D scores. Descriptive analyses stratified by depressive symptoms were also conducted, and the chi-square tests or t-tests were used to describe the distribution of depressive symptoms in categorical or continuous variables. Second, considering this study used a multi-stage sampling design in which students were clustered into classes, generalized linear mixed models were fitted in which classes were treated as groups, and unstandardized β coefficients were reported. Univariable generalized linear mixed models were first conducted to estimate the potential association of PIU or NMUPD with depressive symptoms. Multivariable generalized linear mixed models, in which variables that were significant at the 0.10 level in the univariate analyses or widely reported in the literature were simultaneously incorporated, were performed to test the independent association of PIU or NMUPD with depressive symptoms. Third, multiplicative interaction items were tested by entering a cross-product term for opioid misuse or sedative misuse and PIU along with the main effect terms for each to the multivariable generalized linear mixed models, and p-values for the multiplicative interaction were calculated. Fourth, path models utilizing the maximum likelihood approach were conducted to assess the mediating effects of opioid or sedative misuse on the association between PIU and depressive symptoms. We first ordered the variables as follows: PIU—opioid or sedative misuse—depressive symptoms, and then an alternative model with a different order of the variables were assessed: depressive symptoms—opioid or sedative misuse—PIU. Due to the variables of the CES-D and IAT scores being continuous variables, and the measures of opioid and sedative misuse were categorized, standardized probit coefficients, standardized total effects, and standardized indirect effects were reported, with the bias-corrected 95% confidence intervals (CI) estimated using 1000 bootstrap samples. Path model fit indices were also reported, including comparative fit index (CFI; CFI > 0.90 indicating a good fit), root mean square error of approximation (RMSEA, RMSEA < 0.08 indicating an acceptable fit), and standardized root mean square residual (SRMR; SRMR < 0.08 indicating a good fit) [31,32]. All statistical analyses were conducted using SAS 9.2 (SAS Institute, Inc., Cary, NC, USA) and Mplus version 7.0 (Muthén and Muthén). The percentage of missing data of all relevant variables was less than 0.6, and observations with missing data were eliminated in the generalized linear mixed models and path models. All statistical tests were two-sided, and p-values less than 0.05 were considered statistically significant.

3. Results

The sample characteristics are shown in Table 1. A total of 13.5% of students reported living with others, and 13.9% reported below average HSS. The proportion of students who reported poor family relationships, classmate relations, and relationship with teachers, were 4.1%, 1.6%, and 2.4%, respectively. The mean IAT scores among the total students were 35.8 (SD: 12.8). A total of 0.6% and 0.3% of students reported frequent use of opioids and sedatives, respectively. The mean CES-D scores were 13.6 (SD: 8.7), and 6.7% of the students reported having depressive symptoms. There were significant differences in the CES-D scores among the variables of gender, living arrangement, HSS, academic performance, family relationships, classmate relations, relationships with teachers, opioid misuse, and sedative misuse ($p < 0.001$). Additionally, significant differences emerged between the students with and without depressive symptoms in the distribution of gender, living arrangement, HSS, academic performance, family relationships, classmate relations, relationships with teachers, IAT scores, opioid misuse, and sedative misuse ($p < 0.001$).

Table 1. Sample characteristics stratified by depressive symptoms among 24,345 adolescents.

Variable	Total	CES-D Scores, Mean (SD)	p-Value *	Depressive Symptoms		p-Value *
				Yes	No	
Total	24,345 (100)	13.6 (8.7)		1631 (6.7)	22,714 (93.3)	
Gender						
Boys	12,526 (51.5)	12.9 (8.6)	<0.001	731 (45.0)	11,795 (52.1)	<0.001
Girls	11,732 (48.2)	14.4 (8.8)		892 (55.0)	10,840 (47.9)	
Missing data	87 (0.4)					
Living arrangement						
Living in two-parent family	18,094 (74.3)	13.3 (8.6)	<0.001	1125 (69.1)	16,969 (74.9)	<0.001
Living in a single-parent family	2905 (11.9)	15.0 (9.4)		259 (15.9)	2646 (11.7)	
Living with others	3281 (13.5)	14.3 (8.8)		243 (14.9)	3038 (13.4)	
Missing data	65 (0.3)					
HSS						
Above average	6942 (28.5)	12.1 (8.1)	<0.001	315 (19.3)	6627 (29.3)	<0.001
Average	13,944 (57.3)	13.8 (8.6)		928 (57.0)	13,016 (57.5)	
Below average	3388 (13.9)	16.3 (9.8)		385 (23.6)	3003 (13.3)	
Missing data	71 (0.3)					
Academic performance						
Above average	9195 (37.8)	12.3 (8.5))	<0.001	508 (31.2)	8687 (38.5)	<0.001
Average	7576 (31.1)	13.5 (8.2)		434 (26.7)	7142 (31.6)	
Below average	7448 (30.6)	15.5 (9.3)		685 (42.1)	6763 (29.9)	
Missing data	126 (0.5)					
Family relationships						
Good	19,899 (81.7)	12.6 (8.0)	<0.001	946 (58.1)	18,953 (83.8)	<0.001
Average	3362 (13.8)	17.6 (9.8)		429 (26.3)	2933 (13.0)	
Poor	986 (4.1)	21.5 (11.9)		254 (15.6)	732 (3.2)	
Missing data	98 (0.4)					
Classmate relations						
Good	19,561 (80.3)	12.5 (7.9)	<0.001	899 (55.3)	18,662 (82.6)	<0.001
Average	4274 (17.6)	17.9 (9.7)		580 (35.7)	3694 (16.4)	
Poor	381 (1.6)	26.3 (13.7)		146 (9.0)	235 (1.0)	
Missing data	129 (0.5)					
Relationship with teachers						
Good	15,695 (64.5)	12.1 (7.9)	<0.001	706 (43.6)	14,989 (66.6)	<0.001
Average	7844 (32.2)	16.2 (9.2)		790 (48.8)	7054 (31.4)	
Poor	576 (2.4)	21.2 (12.6)		124 (7.7)	452 (2.0)	
Missing data	230 (0.9)					
IAT scores, Mean (SD)	35.8 (12.8)	NA		49.3 (16.5)	34.8 (11.9)	<0.001
Opioid misuse						
Abstainers	23,822 (97.9)	13.6 (8.7)	<0.001	1559 (95.6)	22,263 (98.0)	<0.001
Experimenters	384 (1.6)	17.3 (10.0)		49 (3.0)	335 (1.5)	
Frequent users	139 (0.6)	19.2 (9.8)		23 (1.4)	116 (0.5)	
Sedative misuse						
Abstainers	24,095 (99.0)	13.6 (8.7)	<0.001	1588 (97.4)	22,507 (99.1)	<0.001
Experimenters	188 (0.8)	17.4 (9.1)		23 (1.4)	165 (0.7)	
Frequent users	62 (0.3)	23.8 (14.6)		20 (1.2)	42 (0.2)	

Note: * t-tests or one-way ANOVA tests were performed to test the differences in CES-D score, and Chi-square tests or t-tests were used to compare the differences in adolescents with and without depressive symptoms; HSS—household socioeconomic status; IAT—internet addiction test; SD–standard deviation; CES-D—Center for Epidemiologic Studies Depression; NA—not applicable or no data available.

Without adjusting for other variables, Model 1 demonstrated that PIU, opioid misuse, and sedative misuse were respectively associated with the increase of depressive symptoms ($p < 0.001$). After adjusting for gender, living arrangement, HSS, academic performance, family relationships, classmate relations, and relationships with teachers, Model 2 showed that PIU was significantly associated with depressive symptoms (unstandardized β estimate = 0.26, 95% CI = 0.25–0.27), frequent use of opioids was positively related to depressive symptoms (unstandardized β estimate = 2.77, 95% CI = 1.90–3.63), and frequent use of sedatives was also related to the elevation of depressive symptoms (unstandardized β estimate = 4.45, 95% CI = 3.02–5.88). Additionally, Model 3 and Model 4 did not find any significant multiplicative interaction item between non-medical use of opioids/sedatives and PIU (Table 2).

As shown in Figure 1 and Table 3, the model including the mediator (opioid misuse or sedative misuse) showed that after adjusting for significant covariates, opioid misuse partially mediated the positive association between PIU and depressive symptoms, and the estimate of the standardized indirect effect was 0.003 (95% CI = 0.001–0.005). The obtained indices suggested that the model fit the data well: CFI = 0.92; RMSEA = 0.042, 95% CI = 0.030–0.055; SRMR = 0.061. However, the results also demonstrated that the adjusted standardized indirect effects of PIU on depressive symptoms through sedative misuse was not significant ($p > 0.05$), indicating that the relationship between PIU and depressive symptoms was not mediated by sedative misuse. The model fit indices indicated that the model fit the data satisfactorily: CFI = 0.89; RMSEA = 0.044, 95% CI = 0.032–0.047; SRMR = 0.052.

Table 2. Association between problematic Internet use, opioid misuse, sedative misuse, and depressive symptoms among adolescents.

Variable	CES-D scores							
	Model 1		Model 2		Model 3		Model 4	
	β Estimate [#] (95% CI)	p-Value	β Estimate [#] (95% CI)	p-Value	β Estimate [#] (95% CI)	p-Value	β Estimate [#] (95% CI)	p-Value
Problematic Internet use (1-score increase)	0.30 (0.29–0.31)	<0.001	0.26 (0.25–0.27)	<0.001	0.26 (0.25–0.27)	<0.001	0.26 (0.25–0.27)	<0.001
Opioid misuse (Ref. = Abstainers)								
Experimenters	3.75 (2.82–4.68)	<0.001	2.77 (1.90–3.63)	<0.001	2.42 (0.19–4.65)	0.034	NA	
Frequent users	5.65 (4.11–7.12)	<0.001	4.45 (3.02–5.88)	<0.001	3.95(−0.32–8.22)	0.071	NA	
Sedative misuse (Ref.= Abstainers)								
Experimenters	3.85 (2.54–5.17)	<0.001	2.86 (1.63–4.09)	<0.001	NA		2.53 (−0.86–5.91)	0.144
Frequent users	10.26 (8.03–12.48)	<0.001	7.18 (5.09–9.26)	<0.001	NA		10.85 (5.15–16.56)	<0.001
Interaction item (opioid misuse)								
Experimenters * Problematic Internet use	NA		NA		−0.02 (−0.07–0.03)	0.502	NA	
Frequent users * Problematic Internet use	NA		NA		−0.04 (−0.13–0.05)	0.387	NA	
Interaction item (sedative misuse)								
Experimenters * Problematic Internet use	NA		NA		NA		−0.01 (−0.09–0.08)	0.884
Frequent users * Problematic Internet use	NA		NA		NA		−0.11 (−0.22–−0.01)	0.086

Note: [#] Unstandardized β coefficient. Model 1: Unadjusted generalized linear mixed models. Model 2: The multivariable generalized linear mixed models were adjusted for gender, living arrangement, HSS, academic performance, family relationships, classmate relations, and relationships with teachers. Model 3: The multivariable generalized linear mixed models simultaneously incorporated the interaction item for opioid misuse and problematic Internet use along with the main effect terms for each, and were adjusted for gender, living arrangement, HSS, academic performance, family relationships, classmate relations, and relationships with teachers. Model 4: The multivariable generalized linear mixed models simultaneously incorporated the interaction item for sedative misuse and problematic Internet use along with the main effect terms for each, and were adjusted for gender, living arrangement, HSS, academic performance, family relationships, classmate relations, and relationships with teachers; Ref.—reference; CES-D—Center for Epidemiologic Studies Depression; NA—not applicable or no data available. * The multiplicative interaction between the two items.

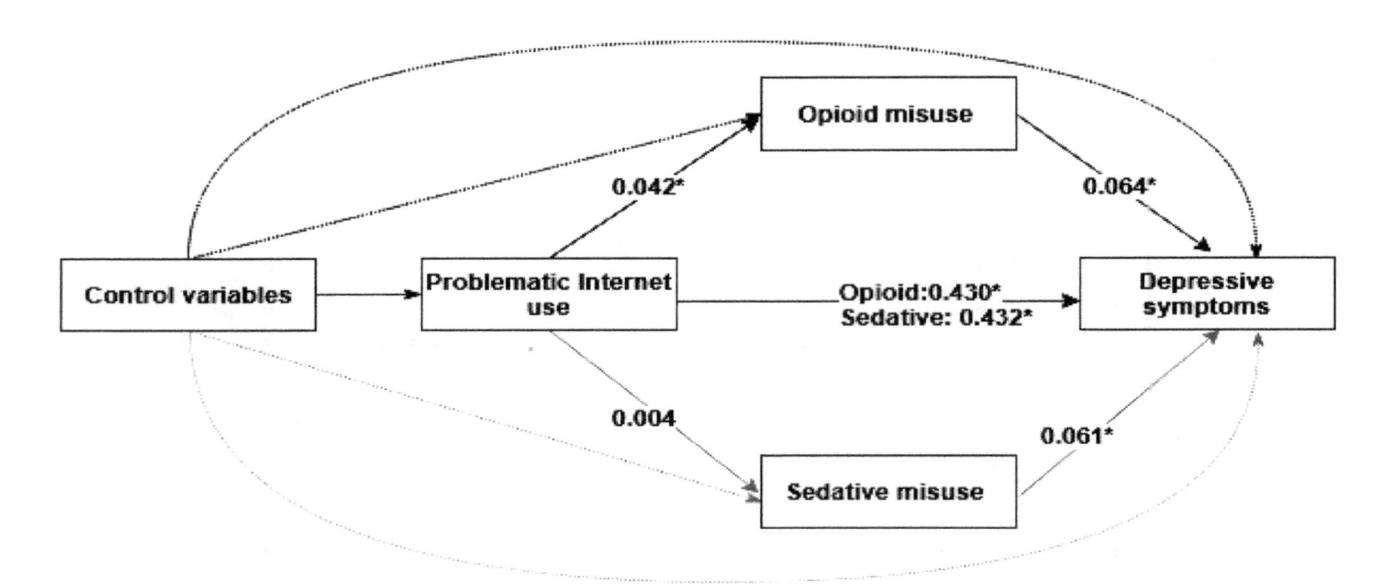

Figure 1. The mediating effects of opioid or sedative misuse on the association betweer. problematic Internet use and depressive symptoms. The solid lines mean the effects between the independent variable, mediator variables, and dependent variable. The dashed lines mean the effects of control variables (gender, living arrangement, HSS, academic performance, family relationships, classmate relations, and relationships with teachers) on the independent variable, mediator variables, and dependent variable.

Table 3. Path analysis showing the effects of problematic Internet use and opioid or sedative misuse on depressive symptoms.

Variable.	Symbol	CES-D Scores	
		Unadjusted Model	Adjusted Model *
		Standardized β Estimate (95% CI)	Standardized β Estimate (95% CI)
Problematic Internet use » Depressive symptoms	Predictor » Outcome	0.437 (0.425–0.449)	0.430 (0.418–0.442)
Opioid misuse » Depressive symptoms	Mediator » Outcome	0.072 (0.058–0.086)	0.064 (0.048–0.080)
Problematic internet use » Opioid misuse	Predictor » Mediator	0.045 (0.033–0.057)	0.042 (0.030–0.054)
Standardized effect			
Indirect		0.003 (0.001–0.005)	0.003 (0.001–0.005)
Total		0.441 (0.429–0.453)	0.430 (0.418–0.442)
Problematic Internet use » Depressive symptoms	Predictor » Outcome	0.4395 (0.4280–0.4518)	0.4318 (0.4202–0.4439)
Sedative misuse » Depressive symptoms	Mediator » Outcome	0.072 (0.058–0.086)	0.061 (0.045–0.077)
Problematic internet use » Sedative misuse	Predictor » Mediator	0.007 (−0.005–0.019)	0.004 (−0.008–0.016)
Standardized effect			
Indirect		0.0005 (−0.002–0.0006)	0.0002 (−0.0018–0.0003)
Total		0.440 (0.428–0.452)	0.432 (0.420–0.444)

Note: * The path models were adjusted for gender, living arrangement, HSS, academic performance, family relationships, classmate relations, and relationships with teachers; CES-D—Center for Epidemiologic Studies Depression.

As shown in Figure 2 and Table 4, the alternative model incorporating the mediator (opioid misuse or sedative misuse) demonstrated that the adjusted indirect effects of depressive symptoms on PIU through opioid misuse were statistically significant (standardized β estimate = 0.002, 95% CI = 0.001–0.002), and the model fit indices were: CFI = 0.91; RMSEA = 0.042, 95% CI = 0.031–0.057; SRMR = 0.063. There were significant standardized indirect effects of depressive symptoms on PIU via sedative misuse (standardized β estimate = 0.001, 95% CI = 0.001–0.001), and the model indices suggested that the model fit the data well: CFI = 0.93; RMSEA = 0.040, 95% CI = 0.029–0.067; SRMR = 0.067. These results suggested that opioid misuse or sedative misuse partially mediated the association of depressive symptoms with PIU, respectively.

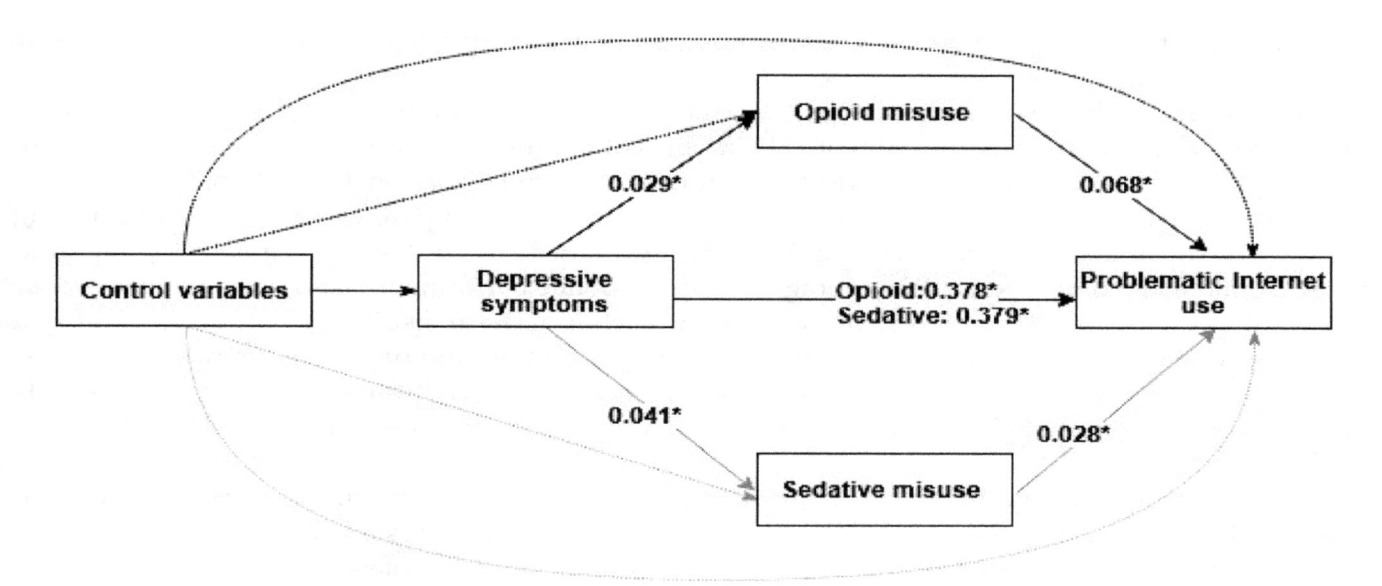

Figure 2. The mediating effects of opioid or sedative misuse on the association between depressive symptoms and problematic Internet use. The solid lines mean the effects between the independent variable, mediator variables, and dependent variable. The dashed lines mean the effects of control variables (gender, living arrangement, HSS, academic performance, family relationships, classmate relations, and relationships with teachers) on the independent variable, mediator variables, and dependent variable.

Table 4. Path analysis showing the effects of depressive symptoms and opioid or sedative misuse on problematic Internet use.

Variable	Symbol	Problematic Internet Use	
		Unadjusted Model	Adjusted Model *
		Standardized β Estimate (95% CI)	Standardized β Estimate (95% CI)
CES-D scores » Problematic Internet use	Predictor » Outcome	0.438 (0.426–0.450)	0.378 (0.366–0.390)
Opioid misuse » Problematic Internet use	Mediator » Outcome	0.076 (0.062–0.090)	0.068 (0.054–0.082)
CES-D scores » Opioid misuse	Predictor » Mediator	0.038 (0.026–0.050)	0.029 (0.017–0.041)
Standardized effect			
Indirect		0.003 (0.001–0.005)	0.002 (0.001–0.002)
Total		0.441 (0.429–0.453)	0.380 (0.368–0.392)
CES-D scores » Problematic Internet use	Predictor » Outcome	0.438 (0.426–0.450)	0.379 (0.367–0.391)
Sedative misuse » Problematic Internet use	Mediator » Outcome	0.039 (0.025–0.053)	0.028 (0.014–0.042)
CES-D scores » Sedative misuse	Predictor » Mediator	0.056 (0.044–0.068)	0.041 (0.029–0.053)
Standardized effect			
Indirect		0.002 (0.001–0.002)	0.001 (0.001–0.001)
Total		0.440 (0.429–0.453)	0.380 (0.368–0.392)

Note: * The path models were adjusted for gender, living arrangement, HSS, academic performance, family relationships, classmate relations, and relationships with teachers; CES-D—Center for Epidemiologic Studies Depression.

4. Discussion

To our knowledge, the present study is the first large-scale study to estimate the direct and indirect association between PIU, opioid or sedative misuse, and depressive symptoms among Chinese adolescents, and to investigate the potential mediating effects of opioid or sedative misuse on the association between PIU and depressive symptoms. This study first found that the mean CES-D scores for the adolescents were13.6 (SD: 8.7), and 6.7% reported having depressive symptoms. These results are parallel with our previous study conducted in 2014 [9], and slightly lower than that described in a prior review revealing a pooled prevalence of depressive symptoms of 24.3% (95% CI, 21.3–27.6%) among adolescents in mainland China [33]. The difference might be related to the variety in the definition of depressive symptoms (i.e., using different measurement scale and cutoff scores), and these results indicate that depressive symptoms among Chinese adolescents are a growing public health problem.

Consistent with previous evidence [9,11], the present study found that there were significant differences in the continuous and categorical variables of depressive symptoms among the groups of gender, living arrangement, HSS, academic performance, family relationships, classmate relations, relationships with teachers, opioid misuse, and sedative misuse. Compared with their corresponding groups, the mean CES-D scores were significantly higher in girls, students living in a single-parent family, students who reported below average HSS or academic performance, and those reporting poor relationships with family members, classmates, or teachers. These results are helpful to identify a profile of adolescents who are vulnerable to depressive symptoms, and particular attention should be paid to the groups with the negative characteristics mentioned above. Moreover, the covariate effects of these variables on the relationship between PIU and depressive symptoms should also be taken into consideration.

In the adjusted generalized linear mixed models without mediation, a positive relationship between depressive symptoms and PIU, opioid misuse, and sedative misuse was found, respectively. First, PIU may increase the risk of depressive symptoms due to adolescents with PIU showing poorer well-being, self-control, and self-esteem, which were reported to be positively associated with psychiatric disorders (including depressive symptoms) [34,35]. Similarly, Park et al. reported that PIU was positively associated with depressive symptoms in Korean adolescents [10]; Dalbudak et al. demonstrated that Internet addiction might increase vulnerability to depressive symptoms in students of Turkey [36]; and Tan et al. found that PIU was significantly related to an increased risk of depressive symptoms among adolescents in Shantou, China [11]. Moreover, the found significant association between opioid or sedative misuse and depressive symptoms might be related to the finding that these drugs may cause negative emotions and urgency, poor concentration, and sleeping problems, which are reported to be associated with an elevated risk of depressive symptoms [17,37]. Adolescents are especially vulnerable to the adverse effects of NMUPD given their still-developing brain [38].

Although there is evidence supporting the role of opioid or sedative misuse in the process through which PIU is related to depressive symptoms, no study before had confirmed the mediating effects of opioid or sedative misuse. Considering mediation analyses require exclusion of an interaction between the exposure and the mediator on the outcome [39], the interaction items between opioid/sedative misuse and PIU on depressive symptoms were first tested, and the results did not find any significant interaction effects. Furthermore, the path models of this study first demonstrated that the association between PIU and depressive symptoms remained significant when opioid or sedative misuse was incorporated as a mediator, and the association above was partially mediated through opioid misuse. These findings were consistent with the theory proposed by Caplan, which showed that PIU might be a reflection of maladaptive cognitions that lead to difficulties with behavioral impulse control and ultimately resulting in adverse outcomes associated with PIU (e.g., NMUPD and depressive symptoms) [18]. Moreover, a possible explanation for the mediating effects of opioid misuse might be that PIU and opioid use may have similarities in biological characteristics [3,15]. PIU may increase the risk of opioid misuse through impaired impulse control [40] and opioid misuse is one of the known factors associated with depressive symptoms [40]. In another aspect, Davis's cognitive–behavioral theory proposed that depressive symptoms may also predispose individuals to develop maladaptive Internet-related cognitions and behaviors that can lead to PIU [19,20]. Moreover, due to the cross-sectional nature of data which may cause bias of the mediating estimates when mediation occurs over time, another path process order was also performed to test the potential the mediating effects opioid or sedative misuse on the association between depressive symptoms and PIU. The present study also demonstrated that opioid and sedative misuse significantly mediated the association of depressive symptoms with PIU, and these results may be related to the finding that adolescents with depressive symptoms may non-medically use opioid or sedatives as a coping strategy to release a negative mood [41], and substance abuse has been reported to be able to predict a high risk of PIU [42]. Taken together, the association between PIU, opioid or sedative misuse, and depressive symptoms might be complicated; for instance, PIU can lead to opioid or sedative misuse and depressive symptoms, which in turn may worsen the problematic Internet use problem among adolescents, and vice versa. The investigation of the mediating effects of opioid or sedative misuse can add evidence for the new understanding of the mechanism of the association between PIU and depressive symptoms.

Based on the findings of the current study, several recommendations for preventing PIU, NMUPD, and depressive symptoms among adolescents are listed below: (1) limiting adolescents' exposure to the Internet for a long time (e.g., playing game); (2) increasing individuals' awareness of the adverse effects of PIU, NMUPD, and depressive symptoms; (3) providing professional health services (e.g., health services provided by clinicians or social workers in the schools or communities) to students who have been involved in PIU, NMUPD, and depressive symptoms. If possible, concomitant treatment for PIU, NMUPD, and depressive symptoms should be considered; and (4) developing a long-term surveillance system to monitor the health-risky behaviors among adolescents in China.

There are several limitations related to this study. First, the use of self-report questionnaires in this study may result in the underestimate of some sensitive data among adolescents (e.g., PIU or NMUPD) for social desirability. Second, due to the cross-sectional nature of the study design, findings should be interpreted with caution, especially regarding the longitudinal indirect and direct effects. Third, because of the school-based study design, the study sample only included students at school, while PIU, NMUPD, or depressive symptoms may be more common among adolescents who were absent from schools. Fourth, PIU and depressive symptoms were measured by the IAT and CES-D scales. Although this measurement of PIU or depressive symptoms has been validated and widely used in previous studies, the answers may still be subjectively biased. Fifth, Axis I comorbidities (such as anxiety or bipolar disorder), which may have an effect on depressive symptoms, were not taken into account in the present study. Despite these limitations, the strength of this study is that it uses a large-scale sample of Chinese adolescents to extend the prior evidence about the association between PIU, opioid or sedative misuse, and depressive symptoms through investigating the mediating effects of opioid or sedative misuse.

5. Conclusions

In conclusion, the present study found that in the models without mediation, PIU and opioid/sedative misuse were positively related to an increased risk of depressive symptoms among adolescents, respectively. Moreover, two path models were conducted to estimate the potential mechanism of the association between PIU, opioid or sedative misuse, and depressive symptoms. The results indicated that the association above might be complex and transactional, and that PIU may elevate the risk of opioid or sedative misuse and depressive symptoms, which in turn could worsen the situation of PIU and vice versa. These study findings have some important implications. Multidisciplinary health intervention programs to prevent adolescents from getting involved in PIU and NMPUD are recommended to be provided, and the concomitant or complex transactional association between PIU, opioid or sedative misuse, and depressive symptoms should be taken into consideration by adolescents, their families and teachers, as well as professional health providers.

Author Contributions: Data curation, L.G., B.F., W.W., T.W., B.X., H.Z. and Y.L.; formal analysis, B.F. and W.W.; funding acquisition, C.L. and L.G.; methodology, L.G.; project administration, C.L. and L.G.; writing—original draft, B.F., W.W. and L.G. All authors have read and agreed to the published version of the manuscript

Acknowledgments: We would like to express our special gratitude and thanks to all the participating schools and students.

References

1. Lin, M.P.; Wu, J.Y.; Chen, C.J.; You, J. Positive outcome expectancy mediates the relationship between social influence and Internet addiction among senior high-school students. *J. Behav. Addict.* **2018**, *7*, 292–300. [CrossRef] [PubMed]

2. An, J.; Sun, Y.; Wan, Y.; Chen, J.; Wang, X.; Tao, F. Associations between problematic internet use and adolescents' physical and psychological symptoms: Possible role of sleep quality. *J. Addict. Med.* **2014**, *8*, 282–287. [CrossRef] [PubMed]

3. Rucker, J.; Akre, C.; Berchtold, A.; Suris, J.C. Problematic Internet use is associated with substance use in young adolescents. *Acta Paediatr.* **2015**, *104*, 504–507. [CrossRef] [PubMed]

4. World Health Organization. Gaming Disoder. Available online: https://www.who.int/features/qa/gaming-disorder/en/ (accessed on 8 December 2019).

5. Tymula, A.; Rosenberg, B.L.; Roy, A.K.; Ruderman, L.; Manson, K.; Glimcher, P.W.; Levy, I. Adolescents' risk-taking behavior is driven by tolerance to ambiguity. *Proc. Natl. Acad. Sci. USA* **2012**, *109*, 17135–17140. [CrossRef] [PubMed]

6. Public Health Implications of Excessive Use of the Internet, Computers, Smartphones and Similar Electronic Devices Meeting report. In *Main Meeting Hall, Foundation for Promotion of Cancer Research National Cancer Research Centre*; World Health Organization: Tokyo, Japan, 2015.

7. Thapar, A.; Collishaw, S.; Pine, D.S.; Thapar, A.K. Depression in adolescence. *Lancet* **2012**, *379*, 1056–1067. [CrossRef]

8. Wesselhoeft, R.; Sorensen, M.J.; Heiervang, E.R.; Bilenberg, N. Subthreshold depression in children and adolescents—A systematic review. *J. Affect. Disord.* **2013**, *151*, 7–22. [CrossRef]

9. Guo, L.; Deng, J.; He, Y.; Deng, X.; Huang, J.; Huang, G.; Gao, X.; Lu, C. Prevalence and correlates of sleep disturbance and depressive symptoms among Chinese adolescents: A cross-sectional survey study. *BMJ Open* **2014**, *4*, e5517. [CrossRef]

10. Park, S.; Hong, K.E.; Park, E.J.; Ha, K.S.; Yoo, H.J. The association between problematic internet use and depression, suicidal ideation and bipolar disorder symptoms in Korean adolescents. *Aust. N. Z. J. Psychiatry* **2013**, *47*, 153–159. [CrossRef]

11. Tan, Y.; Chen, Y.; Lu, Y.; Li, L. Exploring Associations between Problematic Internet Use, Depressive Symptoms and Sleep Disturbance among Southern Chinese Adolescents. *Int. J. Environ. Res. Public Health* **2016**, *13*, 313. [CrossRef]

12. LeClair, A.; Kelly, B.C.; Pawson, M.; Wells, B.E.; Parsons, J.T. Motivations for Prescription Drug Misuse among Young Adults: Considering Social and Developmental Contexts. *Drugs* **2015**, *22*, 208–216. [CrossRef]

13. Center for Behavioral Health Statistics and Quality. *Behavioral Health Trends in the United States: Results from the 2014 National Survey on Drug Use and Health (HHS Publication No. SMA 15-4927, NSDUH Series H-50)*; Substance Abuse and Mental Health Services Administration: Rockville, MD, USA, 2015.

14. Guo, L.; Luo, M.; Wang, W.; Xiao, D.; Xi, C.; Wang, T.; Zhao, M.; Zhang, W.H.; Lu, C. Association between nonmedical use of opioids or sedatives and suicidal behavior among Chinese adolescents: An analysis of sex differences. *Aust. N. Z. J. Psychiatry* **2019**, *53*, 559–569. [CrossRef] [PubMed]

15. Han, D.H.; Hwang, J.W.; Renshaw, P.F. Bupropion sustained release treatment decreases craving for video games and cue-induced brain activity in patients with Internet video game addiction. *Exp. Clin. Psychopharmacol.* **2010**, *18*, 297–304. [CrossRef] [PubMed]

16. Brand, M.; Young, K.S.; Laier, C. Prefrontal control and internet addiction: A theoretical model and review of neuropsychological and neuroimaging findings. *Front. Hum. Neurosci.* **2014**, *8*, 375. [CrossRef] [PubMed]

17. Quello, S.B.; Brady, K.T.; Sonne, S.C. Mood disorders and substance use disorder: A complex comorbidity. *Sci. Pract. Perspect.* **2005**, *3*, 13–21. [CrossRef] [PubMed]

18. Caplan, S.E. Theory and measurement of generalized problematic Internet use: A two-step approach. *Comput. Hum. Behav.* **2010**, *26*, 1089–1097. [CrossRef]

19. Davis, R.A.; Flett, G.L.; Besser, A. Validation of a new scale for measuring problematic internet use: Implications for pre-employment screening. *Cyberpsychol. Behav.* **2002**, *5*, 331–345. [CrossRef]

20. Davis, R.A. A cognitive-behavioral model of pathological Internet use. *Comput. Hum. Behav.* **2001**, *17*, 187–195. [CrossRef]

21. Guo, L.; Luo, M.; Wang, W.X.; Huang, G.L.; Xu, Y.; Gao, X.; Lu, C.Y.; Zhang, W.H. Association between problematic Internet use, sleep disturbance, and suicidal behavior in Chinese adolescents *J. Behav. Addict.* **2018**, *7*, 965–975. [CrossRef]

22. Crockett, L.J.; Beal, S.J. The life course in the making: Gender and the development of adolescents' expected timing of adult role transitions. *Dev. Psychol.* **2012**, *48*, 1727–1738. [CrossRef]

23. Ramo, D.E.; Liu, H.; Prochaska, J.J. Reliability and validity of young adults' anonymous online reports of marijuana use and thoughts about use. *Psychol. Addict. Behav.* **2012**, *26*, 801–811. [CrossRef]

24. Lee, S.W.; Stewart, S.M.; Byrne, B.M.; Wong, J.P.; Ho, S.Y.; Lee, P.W.; Lam, T.H. Factor structure of the Center for Epidemiological Studies Depression Scale in Hong Kong adolescents. *J. Pers. Assess* **2008**, *90*, 175–184. [CrossRef] [PubMed]

25. Radloff, L.S. The use of the Center for Epidemiologic Studies Depression Scale in adolescents and young adults. *J. Youth Adolesc.* **1991**, *20*, 149–166. [CrossRef] [PubMed]

26. Guo, L.; Xu, Y.; Deng, J.; Huang, J.; Huang, G.; Gao, X.; Wu, H.; Pan, S.; Zhang, W.H.; Lu, C. Association Between Nonmedical Use of Prescription Drugs and Suicidal Behavior Among Adolescents. *JAMA Pediatr.* **2016**, *170*, 971–978. [CrossRef]

27. Yang, H.J.; Soong, W.T.; Kuo, P.H.; Chang, H.L.; Chen, W.J. Using the CES-D in a two-phase survey for depressive disorders among nonreferred adolescents in Taipei: A stratum-specific likelihood ratio analysis. *J. Affect. Disord.* **2004**, *82*, 419–430. [CrossRef] [PubMed]

28. Lai, C.M.; Mak, K.K.; Watanabe, H.; Ang, R.P.; Pang, J.S.; Ho, R.C. Psychometric properties of the internet addiction test in Chinese adolescents. *J. Pediatr. Psychol.* **2013**, *38*, 794–807. [CrossRef] [PubMed]

29. Wang, H.; Zhou, X.; Lu, C.; Wu, J.; Deng, X.; Hong, L. Problematic Internet Use in high school students in Guangdong Province, China. *PLoS ONE* **2011**, *6*, e19660. [CrossRef] [PubMed]

30. Young, K.S. *Caught in the Net: How to Recognize the Signs of Internet Addiction and a Winning Strategy for Recovery*; John Wiley & Sons: New York, NY, USA, 1998.

31. Hu, L.; Bentler, P.M. *Evaluating Model Fit*; Sage Publications, Inc.: Thousand Oaks, CA, USA, 1995.

32. Garver, M.S.; Mentzer, J.T. Logistics research methods: Employing structural equation modeling to test for construct validity. *J. Bus Logist* **1999**, *20*, 33–57.

33. Tang, X.; Tang, S.; Ren, Z.; Wong, D. Prevalence of depressive symptoms among adolescents in secondary school in mainland China: A systematic review and meta-analysis. *J. Affect. Disord.* **2019**, *245*, 498–507. [CrossRef]

34. Mei, S.; Yau, Y.H.; Chai, J.; Guo, J.; Potenza, M.N. Problematic Internet use, well-being, self-esteem and self-control: Data from a high-school survey in China. *Addict. Behav.* **2016**, *61*, 74–79. [CrossRef]

35. Ho, R.C.; Zhang, M.W.; Tsang, T.Y.; Toh, A.H.; Pan, F.; Lu, Y.; Cheng, C.; Yip, P.S.; Lam, L.T.; Lai, C.M.; et al. The association between internet addiction and psychiatric co-morbidity: A meta-analysis. *BMC Psychiatry* **2014**, *14*, 183. [CrossRef]

36. Dalbudak, E.; Evren, C.; Aldemir, S.; Coskun, K.S.; Ugurlu, H.; Yildirim, F.G. Relationship of internet addiction severity with depression, anxiety, and alexithymia, temperament and character in university students. *Cyberpsychol. Behav. Soc. Netw.* **2013**, *16*, 272–278. [CrossRef] [PubMed]

37. Pang, R.D.; Farrahi, L.; Glazier, S.; Sussman, S.; Leventhal, A.M. Depressive symptoms, negative urgency and substance use initiation in adolescents. *Drug Alcohol Depend.* **2014**, *144*, 225–230. [CrossRef] [PubMed]

38. Casey, B.J.; Getz, S.; Galvan, A. The adolescent brain. *Dev. Rev.* **2008**, *28*, 62–77. [CrossRef] [PubMed]

39. Lindley, P.; Walker, S.N. Theoretical and methodological differentiation of moderation and mediation. *Nurs. Res.* **1993**, *42*, 276–279. [CrossRef]

40. Yau, Y.H.; Potenza, M.N.; White, M.A. Problematic Internet Use, Mental Health and Impulse Control in an Online Survey of Adults. *J. Behav. Addict.* **2013**, *2*, 72. [CrossRef]

41. Khantzian, E.J. The self-medication hypothesis of substance use disorders: A reconsideration and recent applications. *Harv. Rev. Psychiatry* **1997**, *4*, 231–244. [CrossRef]

42. Lee, Y.S.; Han, D.H.; Kim, S.M.; Renshaw, P.F. Substance abuse precedes Internet addiction. *Addict. Behav.* **2013**, *38*, 2022–2025. [CrossRef]

4

Psychological Risk Factors that Predict Social Networking and Internet Addiction in Adolescents

Montserrat Peris [1], Usue de la Barrera [2], Konstanze Schoeps [3]
and Inmaculada Montoya-Castilla [2,*]

[1] Department of Personality, Evaluation and Psychological Treatments, University of the Basque Country,
    20018 San Sebastian, Spain; montserrat.peris@ehu.eus

[2] Department of Personality, Assessment and Psychological Treatment, Faculty of Psychology,
    University of Valencia, 46010 Valencia, Spain; usue.barrera@uv.es

[3] Department of Psychology, Faculty of Health Sciences, European University of Valencia,
    46010 Valencia, Spain; konstanze.schoeps@universidadeuropea.es

* Correspondence: inmaculada.montoya@uv.es

Abstract: Adolescents' addictive use of social media and the internet is an increasing concern among parents, teachers, researchers and society. The purpose was to examine the contribution of body self-esteem, personality traits, and demographic factors in the prediction of adolescents' addictive use of social media and the internet. The participants were 447 Spanish adolescents aged 13−16 years ($M = 14.90$, $SD = 0.81$, 56.2% women). We measured gender, age, body self-esteem (body satisfaction and physical attractiveness), personality traits (extraversion, neuroticism, disinhibition and narcissism) and social networking and internet addiction (internet addiction symptoms, social media use, geek behaviour, and nomophobia). The effects of gender, age, body self-esteem and personality on the different dimensions of internet addiction were estimated, conducting hierarchical linear multiple regression analysis and a fuzzy-set qualitative comparative analysis (fsQCA). The results evidenced different pathways explaining four types of adolescents' internet addiction: gender and disinhibition were the most relevant predictors of addiction symptoms; gender combined with physical attractiveness best explained social media use; narcissism and neuroticism appear to be the most relevant predictors of geek behaviour; and narcissism was the variable that best explained nomophobia. Furthermore, the advantages and differences between both methodologies (regressions vs. QCA) were discussed.

Keywords: adolescents; internet addiction; social networking; body self-esteem; personality traits; fsQCA models

---

1. Introduction

1.1. Risk of Internet Addiction and Social Media Use

The use of social networking sites and the internet has grown in popularity over the last few decades and new technological tools such as smartphones may have become indispensable today [1,2]. Prevalence rates vary considerably in internet addiction research. Across Europe, recent studies reported prevalence ranging between 4.4% to 13.5% for pathological internet use and between 14.3% and 54.9% for problematic internet use [3]. In Spain, the prevalence of problematic internet users has been estimated to be between 18.5% and 4.9% of pathological internet users [4]. Adolescence is an especially vulnerable period of change and teenagers face the risk of suffering symptoms of addiction as a result of their daily social network use [2]. Traditionally, internet addiction has been analysed in a generalised and global way, however, recent studies suggest the relevance of investigating each subtype of addiction in each particular population [5]. For instance, Peris et al. [6] consider four types of risk behaviour regarding social networking and internet addiction in adolescents on a subclinical level: internet addiction symptoms, social media use, geek behaviour, and nomophobia.

Internet addiction symptoms express the users' urge to continue being connected despite the desire to stop, experiencing unpleasant emotions when they do not succeed. Adolescents, who perceive the constant need to be online, usually present an increased use of social networking sites and the internet. In extreme cases, such behaviour may produce psychological problems that traditionally correspond to substance-related addictions [2]. Addiction symptoms would include sleep disturbance, angry or agitated reaction when forced to disconnect, and loosing track of time while online [6]. Personal characteristics such as gender and age appear to play an essential role in internet addiction [7], however, the results are not conclusive. On the one hand, recent studies report that girls experience higher amount of internet addiction symptoms than boys [4,8,9]. On the other hand, some other studies reveal that boys are more susceptible to addictive online behaviour than girls [10]. With regard to age difference, the results are also inconclusive. On the one hand, some studies report a progressive increase in addiction to the internet with age, enhancing also the negative consequences [11], while other studies report a progressive decrease [12]. On the other hand, there are studies that do not observe any age differences at all [9]. Hence, research investigating the influence of gender and age on internet addiction during adolescence seems warranted.

The aspect of social media use refers to a virtual way of relating with peers, reducing face-to-face interaction. Social networking sites have become a new environment of group socialization for adolescents. Such virtual environments enable the users to create public profiles in an interactive space where they communicate with friends but also with strangers, people they never have contact with outside the network [13]. Excessive use of social networking sites, however, can have negative implications such as negative mood states, concentration problems, and less interest in spending time with friends and family [14]. In relation to gender, it appears that women tend to use smartphones primarily for communication and social media such as Instagram and Facebook [15,16]. On the contrary, other studies have reported that boys are more likely to present problematic social media use than girls [17]. With regard to age difference, studies reveal that the risk and frequency of addictive use of social networking sites decrease as age increases [18].

Geek behaviour refers to a certain habit, which is commonly ascribed to an intense level of interest in the technological field. The term *geek* is widely used among young people in the digital era that is why there is still little literature about the phenomenon. In this study, the term geek behaviour refers to the quality of young people who are passionate about information and communication technologies (ICT), including online social networking. In addition, they usually prefer interacting with their peers through the internet, given the easy access to websites where you can make friends online or look for an online date [19]. Three characteristics have been identified: relating through online games, searching for similar interest groups and/or online eroticism [20]. With regard to gender, research consistently shows that boys engage more frequently in compulsive gaming and gambling [15,21]. Although boys show typically more geek behaviour, some studies have evidenced such behaviour is increasing among girls, too [22]. Furthermore, research stresses that being an adolescent is a well-established risk factor for internet gaming addiction [23].

Nomophobia is conceptualized as the intense fear of being disconnected from smartphone communication on a nonclinical level [24]. Messaging apps have increased nomophobia, especially in teenagers, the age group most affected by this problem. Currently, the accelerating development of smartphones devices and the fact that they are easy to carry around all the time, means that mobile phones are replacing the internet as a primary addictive source [25]. In relation to gender, studies suggest that girls use their smartphones more often than boys and that their use is, therefore, more problematic [16]. Hence, addictive behaviour in boys is associated with gaming apps, while in girls smartphone use is more related to online communication and social interaction [15]. With regard to age, adolescents have been targeted as a group at risk for smartphone addiction [26] and a recent meta-analysis suggests that one in four adolescents presents problematic smartphone use [27].

Social cognitive theory recognizes "personal factors" as potential predictors of internet addiction disorder and nomophobia, considering gender, age, ethnicity or beliefs as the most relevant. However, the contribution of other psychological factors such as self-esteem and personality traits should be considered in order to better understand of such risk behaviour online.

1.2. Body Self-Esteem and the Relationship with Problematic Social Media and Internet Use

Body self-esteem is another psychological variables that has been positively associated with the social networking addiction [28]. The internet is the virtual mirror of the current body image by exposing a manipulated online version with an increased physical and erotic appeal [29]. Frequent social media users have greater body dissatisfaction because they have internalized the model of a thin and long-legged body [30]. On the one hand, physical attractiveness -the emotional dimension of body self-esteem- may correlate positively with social networking and internet addiction [31], while body satisfaction -the cognitive dimension of body self-esteem- may correlate negatively. Recent studies reveal that adolescents who are dissatisfied with their bodies tend to selectively disclose their very positive and attractive features (e.g., their most attractive photographs). Such behaviour may work as a self-preservation strategy that helps to restore their self-confidence and receive positive feedback from their peers, which in turn generates positive feelings about themselves [32]. These idealized self-preservation motivations are positively associated with social networking addiction [33].

On the other hand, body satisfaction seems to be related to social desirability, thus, peers play a decisive role in the matter of public online appearance. Peris et al. [34] reported that an increasing number of adolescents edit their pictures before posting them on social networking sites to improve their image according to how they wish to see themselves and be seen by others. Following this line of research, studies indicate a negative association between adolescent body satisfaction and the use of social networking sites. According to Liu et al. [35], adolescents who are unsatisfied with their body, experience low self-esteem in real life and, therefore, more often seek positive responses through social media. In turn, positive responses from online social interactions may reinforce young people's use of smartphones, enhancing the risk of developing smartphone addiction. If adolescents would receive more positive responses and support in real life, they might refrain from frequent online interactions, even if they have low body satisfaction.

1.3. Personality Traits and the Association with Social Networking and Internet Addiction

In addition to self-esteem, personality has an important bearing on explaining individual differences in problematic internet use [33,36]. One of the most studied personality dimension related to internet addiction is extraversion, which refers to people's varying tendency to be friendly, sociable, and talk active. Studies suggest that there is a positive relationship between being extroverted and an increased risk of internet addiction [37]. Regarding the internet and social media use, they are both strongly and positively related to extraversion [38]. Extraverted individuals use social networking apps to engage in social interaction and they may attain more social resources online. In relation to the geek behaviour, Dieris-Hirche et al. [39] reported that gamers with a problematic internet use scored lower on extraversion and higher on neuroticism than those with non-problematic behaviour. Furthermore, as smartphones allow for the permanent connection demanded by extroverted people, extraversion has been identified as a predictor variable of problematic smartphone use [40]. However, some recent studies did not confirm such relationship [41]. These discrepancies may suggest the importance of a differential conceptualization of social networking and internet addiction in relation to different kinds of risk behaviour.

Another main personality factor is neuroticism, which refers to individual differences in emotional stability and psychological adjustment. Neuroticism has been shown a positive association with problematic internet use [42]. Studies suggest that introverted adolescents show increased online activity when compared with emotionally stable users, which may enhance the risk for internet addiction [27]. Regarding the social aspect of internet use, neurotic adolescents tend to show a more passive behaviour on social networking sites such as posting comments and Likes on other people's profiles, which may represent a way to seek social relationships [33,36,43]. This association can be interpreted in terms of their difficulties to pursue social relationships in real life and poor coping skills with emotional situations [42]. Research on the relationship between neuroticism and geek behaviour is limited. Furthermore, neurotics tend to show an increased or problematic use of online games [39]. With regard to nomophobia, neuroticism appears to predict obsessive smartphone use [44].

Besides extraversion and neuroticism, disinhibition is an other relevant personality domain, which is associated with increased internet addiction symptoms [45]. Research indicates that problematic internet and social media use is linked to different aspects of disinhibited behaviour such as poor self-control, impulsivity and sensation seeking. Disinhibited personality is common among teenagers, but usually decreases with age from adolescence to adulthood, supporting the hypothesis of normative psychological maturation. Apparently, for disinhibited adolescents the internet may represent a useful tool for satisfying their elevated urge of sensation seeking [45] by allowing relief from unpleasant feelings through quick online behaviour without thinking much of the consequences (e.g., by quickly engaging in anonymous virtual relationships) [31]. In view of the relevance of this personality domain related to addictive internet behaviour, it appears negligent that only few studies have included disinhibition as a potential predictor of social networking and internet addiction.

Moreover, narcissism has been related to problematic internet use in adolescence [46]. Narcissism may be understood as a dynamic self-regulation system related to grandiosity, self-absorption and a constant need for external approval. There is evidence to suggest that higher levels of narcissism are linked to an increased risk of social networking and internet addiction [28,37]. Social media use appear to fulfil two basic social needs that may explain the problematic internet use in young people with narcissistic personality: the need for self-presentations through social online profiles featured by pictures, status updates, personal notes, etc.; and the need to belong to a social group seeking repeated approval from their peers [47]. Furthermore, narcissistic teenagers tend to use social media such as Facebook more often because such platforms enable users to create visible profiles, that allow idealized self-promotion in a virtual environment [37]. In addition to problematic social media use, narcissism is strongly associated with smartphone addiction [48].

1.4. Rationale for the Study

Drawing from previous studies, there are psychological risk factors of significant relevance during adolescence such as gender and age, body self-esteem and personality traits, including extraversion, neuroticism, disinhibition and narcissism that predict internet-related addictions [16,21,31,37]. Most studies use a very limited conceptualization of social networking and internet addiction rather than broadening their view and focus on specific addictive behaviours (e.g., [5,45]). To our knowledge, there are no studies that have investigated the combined effects of body self-esteem and personality traits in order to determine different types of risk behaviour regarding the social networking and internet addiction in nonclinical adolescents, involving internet addiction symptoms, social media use, geek behaviour, and nomophobia. Additionally, the role of demographic factors such as gender and age have been extensively studied in relation to adolescent problematic internet use, however with mixed findings [8–10,16]. In addition, most research on social networking and internet addiction has used methodology based on linear regression models (e.g., [1,49]). These models are focused on the individual prediction and do not consider the possibility of different pathways that would lead to the same result [50,51]. In contrast, fuzzy-set qualitative comparative analysis (fsQCA) is a methodology that allows a more in-depth analysis of how a set of causal conditions contribute to a hypothesised outcome [52,53]. QCA is based on the assumption that such outcome depends on a combination of different factors rather than on individual levels of those factors [54,55]. In the field of psychological research, limited studies have used this technique despite it's considerable potential [56].

1.5. Purpose of the Study

The present study aimed to estimate the combined contribution of body self-esteem (body satisfaction and physical attractiveness), personality traits (extraversion, neuroticism, disinhibition and narcissism), and demographic factors (gender and age) in the prediction of four types of adolescent's social networking and internet addiction (internet addiction symptoms, social media use, geek behaviour, and nomophobia). Based on the reviewed research, we hypothesized as follows (1) the primary risk factors that predict internet addiction symptoms will be gender and age (girls of older age), low body satisfaction, and high levels of physical attractiveness, neuroticism, extraversion, disinhibition and narcissism; (2) the potential risk factor of social media use will be gender and age (girls of younger age), low body satisfaction, but high levels of physical attractiveness, neuroticism, extraversion, disinhibition and narcissism; (3) the significant risk factors that predict geek behaviour will be gender (boys), low body satisfaction and extraversion, but high physical attractiveness neuroticism, disinhibition and narcissism; and (4) the main risk factors of nomophobia will be gender (girls), low body satisfaction, but high levels of physical attractiveness, neuroticism, extraversion, disinhibition and narcissism.

2. Materials and Methods

2.1. Participants

The present research involved 447 adolescents aged 13−16 years ($M = 14.90$, $SD = 0.81$). The gender distribution of the sample was equitable (women: $n = 251$; 56.2%). The participants were students from public ($n = 201$; 45%) and private ($n = 246$; 55%) high schools in the Northern Regions of Spain. The following inclusion criteria applied: (a) school board gave their permission to collaborate with the research group; (b) students were not older than 16 years; (c) parents or guardians were asked to sign a written consent to allow adolescents' participation in the research. The simple random probability sampling method has been employed.

2.2. Variables and Instruments

2.2.1. Demographic Variables

Personal data referring to the students' gender, age and high school were collected administrating an ad hoc questionnaire.

2.2.2. Social Networking and Internet Addiction

The social networking and internet addiction was assessed using the Scale of risk of addiction to social media and the internet for adolescents (ERA-RSI) [6]. The scale is composed of 29 items divided into four subscales: internet addiction symptoms, social media use, geek behaviour, and nomophobia. The internet addiction symptoms subscale assesses behaviours of addiction to non-toxic substances (e.g., "I have been losing sleep over social media and watching online shows"; 9 items). The social media use subscale assesses adolescent "online socialization" behaviours (e.g., "I check my friends' profiles"; 8 items). The geek behaviour subscale includes aspects such as joining special interest groups, playing online and role-playing games or having sexual encounters (e.g., "I spend time on social media and the Internet to play online and/or role-playing games"; 6 items). The nomophobia subscale is related to feelings of anxiety and control when using a mobile phone (e.g., "I have a smartphone and I start feeling anxious or distressed when people don't answer immediately to my messages"; 6 items). Participants were asked to rate the items on a 4-point Likert scale (1 = *never or hardly never*; 4 = *many times or almost always*). The reliability indexes were adequate in this sample for the global scale of addiction ($\alpha = 0.90$) and all subscales: internet addiction symptoms ($\alpha = 0.84$), social media use ($\alpha = 0.83$), geek behaviour ($\alpha = 0.69$), nomophobia ($\alpha = 0.80$).

2.2.3. Body Self-Esteem

The body self-esteem was measured with the Body Self-esteem Scale (BSS) [57]. This scale is composed of 26 items and participants evaluate the degree of satisfaction with each part of their body. The first 20 assess body satisfaction, the cognitive dimension of body self-esteem, and are grouped into four body areas: face (e.g., "Are you satisfied with your eyes/mouth?"), upper torso (e.g., "Are you satisfied with your breasts/pectorals?"), lower torso (e.g., "Are you satisfied with your butt?"); and anthropometry (e.g., "Are you satisfied with your height/size?"). The score ranges on a 10-point Likert scale (1 = *very dissatisfied*, 10 = *very satisfied*). Physical attractiveness, the emotional dimension of body self-esteem, is assessed through 6 items and six aspects are evaluated: physically interesting, socially charming, sexy, attractive, sensual and erotic (e.g., "To what extent do you consider yourself a physically attractive person?"). The score ranges on a 10-point Likert scale (1 = *not attractive at all*, 10 = *very attractive*). This scale shows good psychometric properties in the studied sample (Body satisfaction $\alpha = 0.93$; Physical attractiveness $\alpha = 0.93$; Body Self-esteem $\alpha = 0.95$).

2.2.4. Personality Factors

The extraversion and neuroticism dimensions were assessed using NEO Five Factory inventory (NEO-FFI) [58], the brief version of NEO-PI-R. The scale is composed of 60 items distributed equally on five factors (12 items in each factor). Two subscales have been used in the present study: neuroticism (e.g., "I am quite emotionally stable"–inversed item) and extraversion (e.g., "I like having a lot of people around me"). They were chosen for two reasons. First, they are the ones that accumulate the most research with regard to social media and internet use, and second, because it was necessary to reduce the application time due to the fatigue and tiredness. The scale uses a 5-point Likert scale (0 = *strongly disagree*; 4 = *strongly agree*). Both factors have shown suitable reliability in this sample (extraversion: $\alpha = 0.81$; neuroticism: $\alpha = 0.79$).

The disinhibition was evaluated using the Sensation Seeking Scale (SSS-Q) [59], Spanish adaptation [60]. The scale is composed of 40 items, which give rise to 4 subscales (10 items each). We selected the subscale of disinhibition for the aim of our study, given that its content is most relevant for risk behaviour and addiction. The participants provide information about their own disinhibition behaviours (e.g., "I like wild parties without limits"). The adolescents can answer the items *affirmatively* (1) or *negatively* (0). The scale has shown good reliability in this sample ($\alpha = 0.64$).

The narcissism was evaluated using the Narcissistic Personality Inventory (NPI) [61], Spanish adaptation (NP-15) [62]. The scale is composed of 15 items and the narcissism includes facets such as a need for recognition, an exalted and distorted image or a feeling of special status (e.g., "It's very important that others pay attention to me and admire what I do"). The scale uses a 6-point Likert scale (1 = *absolutely false*; 6 = *absolutely true*). The scale has shown adequate reliability in this sample ($\alpha = 0.81$).

2.3. Procedure

The present research was approved by the Ethics Commission for Research with Human Beings (CEISH) of the University of the Basque Country Euskal Herriko Unibersitatea (UPV/EHU), with the registration number CEISH/136/2012/PERIS HERNANDEZ. The declaration of the file was in the Basque Agency of Data Protection with the registration number 2080310015-INA0004. The study applied the ethical principles of the Declaration of Helsinki, the requirements established by the Ethics Commission for Human Research of the University of the Basque Country (UPV) and the State Government, as well as the deontological regulations of the Official College of Psychologists for experimentation on human beings.

First, the headmasters and psychologists of each school were contacted and information about the study and a copy of the research project were provided. Once they accepted to participate, the parents of the adolescents were contacted. An information letter and informed consent was sent to their homes. The informed consent was signed and returned to the school by the adolescent's parents or legal guardians in order to participate. The adolescents were informed about the questionnaires and confidentiality, and they signed the informed consent. The data collection took place in the school classrooms during the tutorial hour. The questionnaires were administered by evaluators with a Degree in Psychology and lasted approximately 40 min.

2.4. Data Analysis

Firstly, descriptive analysis followed by bivariate correlations and linear regression analyses were conducted using the statistical package IBM SPSS V.25 for Windows (IBM Corporation, Foster City, CA, USA). A three-stage hierarchical multiple regression analyses was performed to examine the predictive power of demographic variables (age and gender), body self-esteem (body satisfaction and physical attractiveness), and personality factors (neuroticism, extraversion, disinhibition and narcissism) on social networking and internet addiction. A total of four regression models were carried out, one for each dimension of addiction and predictors were entered in three stages: (a) Gender and age, (b) body self-esteem and (c) personality factors.

Secondly, we performed fuzzy-set qualitative comparative analysis (fsQCA) using the Fs/QCA 3.0 software (University of California, Irvine, CA, USA). Prior to conducting the analysis, we estimated the calibration scores, transformed raw data responses into fuzzy-set responses, and removed missing data. In order to obtain the constructs (variables) and increase the variability, the items of each scale were multiplied [63]. Following the multiplication of the items, the extraversion and neuroticism scales were divided by one hundred to avoid excessively large numbers that the program could not handle. The rest of the variables remained undivided. In addition, each variable was then recalibrated in three categories: percentile 10 (low levels or condition is absent), percentile 50 (intermediate level, condition is neither absent nor present) and percentile 90 (high levels or condition is present) [64]. All scores must range between 0 and 1. Thus, gender and age scores were calibrated manually. Age scores were coded according at four points equidistant between 0 and 1, gender scores were recoded with 0 for boys and 1 for girls. We conducted descriptive analyses with the transformed scores. Finally, necessary and sufficient conditions analyses estimated the combined influence of the demographic variables, body self-esteem and personality factors on high levels of internet addiction symptoms, social media use, geek behaviour and nomophobia. There is no theoretical number of combinations that produces the outcome.

3. Results

3.1. Descriptive Analysis and Relationships Between Variables Studied

Descriptive statistics (means and standard deviations) and correlations between the study variables are displayed in Table 1. Results indicated that age was significantly and in a negative way related to social media use, nomophobia, neuroticism and extraversion, while the associations with disinhibition and narcissism are positive. In general, personality was positively and significant related to social networking and internet addiction. Specifically, disinhibition was associated with the four dimensions of addiction; neuroticism and extraversion were related to internet addiction symptoms, social media use and nomophobia, but not with geek behaviour; and there were a positive association between narcissism and internet addiction symptoms, geek behaviour and nomophobia, but there are not with social media use. With regard to body self-esteem, physical attractiveness was significantly and positively correlated with the four dimensions of addiction to the internet and online social networking, whereas body satisfaction only correlated to internet addiction symptoms and the relationship was negative. As regards the relationship between personality and self-esteem, neuroticism was negatively and significant related to body satisfaction and attraction, whereas extraversion, disinhibition and narcissism were related positively, although there was not relationship between disinhibition and body satisfaction.

Table 1. Bivariate correlations between all variables studied.

	1	2	3	4	5	6	7	8	9	10	11
1. Age	–										
2. IAS	−0.07	–									
3. SMU	−0.17 ***	0.56 ***	–								
4. GB	−0.02	0.29 ***	0.30 ***	–							
5. NP	−0.16 **	0.61 ***	0.55 ***	0.32 ***	–						
6. NT	−0.12 *	0.36 ***	0.29 ***	0.03	0.25 ***	–					
7. EX	−0.11 *	0.12 ***	0.20 ***	0.04	0.09 ***	−0.19 ***	–				
8. DI	0.16 ***	0.40 ***	0.23 ***	0.16 ***	0.23 ***	0.12 **	0.20 ***	–			
9. NA	0.11 *	0.21 ***	0.02	0.18 ***	0.18 ***	0.06	−0.11 *	0.20 ***	–		
10. BS	−0.01	−0.15 ***	−0.02	0.06	−0.03	−0.32 ***	0.20 ***	−0.03	0.10 *	–	
11. PA	0.06	0.13 **	0.11 **	0.15 ***	0.13 **	−0.20 ***	0.25 ***	0.22 ***	0.26 ***	0.66 ***	–
M	14.90	19.05	21.17	9.31	12.62	32.89	46.27	14.73	40.45	6.58	6.18
SD	0.81	5.77	4.86	2.77	4.21	7.31	6.33	2.13	10.13	1.32	1.67

Note. IAS = Internet addiction symptoms. SMU = Social media use. GB = Geek behaviour. NP = Nomophobia. NT = Neuroticism. EX = Extraversion. DI = Disinhibition. NA = Narcissism. BS = Body satisfaction. PA = Physical attractiveness. M = mean. SD = standard deviation. * $p \leq 0.05$. ** $p \leq 0.01$. *** $p \leq 0.001$.

3.2. Demographic and Psychological Predictors of Social Networking and Internet Addiction

Predictive analysis of social networking and internet addiction was conducted with a three-step hierarchical multiple regressions (Table 2).

Regarding the first prediction model, three sets of variables were established, which explained 37% of the variance of adolescents' internet addiction symptoms. In the first step, which included demographic variables, specifically gender and age, explained 9% of the variance. The second next step, which included two dimensions of body self-esteem, accounted for an additional 10% of explained variance. The third and final step included the four dimensions of personality explained an additional 19% of variance. The final regression model indicates that gender, body satisfaction, physical attractiveness, neuroticism, extraversion, disinhibition and narcissism are significant predictors of emotional symptoms.

The second prediction model consisted of three sets of variables, which explained 35% of the variance of social media use. In the first step, gender and age were included and together they explained 23% of the variance. In the second step, the two dimensions of body self-esteem were entered and accounted for a significant increase of 5% of the variance. In the final step, the four personality dimensions were included, which accounted for an additional 10% of variance. In this final model, gender, age, physical attractiveness, neuroticism, extraversion, and disinhibition significantly predicted social media use.

With regard to the third prediction model, the overall regression model was significant but only explained 5% of geek behaviour. Following the same *modus operandi*, demographic variables were included in step 1 explaining 1% of the variance, followed by both dimensions of body self-esteem in step 2 increasing the explained variance by 3% and finally all personality four dimensions were entered in step accounting for an additional 3% of the variance. The resulting model suggested that only disinhibition and narcissism significantly predict geek behaviour.

The forth the prediction model was established in three steps and explained 21% of the variance of nomophobia. Firstly, gender and age were entered in the first step and explained 8% of the variance. Secondly, body satisfaction and physical attractiveness were included in the second step elevating the explained variance by 8%. Thirdly, neuroticism, extraversion, disinhibition and narcissism were added in the third step and together explained an additional 9 % of the variance. In this overall model, gender, age, physical attractiveness, neuroticism, disinhibition and narcissism significantly predicted nomophobia.

Table 2. Results of hierarchical multiple regression analyses.

Variable	Internet Addiction Symptoms				Social Media Use				Geek Behaviour				Nomophobia			
	ΔR^2	ΔF	β	t	ΔR^2	ΔF	β	t	ΔR^2	ΔF	β	t	ΔR^2	ΔF	β	t
Step 1	0.09	21.93 ***			0.23	64.84 ***			0.01	1.62			0.08	20.43 ***		
Gender			0.27	6.50 ***			0.45	10.67 ***			−0.06	−1.08			0.26	5.51 ***
Age			−0.06	−1.45			−0.08	−2.07 *			−0.07	−1.34			−0.14	−3.12 **
Step 2	0.10	28.34 ***			0.05	12.47 ***			0.03	5.77 **			0.05	13.08 ***		
Body satisfaction			−0.18	−3.34 ***			0.04	0.76			−0.04	−0.54			−0.05	−0.87
Physical attractiveness			0.21	3.89 ***			0.11	1.99 *			0.12	1.76			0.16	2.59 **
Step 3	0.19	33.64 ***			0.10	16.51 ***			0.03	3.52 **			0.09	12.66 ***		
Neuroticism			0.23	5.44 ***			0.18	4.16 ***			0.03	0.59			0.15	3.20 ***
Extraversion			0.09	2.11 *			0.15	3.44 ***			0.01	0.18			0.05	1.15
Disinhibition			0.30	7.06 ***			0.20	4.63 ***			0.10	2.02 *			0.17	3.56 ***
Narcissism			0.16	3.93 ***			0.04	1.00			0.13	2.57 *			0.17	3.68 ***
Durbin-Watson		1.27				1.26				1.61				1.33		
R^2		0.37 ***				0.35 ***				0.05 **				0.21 ***		

Note. ΔR^2 = change in R^2; ΔF = change in F; ß = regression coefficient; t = value of t-test statistic; * $p \leq 0.05$. ** $p \leq 0.01$. *** $p \leq 0.001$.

3.3. Combined Contribution of Body Self-Esteem, Personality Traits and Personal Predictors of Social Networking and Internet Addiction

The descriptive statistics of the variables under study and the calibration values were calculated first (Table 3). The dimensions of social networking and internet addiction based on personality, body self-esteem and personal factors were then examined by fuzzy-set QCA. The necessary and sufficient conditions were estimated. On the one hand, the analysis of necessary conditions or variables allows us to determine whether there are any variables that are always required to be present for the prediction of the outcome (in our study, high levels of addiction). For a condition/variable to be necessary, the consistency score must be above 0.90 [51]. The results showed that none of the variables studied have to be considered necessary condition because their consistencies scores were all below 0.90. On the other hand, the sufficient conditions refer to those variables that predict the outcome, but the prediction may be possible without them. All logically possible combinations of the causal conditions are captures in the truth table together with the result of each setting [50]. The analysis provides three types of solutions: a parsimonious one (less restrictive), an intermediate one and a complex one (most restrictive). The literature recommends, therefore, focusing on the intermediate solution [51], which is presented in this study.

Table 3. Descriptive statistics and calibration scores.

	IAS	SMU	GB	NP	NT	EX	DI	NA	BS	PA
Mean	5164.83	6055.23	32.66	181.55	13,973.16	210,162.93	69.35	746,999.25	2261.04	113609.19
Standard deviation	19,216.76	10,541.97	93.71	328.93	54,894.57	336,946.74	112.60	4,809,591.82	1705.54	156,534.70
Minimum	1.00	1.00	1.00	1.00	0.01	0.25	1.00	0.02	21.96	1.00
Maximum	262,144.00	65,536.00	972.00	2304.00	703,125.00	2,441,406.25	1024.00	84,375,000.00	10,000.00	1,000,000.00
Calibration scores										
10	5.60	70.40	1.00	1.00	11.52	6635.52	4.00	6.48	439.84	1896.00
Percentile 50	384.00	1944.00	6.00	48.00	518.40	78,643.20	32.00	2764.80	1837.68	63,504.00
90	10,368.00	15,552.00	72.00	524.80	22,413.31	562,500.00	128.00	813,957.12	4724.43	290,304.00

Note. IAS = Internet addiction symptoms. SMU = Social media use. GB = Geek behaviour. NP = Nomophobia. NT = Neuroticism. EX = Extraversion. DI = Disinhibition. NA = Narcissism. BS = Body satisfaction. PA = Physical attractiveness.

In the social networking and internet addiction, the combination of conditions resulting in high levels of internet addiction symptoms, social media use, geek behaviour and nomophobia were analysed (Table 4). The solutions were found to be adequate, considering that a fsQCA model is acceptable when consistency is above 0.70 [50]. The main three pathways for high levels of all four dimensions of social networking and internet addiction are shown in Table 4.

The solution showed eight pathways, which explained 46% of high levels of internet addiction symptoms. The first pathway was the result of the combined contribution of a high gender score (girl), high age, high disinhibition and high narcissism. The second pathway to predict high levels of internet addiction symptoms was the combined contribution of a high gender score (girl), high neuroticism, high extraversion and high disinhibition and the third was the result of the interaction of a high gender score (girl), high neuroticism, high extraversion, high disinhibition and high narcissism.

The solution showed 12 pathways, which explained 56% of high levels of social media use. The first pathway was the result of the combined contribution of high gender score (girl), high neuroticism and high physical attractiveness. The second pathway was the combined contribution of high gender score (girl), low neuroticism and high disinhibition. The third pathway was the result of the interaction of a high gender score (girl), high age, high extraversion and high physical attractiveness.

The solution showed eight pathways, which explained 33% of high levels of geek behaviour. The first combination was the result of the interaction of a high gender score (girl), high age, high neuroticism, high extraversion, high disinhibition and high narcissism. The second pathway was the result of the combined contribution of high gender score (girl), high age, high neuroticism, high extraversion, high narcissism, high body satisfaction and high physical attractiveness, and the third pathway was the result of the interaction of a low gender score (boy), high neuroticism, high narcissism and low physical attractiveness.

Table 4. Three main pathways for the high levels of social networking and internet addiction.

Frequency Cutoff: 1	High Internet Addiction Symptoms			High Social Media Use			High Geek Behaviour			High Nomophobia		
	Consistency Cutoff: 0.90			Consistency Cutoff: 0.90			Consistency Cutoff: 0.90			Consistency Cutoff: 0.90		
	1	2	3	1	2	3	1	2	3	1	2	3
Gender	●	●	●	●	●	●	●	●	○	●		
Age	●					●	●	●				○
Body satisfaction								●			○	○
Physical attractiveness				●		●		●	○	●		
Neuroticism		●	●	●	○		●	●	●		●	●
Extraversion		●				●	●	●		●	●	
Disinhibition	●	●	●		●		●				●	●
Narcissism	●		●				●	●	●	●	●	●
Raw Coverage	0.24	0.23	0.23	0.29	0.28	0.26	0.13	0.12	0.12	0.21	0.17	0.17
Unique Coverage	0.012	0.044	0.010	0.017	0.020	0.004	0.026	0.015	0.008	0.042	0.028	0.016
Consistency	0.88	0.90	0.91	0.91	0.88	0.91	0.89	0.89	0.89	0.85	0.94	0.90
Overall Solution Coverage			0.46			0.56			0.33			0.41
Overall Solution Consistency			0.86			0.83			0.85			0.85

Note. ● = presence of condition/high levels, ○ = absence of condition/low levels. Gender: ● = girls; ○ = boys. All sufficient conditions are adequate.

Finally, the solution showed 11 pathways, which explained 41% of high levels of nomophobia. The first pathway was the result of the interaction of a high gender score (girl), high extraversion and high narcissism. The second pathway was the result of the interaction of a high neuroticism, high extraversion, high disinhibition, high narcissism, low body satisfaction and high physical attractiveness. The third pathway predicting a high nomophobia was the result of the combined contribution of a low age, high neuroticism, high disinhibition, high narcissism and low body satisfaction.

The solution showed 12 pathways which explained 56% of high levels of social media use. The first pathway was the result of the combined contribution of high gender score (girl), high neuroticism and high physical attractiveness. The second pathway was the combined contribution of high gender score (girl), low neuroticism and high disinhibition. The third pathway was the result of the interaction of a high gender score (girl), high age, high extraversion and high physical attractiveness.

The solution showed eight pathways which explained 33% of high levels of geek behaviour. The first combination was the result of the interaction of a high gender score (girl), high age, high neuroticism, high extraversion, high disinhibition and high narcissism. The second pathway was the result of the combined contribution of high gender score (girl), high age, high neuroticism, high extraversion, high narcissism, high body satisfaction and high physical attractiveness, and the third pathway was the result of the interaction of a low gender score (boy), high neuroticism, high narcissism and low physical attractiveness.

Finally, the solution showed 11 pathways which explained 41% of high levels of nomophobia. The first pathway was the result of the interaction of a high gender score (girl), high extraversion and high narcissism. The second pathway was the result of the interaction of a high neuroticism, high extraversion, high disinhibition, high narcissism, low body satisfaction and high physical attractiveness. The third pathway predicting a high nomophobia was the result of the combined contribution of a low age, high neuroticism, high disinhibition, high narcissism and low body satisfaction.

4. Discussion

Although research on social networking and internet addiction is on the rise, a vast majority of investigations have conceptualized internet addictive as a one-dimensional construct, focusing on problematic or compulsive use rather than specific risk behaviour. We aimed to estimate the combined contribution of body self-esteem (body satisfaction and physical attractiveness), personality traits (extraversion, neuroticism, disinhibition and narcissism), and personal factors (gender and age) in the prediction of four types of adolescents' social networking and internet addiction, involving internet addiction symptoms, social media use, geek behaviour, and nomophobia. Several studies have investigated the relations between addiction to the internet and social networking and several of the variables included within this study [65]; however, the addiction literature using a novel methodological approach by comparing linear regression models with fsQCA models in the prediction of adolescents' internet addiction is sparse. Thus, this study makes an innovative contribution to the addiction literate by evaluating a more comprehensive model of addiction to internet and social media, examine different pathways of variables representing important biologically based personality traits, variables of body self-esteem, which are of special relevance during adolescence and taking into account gender and age differences. The findings extend our understanding of the psychological risk factors of social networking and internet addiction among nonclinical adolescents.

4.1. Risk Factors of Addiction Symptoms

The first hypothesis has been supported by the results from the hierarchical regression and fsQCA models, which showed a significant influence of gender, body self-esteem and personality traits on internet addiction symptoms. Both methodologies match the result that gender and disinhibition were the most relevant predictors of internet addiction symptoms. The regression model suggests that adolescents, more girls than boys, who are more disinhibited, neurotic, narcissistic and extraverted, and experience lower body satisfaction but higher physical attractiveness, present more internet addiction symptoms. The results from fsQCA suggested that the combination of gender (being a girl) and high levels of disinhibition were the most significant predictors of internet addiction symptoms. The two latter in combination with high levels of narcissism, neuroticism and extraversion also predicted an increase in internet addiction symptoms, but to a lesser extent. In contrast to the regression models, results from QCA suggests that body self-esteem does not seem to be an important predictor of internet addiction symptoms, since they have not been included in the three most significant pathways. These findings are in line with recent research, indicating that girls tend to present more addiction symptoms in comparison with boys [8,16]. However, these results are inconsistent with other studies that suggest that boys are more likely to show addictive internet behavior [10]. Evidentially, boys and girls may be at risk of potential internet addiction, but probably for different reasons. While girls are usually more interested in the social interactions over the internet, boys, contrarily, use the internet primarily for online gaming [3]. Furthermore, disinhibition has been the primary psychological risk factor for adolescents' internet addiction symptoms in our study, highlighting the role of impulsive behaviour as a manifestation of poor self-regulating skills in relation to problematic internet use during adolescence [45]. In general, personality factors appear to be more important than body self-esteem in the prediction of internet addiction, matching research finding that have pointed out the important of personality traits in explaining individual differences in symptoms of internet addiction [33,36].

4.2. Risk Factors of Social Media Use

Overall, the second hypothesis is also supported by the results obtained in our study, suggesting that the combination of demographic and psychological variables influence adolescents' problematic social media use. Both regression and QCA models indicate that gender combined with physical attractiveness seem to be the most relevant predictors of social media use. On the one hand, results from the hierarchical regression models revealed that girls more than boys, younger adolescents more than the older ones, with a physically attractive body image and a disinhibited, neurotic and extraverted personality, tend to use social media more often. On the other hand, fsQCA models suggest that there are different pathways to predict the problematic social media use. One of the main pathways shows that girls with higher physical attractiveness in combination with higher neuroticism report more excessive social media use. Another pathway suggests that girls with high levels of disinhibition in combination with low levels of neuroticism also show increased social internet use. A third pathway combines girls of older age with high physical attractiveness and high extraversion, in the prediction of addictive use of social networking sites. These differences may suggest that the combination of personality factors and body self-esteem may vary producing different patterns of risk behaviour. Stressing the role of neuroticism is critical, given that both high and low levels of emotional stability in combination with other psychological risk factors predict social media use. Our findings are relatively conforming with previous studies, which have provided hard evidence that girls use social media more often than boys [8,15]. In a recent study, Escario and Wilkinson (2020) [21] have provided evidence that men and women relate differently to the internet. For instance, while women tend to participate more in social activities, using chat rooms, sending e-mails and visiting social networking sites such as Facebook or Instagram, men spend more time on online games, online gambling, and visit pornographic sites more frequently. Our findings also corroborate previous studies that have reported a positive relationship between adolescents' body image and the use of social media [31]. In fact, teenage girls feel more pressured to present themselves with an idealized physical attractiveness by editing their self-portraits before sharing them in social media, which in turn generates positive feelings by receiving increased external approval, hence, higher risk of social networking addiction [2,7]. With regard to personality factors, our findings were consistent with previous studies, showing that disinhibition, neuroticism and extraversion were positively associated with addictive use of social networking sites [42,45].

4.3. Risk Factors of Geek Behaviour

Additionally, the third hypothesis has been supported by our results in terms of adolescents' geek behaviour, however the predictive capacity of demographic and psychological factors is lower than for the other types, irrespective of the methodology used. The personality factors narcissism and neuroticism appear to be the most relevant predictor of geek behaviour. The results from regression models indicate that high levels of narcissism and disinhibition predict geek behaviour, explaining only a small amount of variance. In fsQCA analysis, the model included more factors than in the other models in order to improve the prediction outcome, producing pathways with many different combinations of variables. For instance, the main pathway suggests that girls of older age with high levels of narcissism, neuroticism, extraversion and disinhibition tend to be geekier. Furthermore, the second pathway shows that girls of older age, who are neurotic, extraverted and narcissistic and experience higher levels of body satisfaction and physical attractiveness, also present more geek behaviour. Lastly, the third pathway indicates that boys with high levels of narcissism and neuroticism combined with an unattractive body image also predict greater geek behaviour. Both boys and girls, especially the older ones, appear to score high on geek behaviour, depending on the combination of several psychological risk factors. In fact, a single dimension of personality traits or body self-esteem is not sufficient in order to explain the individual difference in this type of internet addiction. These unexpected results are, however, compatible with some previous research, which suggests that both boys and girls may present geek behaviour [8]. Traditionally, geek behaviour related to excessive online gaming and gambling has been related to the male gender [15,21,65]. However, girls seem also to be at risk of such behaviour especially related to online eroticism, which is a novel insight regarding current literature. Another important finding of this study is that narcissism and neuroticism are the main predictors of geek behaviour. There is some evidence, that neurotic and introverted adolescents show increased online gaming behaviour [39]. Nevertheless, the role of narcissism in the prediction of geek behaviour has not been established in prior research, thus, our findings may give rise to a new line of research. The strong link between narcissism and geek behaviour may be explained by the "compensatory perspective", which suggest that online gaming might fulfil a compensatory purpose for narcissistic individuals with emotional dysregulation [66]. Regarding the role of body self-esteem, our results are less conclusive. Previous research have associated gamers' body dissatisfaction or negative body attitudes with the exposure to ideal video game bodies [67].

4.4. Risk Factors of Nomophobia

With regard to nomophobia, the results of this study confirm the forth hypothesis, demonstrating a significant impact of demographic factors, body self-esteem and personality traits. However, it should be highlighted that narcissism has been the most influential factor in the prediction of nomophobia in both methodologies. Based on the results of the hierarchical regressions, more girls than boys, younger adolescents more than the older ones, with an attractive body image and a primarily narcissistic, disinhibited and neurotic personality, report higher levels of nomophobia. Similarly, gender and age appear in the primary combinations of fsQCA that predict nomophobia. In addition, low levels of body satisfaction in combination of high levels of physical attractiveness also contribute to the prediction of nomophobia. Even though narcissism is the most significant predictor, high levels of neuroticism, extraversion and disinhibition also appear in two of the three main combinations. In line with previous studies, our findings provide further evidence that personality in general and narcissism specifically are significant predictors of adolescents' nomophobia [28,43]. Results from a recent studies indicate that the link between narcissism and smartphone distress may be explained by increased attention-seeking [48]. One of the characteristics of nomophobia is the constant checking for instant notifications, which may act as reward, but on the other hand, increases the level of anxiety and distress [68]. Hence, the need for affirmation by narcissistic adolescents may encourage greater dependence on social media that manifests itself in increased anxiety or signs of nomophobia. Furthermore, our findings match previous research on the relative effect of demographic variables on nomophobia. On the one hand, girls appear to feel more anxious and insecure regarding their smartphones, and on the other hand, nomophobia levels increase along with age [49]. Finally, our findings suggest different patterns for cognitive versus emotional components of body self-esteem in the prediction of nomophobia [69]. It can be argued that adolescents, who are less satisfied with their body and therefore promote a more attractive image of themselves in social media and internet, tend to feel more anxious and insecure when they are disconnected from their smartphones, similar as the experience of social rejection.

In conclusion, the results of both regression and QCA analyses suggest that demographic variables, body self-esteem and personality traits significantly influence adolescent social networking and internet addiction. On the one hand, girls with a disinhibited personality, in addition to high levels of neuroticism, narcissism and extraversion but to a lesser extend, tend to present more symptoms of internet addiction. Meanwhile, girls, who feel physically attractive and describe themselves as disinhibited and extraverted tend to use social media more often. Neuroticism also seems to be an influence with different patterns: low levels of neuroticism in combination with high levels of disinhibition, or high levels of neuroticism in combination with greater physical attractiveness, predict increased social media use. On the other hand, adolescents, both girls and boys, with high levels of narcissism and neuroticism show greater geek behaviour. The influence of body self-esteem is unclear. Finally, adolescents, mostly girls of younger age, who are less satisfied with their body but show greater physical attractiveness, with high levels of narcissism, and also high levels of neuroticism, extraversion and disinhibition but to a lesser extend, are more likely to present more signs of nomophobia.

4.5. Strengths, Limitations and Further Research

The strengths of this present research are both theoretical and methodological. On the one hand, our study focuses on internet addiction as multidimensional concept rather than a one-dimensional approach. The instrument of measurement of addiction to social media and the internet has been specifically designed for adolescents and contemplates the four different types of addictive online behaviour: (a) symptoms that excessive internet use entails; (b) the use of social networking sites for virtual interactions with peers, due to the fact that at this age peer relationship are more and more important; (c) geek behaviour, which is characterized by an intense level of interest in online gaming and online sexuality typical of adolescence; and (d) finally nomophobia defined as the problematic use of the mobile phone, which starts at early adolescence. On the other hand, the methodological approach is the second strengths of this study. If both methodologies are compared in the prediction of social networking and Internet addiction in adolescence, fsQCA models cover a greater number of factors than regression models. In addition, fsQCA allows for multiple pathways to be estimated by combining the predictors in different ways, depending on the relationships between variables. For these reasons, fsQCA methodology may be considered a complementary analytical approach to traditional regression models.

It is necessary to stress the limitations of the study. With regard to sampling method and size, the sample size was appropriate for conducting multiple regressions and fsQCA, however probability sampling does not guarantee the generalization of the results obtained. It would be recommendable in future research to carry out a cluster-stratified random sampling that includes adolescents from all over the country. With regard to data collection, we believe that self-reports completed by the adolescents were appropriate for the purpose of the study. Future research, however, may use mixed methods (qualitative and quantitative data), multiple reports from parents and peers, which would provide more in-depth information about adolescents' addiction. Finally, one of the main limitations of fsQCA is the limited number of predictor variables that can be included in the analyses. While in regression models an increase in sample size allows an increase in the number of predictors, in fsQCA the maximum number of conditions is invariable.

This research contributes to the study of potential risk factors of social networking and internet addiction in adolescence, regardless of the limitations that has been considered. Moreover, this study offers a more comprehensive conceptualization of internet addiction by identifying four different types of addictive online behaviour in young people and describing the different pathways of variables representing important biologically based personality traits, variables of body self-esteem, which are of special relevance during adolescence and taking into account gender and age differences. Our findings extend previous addiction literature, providing an in-depth analysis of several combinations of psychological and demographic variables that may increase the risk of potential behavioural addictions.

5. Conclusions

The implications of this study are both theoretical and practical. Overall, this study makes a unique contribution to the literature on addictive use of social networking sites and broadens the way for further research that may provide additional evidence towards other adolescent-relevant variables. Such research would provide health professionals with relevant information about individual differences in the four types of social networking and internet addiction, and therefore, enriching their professional experience when working with affected adolescents. Furthermore, from a practical point of view, the findings of our study may help psychotherapists to make decisions on who to prioritize a certain intervention and treatment approach based on the relevance of the reported risk factors such as personality and gender. Such stable characteristics may be detected quickly in adolescents in order to identify those who are most at risk and thus start a preventive intervention at an early stage. Thus, the study of youth internet addiction is essential in order to improve prevention and early intervention. Finally, this study has identified important risk factors that underlie the psychological mechanisms of social networking and internet addiction in adolescents. Stressing the benefits of identifying adolescent internet addiction symptoms, problematic social media use, geek behaviour and nomophobia, through a specific instrument that allows for a multidimensional assessment.

Author Contributions: All authors contributed equivalently to this research. K.S. and I.M.-C. developed and designed the research, supervising the writing of the manuscript; M.P. and U.d.l.B. were in charge of data collection and conducted the formal analysis; M.P. and U.d.l.B. wrote the first draft of the manuscript; and K.S. and I.M.-C. reviewed, edited, and modified the manuscript critically. All authors have read and agreed to the published version of the manuscript.

Acknowledgments: The authors appreciate the participation and support of the secondary schools.

References

1. Buctot, D.B.; Kim, N.; Kim, J.J. Factors associated with smartphone addiction prevalence and its predictive capacity for health-related quality of life among Filipino adolescents. *Child. Youth Serv. Rev.* **2020**, *110*, 104758. [CrossRef]

2. Kuss, D.J.; Griffiths, M.D. Social networking sites and addiction: Ten lessons learned. *Int. J. Environ. Res. Public Health* **2017**, *14*, 311. [CrossRef] [PubMed]

3. Laconi, S.; Kaliszewska-Czeremska, K.; Gnisci, A.; Sergi, I.; Barke, A.; Jeromin, F.; Groth, J.; Gamez-Guadix, M.; Ozcan, N.K.; Demetrovics, Z.; et al. Cross-cultural study of problematicinternet use in nine European countries. *Comput. Human Behav.* **2018**, *84*, 430–440. [CrossRef]

4. Machimbarrena, J.M.; González-Cabrera, J.; Ortega-Barón, J.; Beranuy-Fargues, M.; Álvarez-Bardón, A.; Tejero, B. Profiles of problematic internet use and its impact on adolescents' health-related quality of life. *Int. J. Environ. Res. Public Health* **2019**, *16*, 20. [CrossRef] [PubMed]

5. Fischer-Grote, L.; Kothgassner, O.D.; Felnhofer, A. Risk factors for problematic smartphone use in children and adolescents: A review of existing literature. *Neuropsychiatrie* **2019**, *33*, 179–190. [CrossRef]

6. Peris, M.; Maganto, C.; Garaigordobil, M. Escala de riesgo de adicción-adolescente a las redes sociales e internet: Fiabilidad y validez (ERA-RSI) [Scale of risk of addiction to medias and Internet for adolescents: Reliability and validity (ERA-RSI)]. *Rev. Psic Clin. con Niños y Adolesc* **2018**, *5052*, 30–36.

7. Aparicio-Martínez, P.; Ruiz-Rubio, M.; Perea-Moreno, A.J.; Martínez-Jiménez, M.P.; Pagliari, C.; Redel-Macías, M.D.; Vaquero-Abellán, M. Gender differences in the addiction to social networks in the Southern Spanish university students. *Telemat Inform.* **2020**, *46*, 101304. [CrossRef]

8. Lopez-Fernandez, O. Generalised versus specific internet use-related addiction problems: A mixed methods study on internet, gaming, and social networking behaviours. *Int. J. Environ. Res. Public Health* **2018**, *15*, 2913. [CrossRef]

9. Yudes-Gómez, C.; Baridon-Chauvie, D.; González-Cabrera, J.-M. Cyberbullying and problematic Internet use in Colombia, Uruguay and Spain: Cross-cultural study. *Comunicar* **2018**, *XXXVI*, 49–58. [CrossRef]

10. Munno, D.; Cappellin, F.; Saroldi, M.; Bechon, E.; Guglielmucci, F.; Passera, R.; Zullo, G. Internet addiction disorder: Personality characteristics and risk of pathological overuse in adolescents. *Psychiatry Res.* **2017**, *248*, 1–5. [CrossRef]

11. Gómez, P.; Rial, A.; Braña, T.; Golpe, S.; Varela, J. Screening of problematic internet use among Spanish adolescents: Prevalence and related variables. *Cyberpsychogy Behav. Soc. Netw.* **2017**, *20*, 259–267. [CrossRef] [PubMed]

12. Carbonell, X.; Chamarro, A.; Oberst, U.; Rodrigo, B.; Prades, M. Problematic use of the internet and smartphones in university students: 2006–2017. *Int. J. Environ. Res. Public Health* **2018**, *15*, 475. [CrossRef] [PubMed]

13. Durán, M.; Guerra, J.M. Spanish university students' uses of the social network Tuenti and their addiction levels: The protective role of the positive attitude toward mothers' presence as contact. *Anal. Psicol.* **2015**, *31*, 260–267.

14. Ostovar, S.; Allahyar, N.; Aminpoor, H.; Moafian, F.; Binti, M.; Griffiths, M.D. Internet addiction and its psychosocial risks (depression, anxiety, stress and loneliness) among Iranian adolescents and young adults: A structural equation model in a cross-sectional study. *Int. J. Ment. Health Addict.* **2016**, *14*, 157. [CrossRef]

15. Chen, B.; Liu, F.; Ding, S.; Ying, X.; Wang, L.; Wen, Y. Gender differences in factors associated with smartphone addiction: A cross-sectional study among medical college students. *BMC Psychiatry* **2017**, *17*, 341. [CrossRef] [PubMed]

16. Cimadevilla, R.; Jenaro, C. Impact on psychological health of internet and mobile phone abuse in a spanish sample of secondary students. *Rev. Argentina Clin. Psicol.* **2019**, *XXVIII*, 339–347.

17. Bischof-Kastner, C.; Kuntsche, E.; Wolstein, J. Identifying problematic internet users: Development and validation of the Internet Motive Questionnaire for Adolescents (IMQ-A). *J. Med. Internet Res.* **2016**, *16*, e230. [CrossRef]

18. Brenley, D.B.; Covey, J. Risky behavior via social media: The role of reasoned and social reactive pathways. *Comput. Hum. Behav.* **2018**, *78*, 183–191. [CrossRef]

19. Wiederhold, B.K. VR Online dating: The new safe sex. *Cyberpsychogy Behav. Soc. Netw.* **2016**, *19*, 297–298. [CrossRef]

20. Kokkinakis, A.V.; Lin, J.; Pavlas, D.; Wade, A.R. What's in a name? Ages and names predict the valence of social interactions in a massive online game. *Comput. Hum. Behav.* **2016**, *55*, 605–613. [CrossRef]

21. Escario, J.J.; Wilkinson, A.V. Exploring predictors of online gambling in a nationally representative sample of Spanish adolescents. *Comput. Hum. Behav.* **2020**, *102*, 287–292. [CrossRef]

22. Salonen, A.H.; Alho, H.; Castrén, S. Attitudes towards gambling, gambling participation, and gambling-related harm: Cross-sectional Finnish population studies in 2011 and 2015. *BMC Public Health* **2017**, *17*, 122. [CrossRef] [PubMed]

23. Wittek, C.T.; Finseras, T.R.; Pallesen, S.; Mentzoni, R.A.; Hanss, D.; Molde, H. Prevalence and predictors of video fame addiction: A study based on a national representative sample of gamers. *Int. J. Ment. Health Addict.* **2015**, *14*, 672–686. [CrossRef] [PubMed]

24. King, A.L.; Valença, A.; Nardi, A.E. Nomophobia: The mobile phone in panic disorder with agoraphobia: Reducing phobias or worsening of dependence? *Cogn. Behav. Neurol.* **2010**, *23*, 52–54. [CrossRef]

25. Barnes, S.J.; Pressey, A.D.; Scornavacca, E. Mobile ubiquity: Understanding the relationship between cognitive absorption, smartphone addiction and social network services. *Comput. Hum. Behav.* **2019**, *90*, 246–258. [CrossRef]

26. Cha, S.S.; Seo, B.K. Smartphone use and smartphone addiction in middle school students in Korea: Prevalence, social networking service, and game use. *Health Psychol. Open* **2018**, *5*, 1–15. [CrossRef]

27. Sohn, S.; Rees, P.; Wildridge, B.; Kalk, N.J.; Carter, B. Correction to: Prevalence of problematic smartphone usage and associated mental health outcomes amongst children and young people: A systematic review, meta-analysis and GRADE of the evidence. *BMC Psychiatry* **2019**, *19*, 1–11. [CrossRef]

28. Andreassen, C.S.; Pallesen, S.; Griffiths, M.D. The relationship between addictive use of social media, narcissism, and self-esteem: Findings from a large national survey. *Addict. Behav.* **2017**, *64*, 287–293. [CrossRef]

29. Maganto, C.; Peris, M. La corporalidad de los adolescentes en las redes sociales [The body image in adolescents in social network]. *Cuadernos de Psiquiatría y Psicoterapia del Niño y del Adolescente* **2013**, *55*, 53–62.

30. De Vries, D.A.; Peter, J.; de Graaf, H.; Nikken, P. Adolescents' social network site use, peer appearance-related feedback, and body dissatisfaction: Testing a mediation model. *J. Youth Adolesc.* **2016**, *45*, 211–224. [CrossRef]

31. Peris, M. *Adicción y erotización en las redes sociales e internet: Diseño y estandarización de la batería En-Red-A2* [*Addiction and eroticization in social networks and the internet: Design and standardization of the En-Red-A2 battery*]; Universidad del País Vasco: País Vasco, Spain, 2017.

32. Wang, D. A study of the relationship between narcissism, extraversion, body-esteem, social comparison orientation and selfie-editing behavior on social networking sites. *Personal. Individ. Differ.* **2019**, *146*, 127–129. [CrossRef]

33. Kircaburun, K.; Alhabash, S.; Tosuntaş, Ş.B.; Griffiths, M.D. Uses and gratifications of problematic social media use among university students: A simultaneous examination of the Big Five of personality traits, social media platforms, and social media use motives. *Int. J. Ment. Health Addict.* **2018**, *18*, 525–547. [CrossRef]

34. Peris, M.; Maganto, C.; Arigita, A.; Barrientos, A.; León, A.; Sánchez-Cabrero, R. El derecho al olvido digital la imagen corporal virtual en adolescentes jóvenes. In *Intervención e Investigación en Contextos Clínicos de la Salud*; Pérez-Fuentes, M.C., Molero, M.M., Gázquez, J.J., Martos, A., Barragán, A.B., Simón, M.M., Oropesa, N.F., Pino, R.M., Eds.; ASUNIVEP: Murcia, Spain, 2019; pp. 135–143.

35. Liu, Q.; Sun, J.; Li, Q.; Zhou, Z. Body dissatisfaction and smartphone addiction among Chinese adolescents: A moderated mediation model. *Child. Youth Serv. Rev.* **2020**, *108*, 104613. [CrossRef]

36. Blachnio, A.; Przepiorka, A.; Senol-Durak, E.; Durak, M.; Sherstyuk, L. The role of personality traits in Facebook and internet addictions: A study on Polish, Turkish, and Ukrainian samples. *Comput. Hum. Behav.* **2017**, *68*, 269–275. [CrossRef]

37. Hussain, Z.; Pontes, H.M. Personality, internet addiction, and other technological addictions: A psychological examination of personality traits and technological addictions. In *Psychological, Social, and Cultural Aspects of Internet Addiction*; Bozoglan, B., Ed.; IGI Global: Hershey, PA, USA, 2018; pp. 45–71.

38. Cheng, C.; Wang, H.; Sigerson, L.; Chau, C.I. Do the socially rich get richer? A nuanced perspective on social network site use and online social capital accrual. *Psychol. Bull.* **2019**, *145*, 734–764. [CrossRef]

39. Dieris-Hirche, J.; Pape, M.; te Wildt, B.T.; Kehyayan, A.; Esch, M.; Aicha, S.; Herpertz, S.; Bottel, L. Problematic gaming behavior and the personality traits of video gamers: A cross-sectional survey. *Comput. Hum. Behav.* **2020**, *106*, 106272. [CrossRef]

40. Pivetta, E.; Harkin, L.; Billieux, J.; Kanjo, E.; Kuss, D. Problematic smartphone use: An empirically validated model. *Comput. Hum. Behav.* **2019**, *100*, 105–117. [CrossRef]

41. Mitchell, L.; Hussain, Z. Predictors of problematic smartphone use: An examination of the Integrative Pathways Model and the role of age, gender, impulsiveness, excessive reassurance seeking, extraversion, and depression. *Behav. Sci.* **2018**, *8*, 74. [CrossRef] [PubMed]

42. Marengo, D.; Poletti, I.; Settanni, M. The interplay between neuroticism, extraversion, and social media addiction in young adult Facebook users: Testing the mediating role of online activity using objective data. *Addict. Behav.* **2020**, *102*, 106150. [CrossRef] [PubMed]

43. Lachmann, B.; Sindermann, C.; Sariyska, R.Y.; Luo, R.; Melchers, M.C.; Becker, B.; Cooper, A.J.; Montag, C. The role of empathy and life satisfaction in internet and smartphone use disorder. *Front. Psychol.* **2018**, *9*, 398. [CrossRef]

44. Hussain, Z.; Griffiths, M.D.; Sheffield, D. An investigation into problematic smartphone use: The role of narcissism, anxiety, and personality factors. *J. Behav. Addict.* **2017**, *6*, 378–386. [CrossRef] [PubMed]

45. Gervasi, A.M.; La Marca, L.; Lombardo, E.M.C.; Mannino, G.; Iacolino, C.; Schimmenti, A. Maladaptive personality traits and internet addiction symptoms among young adults: A study based on the alternative DSM-5 model for personality disorders. *Clin. Neuropsychiatry* **2017**, *14*, 20–28.

46. Clancy, E.M.; Klettke, B.; Hallford, D.J. The dark side of sexting—Factors predicting the dissemination of sexts. *Comput. Hum. Behav.* **2019**, *92*, 266–272. [CrossRef]

47. Sarabia, I.; Estévez, A. Sexualized behaviors on Facebook. *Comput. Hum. Behav.* **2016**, *61*, 219–226. [CrossRef]

48. Hawk, S.T.; van den Eijnden, J.J.M.; van Lissa, C.J.; ter Bogt, T.F.M. Narcissistic adolescents' attention-seeking following social rejection: Links with social media disclosure, problematic social media use, and smartphone stress. *Comput. Hum. Behav.* **2019**, *92*, 65–75. [CrossRef]

49. Yildiz Durak, H. Investigation of nomophobia and smartphone addiction predictors among adolescents in Turkey: Demographic variables and academic performance. *Soc. Sci. J.* **2019**, *56*, 492–517. [CrossRef]

50. Eng, S.; Woodside, A.G. Configural analysis of the drinking man: Fuzzy-set qualitative comparative analyses. *Addict. Behav.* **2012**, *37*, 541–543. [CrossRef]

51. Ragin, C.C. *Redesigning Social Inquiry. Fuzzy Sets and Beyond*; University of Chicago Press: Chicago, IL, USA, 2008.

52. Calabuig, F.; Prado-Gascó, V.; Crespo-Hervás, J.; Núñez-Pomar, J.; Añó, V. Predicting future intentions of basketball spectators using SEM and fsQCA. *J. Bus. Res.* **2016**, *69*, 1396–1400. [CrossRef]

53. Legewie, N. An introduction to applied data analysis with Qualitative Comparative Analysis (QCA). *Forum Qual. Soc. Res.* **2013**, *14*, 1–45.

54. De la Barrera, U.; Schoeps, K.; Gil-Gómez, J.-A.; Montoya-Castilla, I. Predicting adolescent adjustment and well-being: The interplay between socio-emotional and personal factors. *Int. J. Environ. Res. Public Health* **2019**, *16*, 4650. [CrossRef]

55. Giménez-Espert M del, C.; Valero-Moreno, S.; Prado-Gascó, V.J. Evaluation of emotional skills in nursing using regression and QCA models: A transversal study. *Nurse Educ. Today* **2019**, *74*, 31–37. [CrossRef] [PubMed]

56. De la Barrera, U.; Villanueva, L.; Prado-Gascó, V. Emotional and personality predictors that influence the appearance of somatic complaints in children and adults. *Psicothema* **2019**, *31*, 407–413. [PubMed]

57. Peris, M.; Maganto, C.; Garaigordobil, M. Escala de Autoestima Corporal: Datos psicométricos de fiabilidad y validez. *Rev. Psicol. Clínica con Niños y Adolesc.* **2016**, *3*, 51–58.

58. Costa, P.T.; McCrae, R.R. *Inventario de Personalidad NEO Revisado (NEO PIR) e Inventario NEO Reducido de Cinco Factores (NEO-FFI)*; TEA Ediciones: Madrid, Spain, 2008.

59. Zuckerman, M.; Eysenck, S.B.G.; Eysenck, H.J. Sensation seeking in England and America: Cross-cultural, age, and sex comparisons. *J. Consult. Clin. Psychol.* **1978**, *46*, 139–149. [CrossRef]

60. Pérez, J.; Torrubia, R. Fiabilidad y validez de la versión española de la Escala de Búsqueda de Sensaciones (Forma V). *Rev. Latinoam Univ.* **1986**, *18*, 7–22.

61. Raskin, R.; Terry, H. Principal-components analysis of the narcissistic personality inventory and further evidence of its construct validity. *J. Pers. Soc. Psychol.* **1988**, *54*, 890–902. [CrossRef]

62. Trechera, J.L.; Millán, G.; Fernández-Morales, E. Estudio empírico del trastorno narcisista de la personalidad (TNP). *Acta Colomb. Psicol.* **2008**, *11*, 25–36.

63. Villanueva, L.; Montoya-Castilla, I.; Prado-Gascó, V. The importance of trait emotional intelligence and feelings in the prediction of perceived and biological stress in adolescents: Hierarchical regressions and fsQCA models. *Stress* **2017**, *20*, 355–362. [CrossRef]

64. Woodside, A.G. Moving beyond multiple regression analysis to algorithms: Calling for adoption of a paradigm shift from symmetric to asymmetric thinking in data analysis and crafting theory. *J. Bus. Res.* **2013**, *66*, 463–472. [CrossRef]

65. Su, W.; Han, X.; Jin, C.; Yan, Y.; Potenza, M.N. Are males more likely to be addicted to the internet than females? A meta-analysis involving 34 global jurisdictions. *Comput. Hum. Behav.* **2019**, *99*, 86–100. [CrossRef]

66. Di Blasi, M.; Giardina, A.; Lo Coco, G.; Giordano, C.; Billieux, J.; Schimmenti, A. A compensatory model to understand dysfunctional personality traits in problematic gaming: The role of vulnerable narcissism. *Personal. Individ. Differ.* **2020**, *160*, 109921. [CrossRef]

67. Matthews, N.L.; Lynch, T.; Martins, N. Real ideal: Investigating how ideal and hyper-ideal video game bodies affect men and women. *Comput. Hum. Behav.* **2016**, *59*, 155–164. [CrossRef]

68. Anshari, M.; Alas, Y.; Sulaiman, E. Smartphone addictions and nomophobia among youth. *Vulnerable Child. Youth Stud.* **2019**, *14*, 242–247. [CrossRef]

69. Peris, M.; Maganto, C.; Kortabarria, L. Body self-esteem, virtual image in social networks and sexuality in adolescent. *Eur. J. Investig. Health Psychol. Educ.* **2013**, *3*, 171–180. [CrossRef]

5

Autonomy Need Dissatisfaction in Daily Life and Problematic Mobile Phone Use: The Mediating Roles of Boredom Proneness and Mobile Phone Gaming

Wei Hong [1], Ru-De Liu [1,*], Yi Ding [2], Rui Zhen [3], Ronghuan Jiang [1] and Xinchen Fu [1]

[1]   Beijing Key Laboratory of Applied Experimental Psychology, National Demonstration Center for Experimental Psychology Education (Beijing Normal University), Faculty of Psychology, Beijing Normal University, Beijing 100875, China; psyhongwei@163.com (W.H.); jrh_psy@163.com (R.J.); fxc_psy@163.com (X.F.)

[2]   Graduate School of Education, Fordham University, New York, NY 10023, USA; yding4@fordham.edu

[3]   Institute of Psychological Sciences, Hangzhou Normal University, Hangzhou 311121, China; zhenrui1206@126.com

*   Correspondence: rdliu@bnu.edu.cn

Abstract: Psychological needs dissatisfaction has been identified as hindering adaptive development, in which autonomy need dissatisfaction, as one core component, may be associated with adolescents' maladaptive online behaviors. Sporadic research has examined the association between autonomy need dissatisfaction and problematic mobile phone use (PMPU). Boredom proneness and mobile phone gaming were suggested to be linked to this association. This study aimed to examine the mediating effects of boredom proneness and mobile phone gaming in the association between autonomy need dissatisfaction and PMPU. A total of 358 secondary school students completed questionnaires at three waves; autonomy need dissatisfaction was measured in time 1 (T1); boredom proneness and mobile phone gaming were measured one year later (time 2, T2); PMPU was measured two years later (time 3, T3). The structural equation model results showed that T1 autonomy need dissatisfaction not only directly predicted T3 PMPU, but also exerted effects via the mediating role of T2 boredom proneness and the chain mediating role of T2 boredom proneness and T2 mobile phone gaming. These findings reveal the unique role of specific psychological need in engaging PMPU, which provides support to targeted interventions, such that promoting autonomy need satisfaction may be an instrumental procedure to prevent adolescents from addiction-like online behaviors.

Keywords: autonomy need dissatisfaction; problematic mobile phone use; boredom proneness; mobile phone gaming; multiple mediation

1. Introduction

Mobile phones, as the most accessible device to connect to the internet, have penetrated every aspect of daily lives, such that they help people obtain information, maintain social connectedness, and entertain themselves [1,2]. According to a national survey in China, there were 897 million mobile phone users as of March 2020, accounting for 99.3% of the Internet users [3]. Some of the users invested an excessive amount of time and resources into their mobile phones. This behavior can be described as problematic mobile phone use (PMPU), which refers to a constellation of emerging addiction symptoms, including cravings, withdrawal, and loss of control [4]. Numerous negative consequences occur after engaging in PMPU. For instance, PMPU has been identified to lead to sleep problems [5,6], poor academic performance and school adjustment [7,8], cognitive failures [6,9], and physical and mental health problems [10–12]. Furthermore, it was found that 10% of British adolescents were problematic users and 20.5% of them were potential problematic users [13]. A recent research showed that the prevalence of PMPU was 29% in young adults from the United Arab Emirates [1]. Such potential hazards and the high prevalence of PMPU stimulate public concerns and gain increasing scholarly attention.

People are active and purposive when engaging on the internet via mobile phones because it can satisfy specific psychological needs, as postulated by uses and gratification theory [14]. This perspective implies that people with unsatisfied needs in daily life tend to use mobile phones as a compensator to cope with the negative life situation. Combined with the model of compensatory internet use [15], this compensatory use of the internet via mobile phones is more likely to result in problematic use and addiction tendencies. A substantial body of literature has revealed that psychological needs dissatisfaction in daily life contributes to pathological Internet use (PIU) [16] and PMPU [17].

Based on self-determination theory, humans have three inherent psychological needs, including the need for autonomy, competence, and relatedness. Deci and Ryan [18] proposed that psychological needs satisfaction is an essential nutriment for psychological growth and wellness; its dissatisfaction hinders self-integrity and lead to problematic outcomes. Given that different needs play different roles in behavior patterns and social functioning [19], an increasing number of studies attempted to differentiate the unique effect of each type of need. One of the very few studies found that only autonomy (not relatedness and competence) need dissatisfaction significantly predicted problematic online behaviors [20]. It is known that autonomy need is described as the need to self-regulate their experiences and actions [21]. That is, when behaviors are volitional and self-endorsed, individuals would experience high levels of autonomy need satisfaction. Stated differently, autonomy need dissatisfaction suggests what individuals do is not congruent with their intrinsic motivation and authentic interests. As a result, ameliorating behaviors, such as engaging on the internet through mobile phones, are activated to compensate for the lack of fulfillment of this kind of need, which increases the probability of problematic use [15]. In short, it seems that autonomy need dissatisfaction is positively associated with PMPU.

Furthermore, autonomy need dissatisfaction as the perceptions of the external environment can be considered to be a distal factor in explaining the etiology of addictive symptoms of PIU; these distal factors exert effects on maladaptive online behaviors via the mediating effects of proximal factors, as postulated in the cognitive-behavioral model of PIU [22]. For instance, boredom proneness results from the external environment without autonomy [23], and servers as a contributor to PMPU [24,25]. Similarly, online gaming, as a specific behavioral response to cope with autonomy need dissatisfaction, is an important predictor of PMPU [26]. These relations indicate that boredom proneness and mobile phone gaming may be potential mediators in the process. However, there has been a lack of empirical research to support this relation. To address this issue, this study aimed to examine the mediating roles of boredom proneness and mobile phone gaming in the association between autonomy need dissatisfaction in daily life and PMPU.

1.1. Boredom Proneness as a Mediator

Boredom proneness may be a potential mediator between autonomy need dissatisfaction and PMPU. Specifically, boredom refers to a general tendency to experience boredom in situations with deficits in interest, meaning, excitement, and challenge [27]. People with autonomy need dissatisfaction have relatively few opportunities to make their own decisions, and have to engage in activities incongruent with their authentic interests [21]. Thus, non-interest-orientated activities may lead to low levels of psychological arousal and high levels of boredom proneness [28]. This notion has been supported by the various findings that psychological needs (including autonomy need) satisfaction/dissatisfaction significantly predicts boredom in sports activities [29], in academic settings [30], and in work domains [31]. In a 2009 study, adolescent soccer athletes who perceived less autonomy reported more boredom experience [23]. Thus, autonomy need dissatisfaction in daily life seems to be positively associated with boredom proneness.

Regarding the second stage of the mediation process, boredom proneness has been identified as a high-risk factor for PIU [32,33] and PMPU [24,34]. Adolescents with high levels of boredom proneness tend to experience low levels of internal motivation and external stimulation [27]. One approach to cope with boredom is to engage in online activities as they may help to increase the feelings of excitement and sensation [32,35]. Chronic and habitual use of this approach would increase the risk of engaging in PIU [32,33]. Similarly, previous research has found that boredom proneness positively predicts PMPU among adolescents [24,34]. Altogether, it appears that autonomy need dissatisfaction is positively associated with boredom proneness, which in turn is positively associated with PMPU.

1.2. Mobile Phone Gaming as a Mediator

Another potential mediator may be mobile phone gaming, because distal causes and proximal factors jointly facilitate an excessive use of specific internet functions (e.g., online gaming), which further leads to behavioral symptoms of PIU [22]. As stated earlier, individuals with autonomy need dissatisfaction may activate ameliorating behaviors to compensate for the deficits in this kind of need. As reviewed by Ryan and Deci [21], a key characteristic of games is providing opportunities for actions. For instance, players are free to choose the types of games and activities that they want to engage in, to decide the avatars and roles, and to fulfill the game missions. Experimental evidence has indicated that the autonomy character of a game would facilitate immersion-related experiences, further increasing enjoyment and decreasing boredom in the game world [36]. In this sense, people who experience autonomy need dissatisfaction might have the motivation to engage in gaming as a way to compensate, thus exhibiting longer game-playtime on a weekly basis [37]. More important, empirical research has found that psychological needs dissatisfaction [38] and autonomy need dissatisfaction [20] in the real world positively predict the excessive use of video games. Thus, autonomy need dissatisfaction appears to be positively associated with frequent mobile phone gaming.

Moreover, when adolescents have a history of mobile phone use for gaming, desirable game experiences (e.g., flow experience in the game world) may encourage them to repeatedly engage in this activity [39]. In the long run, they are more likely to frequently act on mobile phones and become addicted to using mobile phones [40]. In support of this notion, frequent online gaming has been shown to positively predict PIU in cross-sectional research [41] and predict PIU one year later in the longitudinal research [42]. Similarly, Jeong, Kim, Yum and Hwang [26] and Lee, Kim and Choi [40] found that frequent mobile gaming contributed to PMPU. Altogether, it appears that autonomy need dissatisfaction is positively associated with mobile phone gaming, which in turn is positively associated with PMPU.

1.3. A Multiple Mediation Model

The mediating roles of boredom proneness and mobile phone gaming have been advanced to describe the relation between autonomy need dissatisfaction and PMPU wherein boredom proneness was argued to positively associate with frequent mobile phone use [43]. For instance, Chou, et al. [44] found that adolescents with high boredom proneness are more easily to perceive low levels of external stimulation and are more likely to engage in online gaming for self-entertainment. Likewise, Biolcati, Mancini and Trombini [25] supported this finding and found that adolescents with higher boredom proneness reported higher levels of participation in mobile phone gaming in comparison to adolescents with lower boredom proneness.

Taken together, individuals with autonomy need dissatisfaction in the real world cannot voluntarily make choices and engage in activities congruent with their authentic interests [18]. Thus, they are prone to having low intrinsic motivation and exhibit low psychological involvement, which may increase the tendency to experience boredom [21,45,46]. Furthermore, bored individuals are more likely to play mobile games as a compensator of boredom [15]. In this regard, frequent mobile phone gaming increases the risk of problematic use and addictive symptoms [26,40]. Accordingly, it is possible that autonomy need dissatisfaction is indirectly associated with PMPU via the multiple mediating role of boredom proneness and mobile phone gaming.

1.4. The Present Study

According to the above findings, autonomy need dissatisfaction in daily life has been argued to be a contributing factor to PMPU. Autonomy need dissatisfaction as the perceptions of the external environment may exert effects on psychological symptoms via individual characteristics. Based on self-determination theory [18], the model of compensatory internet use [15], and the cognitive-behavioral model of PIU [22], boredom proneness as a dispositional factor can be partially attributed to the lack of autonomy from the external environment; and gaming involved a specific mobile phone usage can be considered as coping strategies. That is, boredom proneness and mobile phone gaming can be postulated as potential mediators to elucidate how autonomy need dissatisfaction was associated with PMPU. Nevertheless, there has been a lack of empirical research, especially using cross-temporal designs, to examine whether autonomy need dissatisfaction is associated with PMPU via the mediating roles of boredom proneness and mobile phone gaming. To this end, we attempted to assess the independent variable in Time 1 (T1), the mediating variables in Time 2 (T2), and the dependent variable in Time 3 (T3). As shown in Figure 1, this study was guided by the following hypotheses:

H1: *T1 autonomy need dissatisfaction in daily life is positively associated with T3 PMPU.*

H2: *T2 boredom proneness mediates the association between T1 autonomy need dissatisfaction and T3 PMPU.*

H3: *T2 mobile phone gaming mediates the association between T1 autonomy need dissatisfaction and T3 PMPU.*

H4: *T1 autonomy need dissatisfaction in daily life is indirectly associated with T3 PMPU through the multiple mediating role of T2 boredom proneness and T2 mobile phone gaming.*

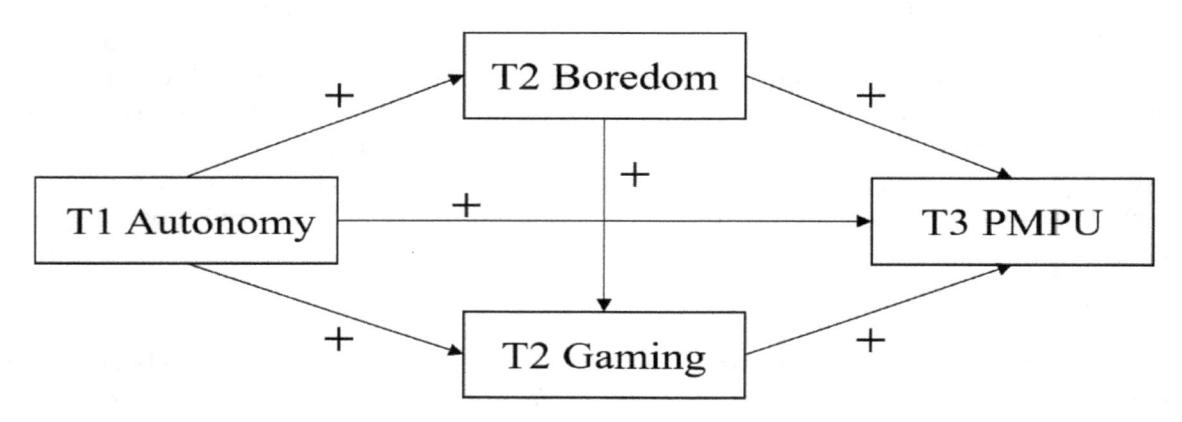

Figure 1. The conceptual model between autonomy need dissatisfaction and PMPU. Note. T1 Autonomy = Autonomy need dissatisfaction in Time 1; T2 Boredom = Boredom proneness in Time 2; T2 Gaming = Mobile phone gaming in Time 2; T3 PMPU = Problematic mobile phone use in Time 3.

2. Materials and Methods

2.1. Participants and Procedures

A sample of 1060 students from a regular secondary school in Beijing, China, was recruited to participate in the first data collection (T1). Due to graduation, 819 students participated in the second data collection (T2) after one year and 358 students participated in the third data collection (T3) after two years. This study focused on the participants who completed the questionnaires at three waves. The sample comprised 154 (43.0%) boys and 204 girls (57.0%). They had an average age of 13.19

years (standard deviation (SD) = 1.44), ranging from 12 to 16 years. Each participant reported having a constant Internet-accessible mobile phone.

This research was approved by the Academic Ethics Committee of the Faculty of Psychology at Beijing Normal University. Before the formal investigation, participants and their parents or legal guardians were provided with written consent forms, which informed them that personal information would be kept confidential and their responses would be used only for research purposes. Additionally, students were informed that they had the right to opt out of the research at any time. The research assistants distributed and collected the self-report questionnaires in the regular classrooms. Data collection took approximately 15 min, and participants were compensated with a small gift (e.g., a pen).

2.2. Measure

2.2.1. Autonomy Need Dissatisfaction

The level of autonomy need dissatisfaction was measured in T1 by the Basic Need Satisfaction in General Scale, which consists of the domains of autonomy, competence, and relatedness needs satisfaction [47]. This scale has been tested and used in the Chinese context [48]. The autonomy subscale contains three negative items (e.g., There is not much opportunity for me to decide for myself how to do things in my daily life), which has been used to assess autonomy need dissatisfaction [49]. Participants rated the items on a 5-point Likert scale (1 = *not at all true*, 5 = *very true*), with higher scores indicating higher levels of autonomy need dissatisfaction. The internal consistency of this scale showed acceptable reliability (Cronbach α = 0.60).

2.2.2. Boredom Proneness

The level of boredom proneness was measured in T2 by the short version of the Boredom Proneness Scale [27]. This scale contains eight items (e.g., I often find myself at "loose ends," not knowing what to do) with one-dimensional structure. Participants rated the items on a 7-point Likert scale (1 = *strongly disagree*, 7 = *strongly agree*), with higher scores indicating higher levels of boredom proneness. The internal consistency of this scale showed satisfactory reliability (Cronbach α = 0.94).

2.2.3. Mobile Phone Gaming

The measure of mobile phone gaming in T2 was adapted from the Chinese Internet Usage Questionnaire [50] and the Mobile Phone Use Patterns Questionnaire [43]. In total, there were 10 items regarding Internet use and 17 items regarding mobile phone use. After instructing "according to your daily routine, ... ", only one item (i.e., I play mobile games on my phone) was used to assess the mobile phone gaming frequency on a daily basis. Participants rated the items on a 5-point Likert scale (1 = *never*, 5 = *always*), with higher scores indicating more frequent use for mobile games.

2.2.4. Problematic Mobile Phone Use (PMPU)

Participants' severity of PMPU was assessed in T3 by the short version of the Mobile Phone Problem Use Scale [51], which has been validated in the Chinese context and showed good validity and reliability [17,52]. This scale contains 10 items (e.g., I find it difficult to switch off my mobile phone) with five aspects, including craving, withdrawal, peer dependence, loss of control, and negative life consequences. Participants rated the items on a 5-point Likert scale (1 = *strongly disagree*, 5 = *strongly agree*), with higher scores indicating more severe PMPU. The internal consistency of this scale showed satisfactory reliability (Cronbach's α = 0.87).

2.3. Data Analyses

Means, standard deviations, and Pearson correlations were calculated using SPSS 19.0. The hypothesized multiple mediation model was tested by structural equation modeling (SEM) using Mplus 7.1 [53]. The model was evaluated by following model fit indices: the chi-square values ($\chi 2$), the comparative fit index (CFI), the Tucker–Lewis fit index (TLI), the root mean square error of approximation (RMSEA), and the standardized root mean square residual (SRMR). The CFI and TLI at 0.90 or above, and the RMSEA and SRMR at 0.08 or lower, indicate that the model is acceptable [54].

3. Results

3.1. Descriptive Statistics and Correlations

Means, standard deviations, and Pearson correlations are presented in Table 1. As shown, autonomy need dissatisfaction was significantly and positively correlated with boredom proneness and PMPU, but it was not correlated with mobile phone gaming. Furthermore, each two elements of boredom proneness, mobile phone gaming, and PMPU had a positive association.

Table 1. Means, standard deviations, and correlations among the main variables.

Variables	M	SD	1	2	3	4
1 T1 Autonomy	2.91	0.84	-			
2 T2 Boredom	3.82	1.33	0.32 ***	-		
3 T2 Gaming	3.24	1.17	0.06	0.19 ***	-	
4 T3 PMPU	2.70	0.76	0.25 ***	0.27 ***	0.21 ***	-

Note. T1 Autonomy = Autonomy need dissatisfaction in Time 1; T2 Boredom = Boredom proneness in Time 2; T2 Gaming = Mobile phone gaming in Time 2; T3 PMPU = Problematic mobile phone use in Time 3; *** $p < 0.001$.

3.2. Examinations of the Measurement Model

Before testing the hypothesized model by SEM, it was necessary to examine the measurement model. According to the recommendation from Wu and Wen [55], autonomy need dissatisfaction could be loaded by the three observed items; boredom proneness that has eight items with one-dimensional structure could be parceled into three indicators; mobile phone gaming with only one item could be loaded by the one item; PMPU with five aspects could be loaded by the five substructures. Altogether, the CFA results of the measurement model showed a good model fit: $\chi^2/df = 3.17$, CFI = 0.95, TLI = 0.93, RMSEA = 0.08, SRMR = 0.05, in that all the loadings on latent variables were significant ($p < 0.001$).

3.3. Examinations of the Structural Model

As hypothesized, a multiple model with T1 autonomy need dissatisfaction as the independent variable, T2 boredom proneness and mobile phone gaming as the mediators, and T3 PMPU as the dependent variable was established. The SEM results showed a good model fit: $\chi^2/df = 3.15$, CFI = 0.94, TLI = 0.92, RMSEA = 0.05, SRMR = 0.05. As shown in Figure 2, T1 autonomy need dissatisfaction significantly predicted T3 PMPU. Similarly, T1 autonomy need dissatisfaction positively predicted T2 boredom proneness, which in turn positively predicted T3 PMPU. However, T1 autonomy need dissatisfaction did not predict T2 mobile phone gaming, although T2 mobile phone gaming positively predicted T3 PMPU.

To further examine the significance of the indirect effects, bias-corrected bootstrap tests derived with 1000 samples were used. That the 95% confidence interval did not contain zero indicated statistical significance [56]. As shown in Table 2, T1 autonomy need dissatisfaction positively predicted T3 PMPU, supporting H1. Furthermore, T2 boredom proneness significantly mediated the association between T1 autonomy need dissatisfaction and T3 PMPU, supporting H2. Whereas, mobile phone gaming did not mediate the association between T1 autonomy need dissatisfaction and T3 PMPU, rejecting H3. Additionally, the chain of T2 boredom proneness and T2 mobile phone gaming significantly mediated the association between T1 autonomy need dissatisfaction and T3 PMPU, supporting H4.

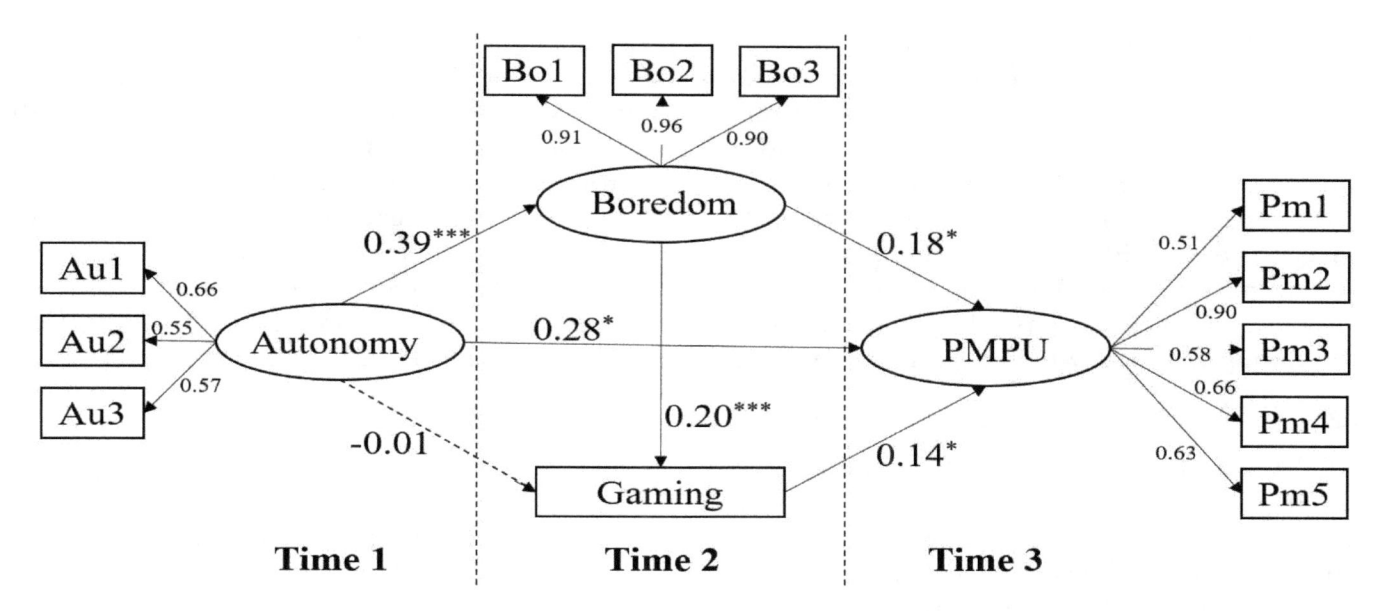

Figure 2. The mediation model of the association between T1 autonomy need dissatisfaction and T3 PMPU. Note. All the loadings on latent variables were significant ($p < 0.001$). Autonomy = Autonomy need dissatisfaction, Boredom = Boredom proneness, Gaming = Mobile phone gaming, PMPU = Problematic mobile phone use. * $p < 0.05$, *** $p < 0.001$.

Table 2. Bias-corrected bootstrap tests on the direct and indirect effects.

Paths	Standardized(β)	95% Confidence Interval		Hypotheses
		Low	High	
T1 Autonomy → T3 PMPU	0.277	0.112	0.443	Supporting H1
T1 Autonomy → T2 Boredom → T3 PMPU	0.069	0.007	0.013	Supporting H2
T1 Autonomy → T2 Gaming → T3 PMPU	−0.001	−0.024	0.022	Rejecting H3
T1 Autonomy → T2 Boredom → T2 Gaming → T3 PMPU	0.011	0.001	0.025	Supporting H4

Note. T1 Autonomy = Autonomy need dissatisfaction in Time 1; T3 PMPU = Problematic mobile phone use in Time 3; T2 Boredom = Boredom proneness in Time 2; T2 Gaming = Mobile phone gaming in Time 2.

4. Discussion

This study focused on autonomy need dissatisfaction and examined its potential effect on PMPU. Boredom proneness and mobile phone gaming were suggested to be incorporated into this association to elucidate the underlying mechanism. Based on three-wave data, the SEM model results showed that T1 autonomy need dissatisfaction not only directly predicted T3 PMPU, but also exerted effects on T3 PMPU via the mediating role of T2 boredom proneness and via the chain mediating role of T2 boredom proneness and T2 mobile phone gaming. Altogether, the findings provide empirical evidence to support the relation between specific psychological need and PMPU, which lends further insight into targeted prevention and interventions of problematic online behaviors.

4.1. Autonomy Need Dissatisfaction, Boredom Proneness, and PMPU

This study demonstrated that T1 autonomy need dissatisfaction directly predicted T3 PMPU, it also indirectly predicted T3 PMPU through the mediating role of T2 boredom proneness. According to self-determination theory [18], adolescents with autonomy need dissatisfaction have few opportunities to volitionally make choices and self-organize actions in daily life. Thus, they may have to participate in activities with little intrinsic motivation, which increases a tendency to experience boredom [29,45]. For instance, they may execute what others compel them to do, such as participating in extracurricular courses that are arranged by their parents. In this sense, they are more likely to experience boredom.

This finding was consistent with the previous studies that the higher levels of autonomy need dissatisfaction that adolescents perceive, the more likely they would experience boredom [31].

Furthermore, bored adolescents are more likely to seek external stimulation to cope with boredom [27], and thus they may spend much time and resources on the internet (or via mobile phones), which further increases the risk of problematic behaviors, including PIU [32,33] and PMPU [24]. Altogether, adolescents with autonomy need dissatisfaction cannot freely make decisions and volitionally engage in what they are interested in, which chronically contributes to boredom proneness. These bored adolescents are more likely to frequently act on mobile phones, leading to problematic use. Thus, it seems that autonomy need dissatisfaction in daily life gives rise to boredom proneness, which in turn increases the risk of subsequent PMPU.

4.2. Autonomy Need Dissatisfaction, Mobile Phone Gaming, and PMPU

This study showed that T1 autonomy need dissatisfaction did not predict T2 mobile phone gaming although T2 gaming positively predicted T3 PMPU. This finding weakly supported the mediating role of mobile phone gaming in the mediation process because the first stage was not significant. One possibility may be that psychological need dissatisfaction plays a double-edged role in determining online gaming [37]. As mentioned earlier, games that provide adolescents with opportunities for actions can assist in compensating for unsatisfied autonomy need in the real world [21,57]. Therefore, adolescents with autonomy need dissatisfaction may resort to the internet (or via mobile phones) to compensate for this dissatisfaction [15]. For instance, when individuals feel psychologically pressured and constrained, they would use mobile phones for gaming to alleviate these undesirable feelings as a way to compensate because they are free to do whatever they want in the game world. This perspective implies that the higher levels of autonomy need dissatisfaction that adolescents perceive, the more frequent mobile phone gaming they would engage in [38].

Nevertheless, adolescents with autonomy need dissatisfaction have few opportunities to decide for themselves even though they may think that gaming is tempting [39,47]. Specifically, adolescents with autonomy need dissatisfaction may be under the restrictions of their parents, particularly when engaging in mobile phone gaming. This perspective suggests that the higher levels of autonomy need dissatisfaction that adolescents perceive, the fewer opportunities they might have to play mobile games. Taken these two perspectives together, the former compensatory effect (i.e., autonomy need dissatisfaction motivates mobile gaming as a compensator) may neutralize the later restriction effect (i.e., autonomy need dissatisfaction indicates few opportunities for mobile gaming). Thus, it is not surprising that autonomy need dissatisfaction in daily life was weakly associated with mobile phone gaming. Future studies are warranted to further examine the complicated association between autonomy need dissatisfaction and online gaming.

4.3. A Multiple Mediation Model

One intriguing finding was that the chain of T2 boredom proneness and T2 mobile phone gaming significantly mediated T1 autonomy need dissatisfaction and T3 PMPU. Consistent with the etiology of addictive symptoms of PIU [22], psychological needs dissatisfaction as a distal factor exerts effects on addiction tendencies through the mediating variables (i.e., boredom proneness and mobile phone gaming). Specifically, adolescents with autonomy need dissatisfaction in real life tend to have relatively fewer opportunities to make decisions; thus, they may have to engage what is not congruent with their authentic interests [47]. For instance, the parents of Chinese students may arrange for them to engage in repetitive and monotonous academic activities. In a long run, they may possess low levels of intrinsic motivation and exhibit high levels of boredom proneness. Concurring with the earlier findings [25,44], bored adolescents may engage in online gaming to alleviate boredom as they can obtain external stimulation and gain flow experiences when fully involving in gaming [39]. For instance, participants reported that they played a kind of multiplayer online battle arena game named *Arena of Valor* on mobile phones because they felt that doing so can swipe away boring time. Additionally, mobile phone gaming has been identified as a high-risk factor for PMPU [26,40]. That is, adolescents who frequently engage in mobile phone gaming are at risk in developing problematic use and nurturing addiction tendencies. Taken together, it seems that autonomy need dissatisfaction in daily life positively predicts boredom proneness that contributes to frequent mobile phone gaming, which in turn leads to subsequent PMPU.

4.4. Limitations, Future Directions, and Implications

There are several limitations of this study. First, self-reported data may produce response bias although there was no serious common method bias using Harman's single factor test [58]. Future studies could record time of generalized use and gaming on mobile phones, which may provide objective data and enhance reliability and validity. Second, the reliability of the measure of autonomy need dissatisfaction appeared to be somewhat low although it has been used in several studies [47–49]. Thus, this scale should be further improved in future research. Third, this study recruited secondary school students only from a regular secondary school; therefore, generalization of the conclusions to other groups should be made with caution. Future studies could focus on adults and/or clinical groups, which may contribute to a broader application of these findings. Fourth, the mediating effects seemed to be relatively small, however small effects can assist in developing theories when the findings support the theoretical hypotheses [59]. In addition, small effects should not be disregarded because they might be accumulated to generate large effects with the changing conditions [60]. In this digital age in particular, the use of mobile phones has exponentially grown and corresponding problems (e.g., addiction tendencies) have been increasing and appear severe, thus possibly leading to large effects on PMPU in future studies.

Despite the limitations, notable implications are twofold. From a theoretical perspective, this study was the first of its kind to use a cross-temporal design and to exclusively examine the effect of autonomy need dissatisfaction on subsequent PMPU. On the one hand, this study focused on the role of specific need (i.e., autonomy need), instead of psychological needs as a single entity, in explaining maladaptive online behaviors. On the other hand, boredom proneness as an individual characteristic and gaming as possible coping strategies helped to elucidate the potential etiology of addiction-like symptoms associated with mobile phone use in the framework of self-determination. These findings based on the three-wave data revealed that autonomy need dissatisfaction not only directly predicted subsequent PMPU, but also exerted indirect effects via the mediating roles of boredom proneness and mobile phone gaming. These findings help to develop a better understanding of the formation process of PMPU, which provides support for prevention and intervention programs. For instance, excessive parental restrictions on children's online behaviors (e.g., limiting use time, monitoring online content) may backfire because these children perceive autonomy need dissatisfaction and may increase addiction-like tendencies [61,62]. In contrast, we recommend that families and schools provide adolescents with a certain degree of autonomy and encourage adolescents to self-organize their behaviors, which can reduce their tendencies to experience boredom. Accordingly, these less-bored adolescents are less likely to engage in high-frequency game play, thus decreasing the risk of engaging in PMPU. Additionally, families and school personnel could try to purposefully increase diverse activities to avoid boredom from adolescents, as well as to guide adolescents to increase appropriate mobile phone use and decrease excessive mobile gaming, which may be instrumental to prevent from addiction-like online behaviors.

5. Conclusions

This is one of very few studies to focus on the association between autonomy need dissatisfaction in daily life and PMPU. With boredom proneness and mobile phone gaming introduced, the mediation model may contribute to explaining the potential mechanism of this association. Based on three-wave data, the results showed that T1 autonomy need dissatisfaction not only directly predicted T3 PMPU, but also exerted effects on T3 PMPU via the mediating role of T2 boredom proneness and via the chain mediating role of T2 boredom proneness and T2 mobile phone gaming. Altogether, these findings reveal the unique role of specific psychological need satisfaction in PMPU, which suggests that promoting autonomy need satisfaction may prevent adolescents from mobile phone addiction.

Author Contributions: Conceptualization, W.H. and R.-D.L.; Formal analysis, W.H.; Funding acquisition, R.-D.L.; Investigation, R.Z., R.J. and X.F.; Project administration, R.-D.L.; Supervision, R.-D.L.; Validation, R.-D.L. and Y.D.; Writing—original draft, W.H.; Writing—review and editing, W.H. and Y.D. All authors have read and agreed to the published version of the manuscript.

Acknowledgments: We appreciated the support from the participating schools' students and teachers.

References

1.   Vally, Z.; El Hichami, F. An examination of problematic mobile phone use in the United Arab Emirates: Prevalence, correlates, and predictors in a college-aged sample of young adults. *Addict. Behav. Rep.* **2019**, *9*, 100185. [CrossRef] [PubMed]

2.   Elhai, J.D.; Dvorak, R.D.; Levine, J.C.; Hall, B.J. Problematic smartphone use: A conceptual overview and systematic review of relations with anxiety and depression psychopathology. *J. Affect. Disord.* **2017**, *207*, 251–259. [CrossRef] [PubMed]

3.   CNNIC. The 45th China Statistical Report on Internet Development. 2020. Available online: http://www.cnnic.net.cn/hlwfzyj/hlwxzbg/hlwtjbg/202004/P020200428596599037028.pdf (accessed on 28 April 2020).

4.   Bianchi, A.; Phillips, J.G. Psychological predictors of problem mobile phone use. *Cyberpsychol. Behav.* **2005**, *8*, 39–51. [CrossRef] [PubMed]

5.   Liu, Q.Q.; Zhou, Z.K.; Yang, X.J.; Kong, F.C.; Niu, G.F.; Fan, C.Y. Mobile phone addiction and sleep quality among Chinese adolescents: A moderated mediation model. *Comput. Hum. Behav.* **2017**, *72*, 108–114. [CrossRef]

6.   Hong, W.; Liu, R.-D.; Ding, Y.; Sheng, X.; Zhen, R. Mobile phone addiction and cognitive failures in daily life: The mediating roles of sleep duration and quality and the moderating role of trait self-regulation. *Addict. Behav.* **2020**, *107*, 106383. [CrossRef] [PubMed]

7.   Seo, D.G.; Park, Y.; Kim, M.K.; Park, J. Mobile phone dependency and its impacts on adolescents' social and academic behaviors. *Comput. Hum. Behav.* **2016**, *63*, 282–292. [CrossRef]

8.   Jun, S. Longitudinal influences of depressive moods on problematic mobile phone use and negative school outcomes among Korean adolescents. *Sch. Psychol. Int.* **2019**, *40*, 294–308. [CrossRef]

9.   Hadlington, L.J. Cognitive failures in daily life: Exploring the link with internet addiction and problematic mobile phone use. *Comput. Hum. Behav.* **2015**, *51*, 75–81. [CrossRef]

10.   Chen, L.; Yan, Z.; Tang, W.; Yang, F.; Xie, X.; He, J. Mobile phone addiction levels and negative emotions among Chinese young adults: The mediating role of interpersonal problems. *Comput. Hum. Behav.* **2016**, *55*, 856–866. [CrossRef]

11.   Kim, E.; Cho, I.; Kim, E.J. Structural equation model of smartphone addiction based on adult attachment theory: Mediating effects of loneliness and depression. *Asian Nurs. Res.* **2017**, *11*, 92–97. [CrossRef]

12.   Asante, K.O.; Nyako, J. The physical and behavioural consequences of Facebook use among university students. *Mediterr. J. Soc. Sci.* **2014**, *5*, 774–781. [CrossRef]

13.   Lopez-Fernandez, O.; Honrubia-Serrano, L.; Freixa-Blanxart, M.; Gibson, W. Prevalence of problematic mobile phone use in British adolescents. *Cyberpsychol. Behav. Soc. Netw.* **2014**, *17*, 91–98. [CrossRef] [PubMed]

14.   Katz, E.; Blumler, J.; Gurevitch, M. Utilization of mass communication by the individual. In *The Uses of Mass Communications: Current Perspectives on Gratifications Research*; Katz, E., Blumler, J., Eds.; Sage: Beverly Hills, CA, USA, 1974; pp. 19–32.

15.   Kardefelt-Winther, D. A conceptual and methodological critique of internet addiction research: Towards a model of compensatory internet use. *Comput. Hum. Behav.* **2014**, *31*, 351–354. [CrossRef]

16.   Liu, Q.X.; Fang, X.Y.; Wan, J.J.; Zhou, Z.K. Need satisfaction and adolescent pathological internet use: Comparison of satisfaction perceived online and offline. *Comput. Hum. Behav.* **2016**, *55*, 695–700. [CrossRef]

17.   Hong, W.; Liu, R.-D.; Oei, T.-P.; Zhen, R.; Jiang, S.; Sheng, X. The mediating and moderating roles of social anxiety and relatedness need satisfaction on the relationship between shyness and problematic mobile phone use among adolescents. *Comput. Hum. Behav.* **2019**, *93*, 301–308. [CrossRef]

18. Deci, E.L.; Ryan, R.M. The "what" and "why" of goal pursuits: Human needs and the self-determination of behavior. *Psychol. Inq.* **2000**, *11*, 227–268. [CrossRef]

19. Chen, B.; Vansteenkiste, M.; Beyers, W.; Boone, L.; Deci, E.L.; Van der Kaap-Deeder, J.; Duriez, B.; Lens, W.; Matos, L.; Mouratidis, A.; et al. Basic psychological need satisfaction, need frustration, and need strength across four cultures. *Motiv. Emot.* **2014**, *39*, 216–236. [CrossRef]

20. Mills, D.J.; Milyavskaya, M.; Heath, N.L.; Derevensky, J.L. Gaming motivation and problematic video gaming: The role of needs frustration. *Eur. J. Soc. Psychol.* **2018**, *48*, 551–559. [CrossRef]

21. Ryan, R.M.; Deci, E.L. *Self-Determination Theory: Basic Psychological Needs in Motivation, Development, and Wellness*; Guilford Publications: New York, NY, USA, 2017.

22. Davis, R.A. A cognitive-behavioral model of pathological internet use. *Comput. Hum. Behav.* **2001**, *17*, 187–195. [CrossRef]

23. Alvarez, M.S.; Balaguer, I.; Castillo, I.; Duda, J.L. Coach autonomy support and quality of sport engagement in young soccer players. *Span. J. Psychol.* **2009**, *12*, 138–148. [CrossRef]

24. Ksinan, A.J.; Mališ, J.; Vazsonyi, A.T. Swiping away the moments that make up a dull day: Narcissism, boredom, and compulsive smartphone use. *Curr. Psychol.* **2019**. Published online. [CrossRef]

25. Biolcati, R.; Mancini, G.; Trombini, E. Proneness to boredom and risk behaviors during adolescents' free time. *Psychol. Rep.* **2018**, *121*, 303–323. [CrossRef] [PubMed]

26. Jeong, S.H.; Kim, H.; Yum, J.Y.; Hwang, Y. What type of content are smartphone users addicted to?: SNS vs. games. *Comput. Hum. Behav.* **2016**, *54*, 10–17. [CrossRef]

27. Struk, A.A.; Carriere, J.S.; Cheyne, J.A.; Danckert, J. A short boredom proneness scale: Development and psychometric properties. *Assessment* **2015**, *24*, 346–359. [CrossRef] [PubMed]

28. Farmer, R.; Sundberg, N.D. Boredom proneness: The development and correlates of a new scale. *J. Pers. Assess.* **1986**, *50*, 4–17. [CrossRef] [PubMed]

29. González, L.; Castillo, I.; Balaguer, I. Exploring the role of resilience and basic psychological needs as antecedents of enjoyment and boredom in female sports. *Rev. Psicodidáctica* **2019**, *24*, 131–137.

30. Sulea, C.; van Beek, I.; Sarbescu, P.; Virga, D.; Schaufeli, W.B. Engagement, boredom, and burnout among students: Basic need satisfaction matters more than personality traits. *Learn. Individ. Differ.* **2015**, *42*, 132–138. [CrossRef]

31. Van Hooff, M.L.M.; Van Hooft, E.A.J. Boredom at work: Towards a dynamic spillover model of need satisfaction, work motivation, and work-related boredom. *Eur. J. Work Organ. Psychol.* **2016**, *26*, 133–148. [CrossRef]

32. Skues, J.; Williams, B.; Oldmeadow, J.; Wise, L. The effects of boredom, loneliness, and distress tolerance on problem internet use among university students. *Int. J. Ment. Health Addict.* **2015**, *14*, 167–180. [CrossRef]

33. Nichols, L.A.; Nicki, R. Development of a psychometrically sound internet addiction scale: A preliminary step. *Psychol. Addict. Behav.* **2004**, *18*, 381–384. [CrossRef]

34. Leung, L. Linking psychological attributes to addiction and improper use of the mobile phone among adolescents in Hong Kong. *J. Child. Media* **2008**, *2*, 93–113. [CrossRef]

35. Lin, C.H.; Yu, S.F. Adolescent internet usage in Taiwan: Exploring gender differences. *Adolescence* **2008**, *43*, 317–331. [PubMed]

36. Kim, K.; Schmierbach, M.G.; Bellur, S.; Chung, M.Y.; Fraustino, J.D.; Dardis, F.; Ahern, L. Is it a sense of autonomy, control, or attachment? Exploring the effects of in-game customization on game enjoyment. *Comput. Hum. Behav.* **2015**, *48*, 695–705. [CrossRef]

37. Mills, D.J.; Allen, J.J. Self-determination theory, internet gaming disorder, and the mediating role of self-control. *Comput. Hum. Behav.* **2020**, *105*, 106209. [CrossRef]

38. Scerri, M.; Anderson, A.; Stavropoulos, V.; Hu, E. Need fulfilment and internet gaming disorder: A preliminary integrative model. *Addict. Behav. Rep.* **2019**, *9*, 100144. [CrossRef]

39. Leung, L. Exploring the relationship between smartphone activities, flow experience, and boredom in free time. *Comput. Hum. Behav.* **2020**, *103*, 130–139. [CrossRef]

40. Lee, H.; Kim, J.W.; Choi, T.Y. Risk factors for smartphone addiction in Korean adolescents: Smartphone use patterns. *J. Korean Med. Sci.* **2017**, *32*, 1674–1679. [CrossRef]

41. Škařupová, K.; Ólafsson, K.; Blinka, L. The effect of smartphone use on trends in European adolescents' excessive internet use. *Behav. Inf. Technol.* **2015**, *35*, 68–74. [CrossRef]

42. van Rooij, A.J.; Schoenmakers, T.M.; van de Eijnden, R.J.; Van de Mheen, D. Compulsive internet use: The role of online gaming and other internet applications. *J. Adolesc. Health* **2010**, *47*, 51–57. [CrossRef]

43. Hao, Z.; Jin, L.; Li, Y.; Akram, H.R.; Saeed, M.F.; Ma, J.; Ma, H.; Huang, J. Alexithymia and mobile phone addiction in Chinese undergraduate students: The roles of mobile phone use patterns. *Comput. Hum. Behav.* **2019**, *97*, 51–59. [CrossRef]

44. Chou, W.J.; Chang, Y.P.; Yen, C.F. Boredom proneness and its correlation with internet addiction and internet activities in adolescents with attention-deficit/hyperactivity disorder. *Kaohsiung J. Med. Sci.* **2018**, *34*, 467–474. [CrossRef] [PubMed]

45. Mcleod, C.R.; Vodanovich, S.J. The relationship between self-actualization and boredom proneness. *J. Soc. Behav. Pers.* **1991**, *6*, 137–146.

46. Pekrun, R.; Goetz, T.; Daniels, L.M.; Stupnisky, R.H.; Perry, R.P. Boredom in achievement settings: Exploring control–value antecedents and performance outcomes of a neglected emotion. *J. Educ. Psychol.* **2010**, *102*, 531–549. [CrossRef]

47. Johnston, M.M.; Finney, S.J. Measuring basic needs satisfaction: Evaluating previous research and conducting new psychometric evaluations of the basic needs satisfaction in general scale. *Contemp. Educ. Psychol.* **2010**, *35*, 280–296. [CrossRef]

48. Shen, C.X.; Liu, R.D.; Wang, D. Why are children attracted to the internet? The role of need satisfaction perceived online and perceived in daily real life. *Comput. Hum. Behav.* **2013**, *29*, 185–192. [CrossRef]

49. Wang, C.; Hsu, H.C.K.; Bonem, E.M.; Moss, J.D.; Yu, S.; Nelson, D.B.; Levesque-Bristol, C. Need satisfaction and need dissatisfaction: A comparative study of online and face-to-face learning contexts. *Comput. Hum. Behav.* **2019**, *95*, 114–125. [CrossRef]

50. Shen, C.X.; Liu, R.D.; Wang, D. The relationship between internet use and children's loneliness: A moderating effect of personality. *J. Psychol. Sci.* **2013**, *36*, 1140–1145. (In Chinese)

51. Foerster, M.; Roser, K.; Schoeni, A.; Röösli, M. Problematic mobile phone use in adolescents: Derivation of a short scale MPPUS-10. *Int. J. Public Health* **2015**, *60*, 277–286. [CrossRef]

52. Liu, R.D.; Hong, W.; Ding, Y.; Oei, T.P.; Zhen, R.; Jiang, S.; Liu, J. Psychological distress and problematic mobile phone use among adolescents: The mediating role of maladaptive cognitions and the moderating role of effortful control. *Front. Psychol.* **2019**, *10*, 1589. [CrossRef]

53. Cheung, M.W.L. Comparison of approaches to constructing confidence intervals for mediating effects using structural equation models. *Struct. Equ. Modeling* **2007**, *14*, 227–246. [CrossRef]

54. Wen, Z.L.; Hau, K.T.; Marsh, H.W. Structural equation model testing: Cutoff criteria for goodness of fit indices and chi-square test. *Acta Psychol. Sin.* **2004**, *36*, 186–194. (In Chinese)

55. Wu, Y.; Wen, Z. Item parceling strategies in structural equation modeling. *Adv. Psychol. Sci.* **2011**, *19*, 1859–1867. (In Chinese)

56. MacKinnon, D.P.; Lockwood, C.M.; Williams, J. Confidence limits for the indirect effect: Distribution of the product and resampling methods. *Multivar. Behav. Res.* **2004**, *39*, 99–128. [CrossRef] [PubMed]

57. Allen, J.J.; Anderson, C.A. Satisfaction and frustration of basic psychological needs in the real world and in video games predict internet gaming disorder scores and well-being. *Comput. Hum. Behav.* **2018**, *84*, 220–229. [CrossRef]

58. Zhou, H.; Long, L. Statistical remedies for common method biases. *Adv. Psychol. Sci.* **2004**, *12*, 942–950. (In Chinese)

59. Gall, M.D.; Gall, J.P.; Borg, W.R. *Educational Research: An Introduction*, 8th ed.; Pearson: Boston, MA, USA, 2007.

60. Ellis, P.D. *The Essential Guide to Effect Sizes—Statistical Power, Meta-Analysis, and the Interpretation of Research Results*; Cambridge University Press: New York, NY, USA, 2010.

61. Hefner, D.; Knop, K.; Schmitt, S.; Vorderer, P. Rules? Role model? Relationship? The impact of parents on their children's problematic mobile phone involvement. *Media Psychol.* **2018**, *22*, 82–108. [CrossRef]

62. Fu, X.; Liu, J.; Liu, R.D.; Ding, Y.; Wang, J.; Zhen, R.; Jin, F. Parental monitoring and adolescent problematic mobile phone use: The mediating role of escape motivation and the moderating role of shyness. *Int. J. Environ. Res. Public Health* **2020**, *17*, 1487. [CrossRef]

6

The Prevalence of E-Gambling and Problem of E-Gambling in Poland

Bernadeta Lelonek-Kuleta *, Rafał P. Bartczuk, Michał Wiechetek, Joanna Chwaszcz and Iwona Niewiadomska

Institute of Psychology, The John Paul II Catholic University of Lublin, 20-950 Lublin, Poland; bartczuk@kul.lublin.pl (R.P.B.); wiechetek@kul.lublin.pl (M.W.); chwaszcz@kul.lublin.pl (J.C.); pfrau@kul.lublin.pl (I.N.)
* Correspondence: bernadetalelonek@kul.lublin.pl

Abstract: This study estimated the levels of involvement in e-gambling and problem e-gambling in Poland and identified selected sociodemographic variables associated with e-gambling activities. The study was conducted using a representative sample of the adult inhabitants of Poland ($n = 2000$). The survey contained questions measuring three aspects of gambling (involvement in e-gambling, types of e-gambling activity, and problematic e-gambling). Results suggested that 4.1% of respondents were involved in e-gambling and 26.8% of them could be classified as problem gamblers. The most popular e-gambling games were lotteries and sports betting. Gender, age, size of city of residence, level of education, and income were identified as significant predictors of involvement in e-gambling. The results indicated that men, younger people, and people who earnt less were more often involved in e-gambling. Having children, playing online scratch cards, and online sport betting—but not online lotteries—turned out to be typical for problem online gamblers. The prevalence of problem gambling among Polish e-gamblers suggests that extended research in this area is needed.

Keywords: e-gambling; e-gambling prevalence; forms of e-gambling; problem e-gambling

1. Introduction

The involvement of societies in gambling is a subject that has interested researchers for many years [1,2]. Gambling, as an entertainment form permitted for adults, involves a game in which there is a valuable stake, the result of which partially depends on chance, and it interests the representatives of social sciences mostly due to the potential damages that the activity can cause if specific circumstances arise. In 2013, in the 5th edition of the Diagnostic and Statistical Manual of Mental Disorders (DSM-5), pathological gambling was included in the group of non-substance related disorders (in section: Substance-Related and Addictive Disorders), which made the scientific world admit that pathological gambling and substance addiction have common development mechanisms and analogous symptoms [3]. The World Health Organisation included gambling disorder in the section "Disorders" due to substance use or addictive behaviours in the 11th edition of the International Classification of Diseases (ICD) classification. It is noteworthy that WHO distinguishes two categories of this disorder, including: 6C50.0 gambling disorder, predominantly offline, and 6C50.1 gambling disorder, predominantly online [4]. The development of addiction is most often described in four stages, common for substance and behavioural addictions. Taking the example of exercise addiction, they are as follows: recreational exercise, at-risk exercise, problematic exercise, and exercise addiction [5]. The traditional description of the gambling disorder has included four phases: the reaction to winning, losing, desperation, and hopelessness [6]. The next distinguished phases are accompanied by an increasing intensity of problems resulting from involvement in a given activity, progressive concentration and loss of control. According to researchers, the social consequences of gambling abuse include decreased productivity, social welfare costs resulting from absence from work [7], loss of jobs, early retirement, and even an increase in mortality resulting from suicidal tendencies occurring at advanced stages of gambling addiction [8,9]. Social detriments are also considered in the context of elevated distress and social isolation resulting from gambling [10].

Despite the long tradition of research on the involvement in gambling and problem gambling, a new phenomenon that has very quickly caused concern among the specialists emerged in the recent decades—online gambling [11]. Studies on online gambling have led many researchers to conclude that it has higher addictive potential than any other type of gambling [12–16]. Although results that do not confirm the higher addictive potential of online gambling do exist, most studies confirm this phenomenon [17,18]. Its high addictive potential is further confirmed by the higher rate of gambling addiction among online gamblers than among those who gamble in the traditional form [16,19,20]; this increase may even be three to five times higher [21]. The studies conducted by Effertz et al. on a representative group of 15,023 Germans showed that replacing 10% of offline gambling with online gambling increased the risk of becoming a problem gambler by 8.8–12.6% [22].

As for the increase in problem gambling among online players, the results of international studies conducted by McCormack among 1119 gamblers showed that 14% met the Problem Gambling Severity Index (PGSI) criteria for problem gambling, 29% met the criteria for moderate risk gambling, 32.7% met the criteria for problem gambling at a low level, and 24.3% did not show symptoms indicating problems resulting from gambling [23].

Why online gambling is more addictive remains uncertain; does it result from its higher accessibility, or, perhaps, from the nature of the Internet as a medium via which players gamble? [17,18]. Some studies have reported a lower percentage of addicted gamblers among "pure" online gamblers in comparison with "pure" offline gamblers [18]. Studies have, however, determined certain factors increasing the addictive potential of online gaming, including the games' structure, which consists of, among other things, directness, accessibility, and ease of betting, all of which are particularly dangerous for young gamblers [24]. These factors are said by other gamblers, to have addictive potential. For example, Griffiths et al. also indicated factors related to the games' structure—the directness of reinforcement, the speed of their course, and the frequency of game appearance—but also situational factors, such as accessibility and availability—which other researchers have also confirmed [25–29].

Online gambling seems to be more attractive for various reasons. It offers gamblers additional profits from gambling compared to offline gambling. First and foremost, gamblers can play whenever and wherever they choose (at home or work), which is associated with a high level of comfort and low access costs: players do not need to travel to certain locations, dedicate their time, and so forth [12]. Gamblers also save time because they can play several games simultaneously, which accelerates the course of online games [30,31]. The basic benefit of online gambling is anonymity, which seems to be particularly desirable for certain types of users [32,33].

Recent studies on involvement in online gambling have mainly focused on identifying the risk factors of problem gambling. The studies conducted by Effertz et al. on a representative group of Germans indicated that the risk of problem gambling decreases with higher levels of education and increases in the case of men; people who are unemployed, single, and divorced (respectively); and among migrants [22]. Effertz et al. also noticed that the risk of problem online gambling is the highest among heavy Internet users. Scientists have also drawn attention to the correlation between the type of game and problem gambling. For example, McCormack et al. observed that the risk of problem online gambling was significantly higher among people who gamble regularly and play online betting games, online slot machines, and online roulette, compared to gamblers who do not play regularly. In addition, persons who regularly played two or more types of online games were also at considerably greater risk of developing problem gambling than those who played one game only [23]. Other studies [34] have also highlighted the correlation between the number of the gambling accounts a gamer has, increased involvement in gambling, and increased intensity of problem gaming [35]. In the McCormack studies, people who regularly played only online poker were at lower risk of problem gambling than people who did not play poker regularly, but played other games as well, which is in line with the results of other studies [36]. Although the results suggest that there is a correlation between multi-gambling and problem gambling, researchers have emphasised the shortage of studies in the area [23].

There are few studies on gender differences in online gambling involvement. For example, studies conducted in Ireland have shown that women prefer online games that are more acceptable socially, such as lotteries or scratch cards [37]. Scratch cards are also the game type that women tend to become addicted to, which has also been highlighted by other researchers [32]. Women, on average, play for a shorter period of time (an average of two years for women and seven years for men), and spend less time gambling online than men (1 h per session, compared to 3 h for men).

Legal regulations are another aspect that has also been regarded as significant in recent studies on online gambling, particularly concerning the involvement of citizens in gambling. In his 2016 study, which included 1277 pathological gamblers undergoing addiction treatment, Chóliz discovered significant changes that occurred between 2012 (when online gambling was legalised in Spain) and the turn of 2014/2015. First and foremost, the number of people entering treatment due to pathological gambling in the studied facilities quadrupled. Also, most importantly, patients indicated online gambling as the source of their problems ten times more often than in 2012 (from 2.53% in 2012 to 24.21% in 2014/2015). For a comparison, the number of people indicating slot machines as the main source of their problems decreased (from 80.26% to 65.71%). These results seem particularly important in the context of the tendency to legalise online gambling and liberalise access to it, which has been observed by the specialists [38,39]. Moreover, researchers have also noted that using legal websites for online gambling causes less gambling-related damage [40], and a higher percentage of problem gambling occurs in populations in which legal regulations for online gambling are less restrictive [41].

The gambling market in Poland is regulated by the Act of 19 November 2009 on online gambling, which has so far been amended several times. In light of the Act of 15 December 2016 amending the Act on gambling, online gambling—with the exclusion of pari-mutuel betting and promotional lotteries—is subject to state monopoly [42]. Online games subject to state monopoly are organised by Totalizator Sportowy—a company owned by the State Treasury (Warsaw, Poland). The first online gambling games were introduced by Totalizator Sportowy in December 2018 and included a number of lotteries and games offered by the only legal online casino in Poland—slot machines, roulette, and card games for money. Legal online betting games are currently offered by nine private operators. Until 2017, when Poland tightened its restrictions on the betting market, introducing the possibility of blocking illegal domains, 90% of the industry belonged to the grey market [43].

Due to the relatively recent regulation of online gambling in Poland, there have thus far been no studies on the matter. It is worth noting that the longer tradition of research in Poland on addiction to slot machines resulted in the regulation of the market for these games [44]. The first study to estimate the involvement of Polish people in online gambling, and problem involvement in the activity and its determinants, was therefore, undertaken.

2. Materials and Methods

2.1. Participants

This study was conducted on a nationwide sample of 2000 adult Poles. The sample was representative and randomly selected on the basis of PESEL (Personal Identification Number). The distribution of gender, age, education, the size of place of residence, the region, and the number of people in the household were controlled. The Polish population was layered according to 9 geographical macro-regions, and then, in each of them, the localities were layered into 7 layers, according to size; the municipalities with probabilities proportional to the number of residents older than 18 years of age were randomly selected. Within the framework of each selected municipality, 6 interviews with randomly selected respondents were carried out. The respondents in municipalities were at first selected by means of drawing households proportionally to the number of household members according to the PESEL census records. Upon visiting a selected household, the interviewers selected the respondents using the Kish grid and then conducted computer-assisted personal interviews with them. If conducting the interview with the person from the list was not possible, the interviewer would look for a person of the same age and gender in the same town. The study was carried out by the GfK Polonia, the Polish branch of a well-known international public opinion research institute (GfK SE, Nuremberg, Germany), which also ensured the anonymity and uniformity of testing.

2.2. Measures

2.2.1. E-Gambling

The questionnaire consisted of questions regarding use of online gambling games, frequency, frequency of online gambling, time duration of a single session, and money spent on online gambling. In the first question, the respondent was asked to select the online games on which they have bet money at least once within the last 12 months. The list included 11 categories: online lottery (i.e., receipt lottery), online scratch cards, slot machines and other gambling machines on the Internet, online card games for money, other online casino games (i.e., roulette, dice), Totalizator Sportowy number games via the Internet, other online number games (i.e., bingo), online arcade games for money, online sports betting (including "fantasy sports"), online betting on e-sport or online virtual sports, and online betting on financial markets (i.e., stock exchange, FOREX, binary options). A memory-activating filtering statement was posed: "I am certain that I have not made online cash bets within the last 12 months." The question regarding e-gambling frequency was: How often, within the last 12 months, have you gambled online? (1 = everyday; 2 = several times a week, but not every day; 3 = once a week; 4 = several times a month but more rarely than once a week; 5 = once a month; 6 = several times a year, but more rarely than once a month). The question regarding the time duration of a single session was: How much time did one session of the game usually take? (1 = less than 15 min; 2 = from 15 to 30 min; 3 = from 31 min to an hour; 4 = from over an hour to 2 h; 5 = from over 2 h to 3 h; 6 = more than 3 h). The question regarding spending was open: "How much money exactly have you spent on online gambling within the last 4 months?"

2.2.2. Problem E-Gambling

The Brief Biosocial Gambling Screen (BBGS), adapted to Polish by Niewiadomska et al., was adjusted to the assessment of problem e-gambling [45,46]. It contains three questions about gambling and has been shown to have good screening properties for the criteria of problem gambling compliant with DSM-5 [47]. Each of the questions could be answered with either "Yes" or "No." The risk of problem gambling cut-off at endorsing one symptom is the best indicator of gambling disorder, taking into account that sensitivity and negative predictive value are most important for identifying individuals who potentially need treatment [45,47]. The psychometric properties of the Polish adaptation of BBGS were tested on a representative sample of high school students of the Lublin province. The criterion was fulfilment of at least 5 DSM-IV criteria of pathological hazard, measured by self-report. Sensitivity was 0.82, and specificity was 0.96 [46]. Because not distinguishing by a measure of problem gambling between forms of gambling (online versus offline) is a potentially confounding issue [48], we adjusted the BBGS for the purposes of the current study by rewording the questions in the BBGS to refer to online gambling. The final versions of the questions used in this study were as follows: Within the last 12 months, have you felt powerless, irritated, or anxious when you were trying to quit or limit online gambling? Within the last 12 months, have you tried to keep the fact that you are gambling online from your family and friends? Have you had financial trouble resulting from online gaming, because of which you had to ask your family, friends, or social services for financial support within the last 12 months?

2.2.3. Sociodemographic Variables

Information on the sociodemographic profiles of the respondents was obtained from data collected by the interviewer and from the questionnaire. The sociodemographic questions were answered by 2000 people. Their average age was 45.61 years (SD = 18.456, minimum = 18, maximum = 94). Table 1 presents the sociodemographic descriptive statistics.

Table 1. Descriptive statistics for the sociodemographic variables for the test group ($n = 2000$).

Variable	Category	n	%
Gender	Male	964	48.2
	Female	1036	51.8
Place of residence	countryside	815	40.8
	town of up to 20,000 residents	263	13.1
	town of 20,000–50,000 residents	213	10.7
	town of 50,000–100,000 residents	163	8.2
	town of 100,000–00,000 residents	151	7.6
	city of 200,000–500,000 residents	182	9.1
	city of more than 500,000 residents	212	10.6
Education	primary	481	24.0
	basic vocational	469	23.4
	secondary	683	34.1
	higher	368	18.4
Frequency of Internet use	nearly every day	1209	60.5
	at least once in a month	276	13.8
	less frequently or does not use at all.	514	25.7
Monthly household income	up to PLN 2000	156	7.8
	PLN 2000–2999	231	11.5
	PLN 3000–4499	487	24.4
	PLN 4500 and above	1125	56.3
Children living in the same household	Yes	268	63.4
	No	732	36.6

Note: PLN—Polish zloty; 1€ ≈ 4.3 PLN.

2.3. Data Analysis

All statistical analyses were performed using IBM SPSS version 24 software [49]. We used methods and statistics appropriate to the types of measurement scale and the specific parameters applied. Categorical data are presented as frequencies and percentages, and group comparisons were made using the χ^2-test. We used logistic regression (enter method and simple contras, with the reference category first) to identify the variables that best predict involvement in e-gambling.

3. Results

3.1. Popularity of Gambling and Types of Games

The results obtained indicate that 83 (4.1%; 95% CI (3.3%, 5.1%)) of the 2000 respondents surveyed in the last 12 months have made monetary bets using online gambling services. Most respondents played Totalizator Sportowy lotteries, online sports betting, sports betting concerning e-sport or virtual sport, and online card games for money. Online slot and gambling machines and online betting on the financial markets were used least frequently. None of the respondents indicated using online arcade games for money (Table 2).

Table 2. Prevalence of forms of online gambling ($N = 2000$).

Game Type	n	%	95% CILL	95% CIUL
Totalizator Sportowy lotteries	41	2.0	1.5	2.7
Online sports betting (including "fantasy sports")	19	1.0	0.6	1.4
Online betting on e-sports or online virtual sports	11	0.6	0.3	0.9
Online card games for money	10	0.5	0.3	0.9
Online scratch cards	6	0.3	0.1	0.6
Other online casino games (e.g., roulette, dice)	5	0.2	0.1	0.5
Internet lottery (e.g., receipt lottery)	4	0.2	0.1	0.5
Other online lotteries (e.g., bingo)	4	0.2	0.1	0.5
Slot machines or other online gambling machines	1	0.1	0.0	0.2
Online betting on financial markets	1	0.1	0.0	0.2
Online arcade games for money	0	0.0	0.0	0.0

Note: 95% CILL: 95% confidence interval lower limit; 95% CIUL: 95% confidence interval upper limit.

3.2. Sociodemographic Variables Associated with Online Gambling

Logistic regression was used to assess the factors associated with involvement in online gambling (cf. Table 3). The dependent variable had two categories (1—gambling versus 0—not using online gambling services in the last twelve months). Age, gender, population of the place of residence, education, income level, having children, and frequency of Internet use were considered as independent variables. The factors that significantly explained involvement in online gambling were: gender, age, population of the place of residence, education, and monthly family income. Men were more likely to be involved in gambling activities than women. In terms of age, the youngest group (up to age 29) was significantly more likely to be involved in online gambling than older people (over 50). Analysing the size of the place of residence, people living in the countryside were significantly different from those living in towns with 20,000–100,000 residents and those coming from cities of 200,000–500,000 residents. Online gambling activity was much less frequent among people living in towns or cities compared to people living in the countryside. Higher online gambling activity could also be seen among people with primary education compared to those with vocational education. Monthly income was also an important factor explaining involvement in online gambling. People with low monthly incomes were much more likely to devote their time to online gambling than those earning more than PLN 3000. Frequency of Internet use was also an element co-existing with online gambling activity. Individuals using the Internet more frequently were also inclined to become more involved in online gambling.

Table 3. An explanatory model of e-gambling ($n = 2000$).

Variables	B	SE	Wald	df	p	Exp(B)	95% CI for EXP(B)	
							Lower	Upper
Gender: (ref.: male)	−1.129	0.282	16.055	1	<0.001	0.323	0.186	0.562
Age: (ref.: 15–29 years of age)			21.002	5	0.001			
30–39	−0.527	0.367	2.067	1	0.150	0.590	0.288	1.211
40–49	0.414	0.319	1.685	1	0.194	1.513	0.810	2.829
50–59	−2.904	1.004	8.366	1	0.004	0.055	0.008	0.392
60–69	−1.392	0.681	4.178	1	0.041	0.249	0.065	0.944
70 and above	−2.135	1.166	3.353	1	0.067	0.118	0.012	1.162
Population of the place of residence: (ref.: countryside)			15.507	6	0.017			
town of up to 20,000 residents	0.072	0.377	0.036	1	0.849	1.074	0.513	2.248
town of 20,000–50,000 residents	−1.266	0.559	5.125	1	0.024	0.282	0.094	0.844
town of 50,000–100,000 residents	−1.103	0.580	3.615	1	0.057	0.332	0.106	1.035
town of 100,000–200,000 residents	−0.649	0.509	1.625	1	0.202	0.523	0.193	1.417
city of 200,000–500,000 residents	−4.465	2.268	3.876	1	0.049	0.012	0.000	0.980
city of more than 500,000 residents	0.307	0.379	0.659	1	0.417	1.360	0.647	2.855
Education: (ref.: primary)			14.184	3	0.003			
basic vocational	−1.851	0.547	11.450	1	0.001	0.157	0.054	0.459
secondary	−0.189	0.327	0.335	1	0.563	0.828	0.436	1.570
higher	0.244	0.378	0.415	1	0.519	1.276	0.608	2.675
Children living in the same household: [ref.: no children]	0.260	0.289	0.809	1	0.368	1.297	0.736	2.283
Household net income: (ref.: up to PLN 2000)			24.876	3	0.000			
PLN 2000–2999	−1.105	0.580	3.630	1	0.057	0.331	0.106	1.032
PLN 3000–4499	−1.732	0.532	10.593	1	0.001	0.177	0.062	0.502
PLN 4500 and above	−2.405	0.517	21.649	1	0.000	0.090	0.033	0.249
Internet use: (ref.: nearly every day)			5.077	2	0.079			
at least once in a month	−0.128	0.481	0.071	1	0.789	0.880	0.343	2.256
less frequently or does not use at all	−1.758	0.782	5.054	1	0.025	0.172	0.037	0.798
constantly	−4.682	0.450	108.157	1	0.000	0.009		

Note: Overall model evaluation: Likelihood ratio test: $\chi^2(21) = 167.916$; $p < 0.001$; Cox and Snell $R^2 = 0.081$; Nagelkerke's $R^2 = 0.276$.

3.3. Prevalence of Problem Gambling among Players and Related Factors

Out of the 83 people who participated in online gambling, 22 (26.8%; 95% CI (17.9%, 36.7%)) were at risk of becoming problem gamblers. This group consisted of respondents who provided at least one affirmative answer on the BBGS scale. In order to determine the characteristics of problem online gamblers, we compared them to non-problematic gamblers in respect of sociodemographic variables using the chi-square test (cf. Table 4).

A comparison between gamblers at risk of becoming problem gamblers and those who were not at such risk indicated several differentiating variables (cf. Table 4). These included having children and choice of online e-gambling services. Individuals who manifested symptoms of problem use of e-gambling more frequently had children than those with no symptoms of problem gambling. PeGs were also less active in playing Totalizator Sportowy lotteries and more often used online sports betting (including fantasy sports) and online scratch cards.

Table 4. Comparison of sociodemographic variables between non-problem online gamblers (NPeG, n = 61) and problem online gamblers (PeG, n = 22).

Variables	NPeG		PeG		χ^2	p
	n	%	n	%		
Gender:					0.381	0.537
Male	45	75	15	68.2		
Female	15	25	7	31.8		
Age:					8.993	0.109
15–29	34	55.7	6	28.6		
30–39	10	16.4	3	14.3		
40–49	14	23.0	10	47.6		
50–59	1	1.6	0	0		
60–69	1	1.6	2	9.5		
70 and above	1	1.6	0	0		
Population of the place of residence:					5.320	0.503
countryside	25	41.7	14	60.9		
town of up to 20,000 residents	9	15.0	2	8.7		
town of 20,000–50,000 residents	3	5.0	1	4.3		
town of 50,000–100,000 residents	4	6.7	0	0		
town of 100,000–200,000 residents	5	8.3	0	0		
city of 200,000–500,000 residents	0	0	0	0		
city of more than 500,000 residents	14	23.3	6	26.1		
Education:					4.871	0.181
primary	16	26.2	11	50.0		
basic vocational	4	6.6	1	4.5		
secondary	22	36.1	7	31.8		
higher	19	31.1	3	13.6		
Children living in the same household:	24	40.0	15	68.2	5.126	0.022
Household net income:					3.540	0.316
up to PLN 2000	7	11.7	4	19.0		
PLN 2000–2999	8	13.3	1	4.8		
PLN 3000–4499	20	33.3	4	19.0		
PLN 4500 and above	25	41.7	12	57.1		
Internet use:					1.151	0.562
nearly every day	52	85.2	20	90.9		
at least once in a month	6	9.8	2	9.1		
less frequently or does not use at all.	3	4.9	0	0		
Types of online gambling services:						
Internet lottery	2	3.3	2	9.1	1.150	0.284
Online scratch cards	2	3.3	3	13.6	2.984	0.084
Slot machines or other online gambling machines	1	1.7	0	0	0.371	0.542
Online card games for money	8	13.1	2	9.1	0.247	0.619
Other online casino games (e.g., roulette, dice)	5	8.2	0	0	1.919	0.166
Totalizator Sportowy lotteries	36	59.0	5	21.7	9.289	0.002
Other online lotteries (e.g., bingo)	3	5.0	1	4.5	0.007	0.933
Online arcade games for money	0	0	0	0.0	-	-
Online sports betting (including "fantasy sports")	11	18.3	8	36.4	2.940	0.086
Online betting on e-sports or online virtual sports	10	16.7	1	4.5	2.036	0.154
Online betting on financial markets	1	1.6	0	0	0.365	0.546

Note: PeG—problem online gamblers; NPeG—non-problem online gamblers.

4. Discussion

The results of our study allowed us to determine the extent of the involvement of adult Poles in online gambling. First, it is worth mentioning that the first legitimate online gambling games in Poland were sports betting services, first organised in 2012. The provision of other online gambling services was regulated only by the 2016 Act, under which the provision of other online games is subject to a state monopoly [42]. It should be noted that, in practice, these games were made available on the market only in December 2018, which highlights the specificity of the e-gambling market in Poland and sheds light on the results of this study, which was conducted in December 2018. The lotteries organised by Totalizator Sportowy proved to be the most popular online and offline gambling games, having been the most common type of such games for Poles [50]. It is worth noting here that these games, covered by the state monopoly, may be advertised in public media, which significantly increases their potential accessibility compared to other types of gambling games, the advertising of which is prohibited by law. The second most popular games included sports betting and betting related to e-sports and virtual sports, the popularity of which may be explained by the relatively long history of this type of online gambling in Poland. The popularity of gambling reflects, to a large extent, the cultural specificity or legal regulations of a given country concerning the availability of games. For example, the most popular online gambling game in France is, among others, horse race betting, which illustrates the long-standing tradition of what is considered to be a national sport in France [51]. In Poland, football plays a similar role. The relatively high interest of Poles in e-sports or online virtual sports betting is a new trend. This phenomenon has not yet been assessed, so it is difficult to estimate the extent to which there is an upward trend or whether the behaviour has been long-standing. Taking into account the novelty of the phenomenon of e-sports betting, not only in Poland but also worldwide (e.g., this phenomenon was included in the national survey "e-Games France 2017" for the first time only in 2017), an upward trend may be expected [51]. The interest of Poles in such betting even exceeds the popularity of online card games, which is fourth in terms of popularity. The interest in online gambling as a whole seems to be low in Poland. During the 12-month period prior to the survey, 4.1% of adult Poles made an online bet, which is a very small percentage compared to the 37.1% of Poles engaged in offline gambling during the same period [48]. It is worth mentioning that, in the latest epidemiological study on behavioural addictions in Poland, only 1.2% of Poles declared that they had gambled online in the past year. However, it is also significant that, in this study, the category of online gambling was only one among nine categories of offline gambling.

Due to the fact that this was the first study on e-gambling in Poland, we were interested in determining which individuals choose this form of entertainment most often. The results showed that e-gambling was more popular with men than women, and that interest decreases with age. These data are confirmed by studies conducted in other countries [26,37]. Additionally, online gambling was more popular among those with incomes lower than the national average salary than those with incomes equal to or higher than the national average wage. Involvement in online gambling also decreased with the decline in daily Internet use. This phenomenon was all the more alarming because, in light of the Effertz study, the risk of problem online gambling is largest among highly engaged Internet users [22], which was confirmed by the research of Rémond and Romo [52]. The results obtained are in line with other studies, which show that the popularity of online gambling in the West is attributable, among other things, to low access costs—the gambler does not need to travel to the place where the game is played or devote time to such travel [12]. This makes online gambling more accessible from an economic point of view, and therefore more likely to be selected by people with lower socioeconomic status. Other researchers have also emphasised that accessibility and availability are the factors contributing to increased involvement in online gambling [25–29].

Finally, we were interested in the extent to which problem gambling was exacerbated among online gamblers. The study results showed that 26.8% of gamblers had symptoms indicating a probable gambling addiction on the basis of the BBGS scale. These results reveal that the risk of gambling addiction is higher among Polish online gamblers than among gamblers in general (both online and offline). In light of the latest results of a national survey conducted by the Centre for Public Opinion Research (CBOS: Centrum Badania Opinii Społecznej) on behavioural addictions, 7.7% of all gamblers show a low addiction risk, 0.9% of them a moderate risk level and 0.9% of gamblers are problem gamblers, making a total of 9.5% of gamblers at risk of addiction [53]. It should be mentioned, however, that the CBOS survey was conducted using the Canadian Problem Gambling Index (CPGI) scale.

Relating the results obtained in our study to other studies, a convergence may be observed. International online gambling studies have showed, for instance, that 14% of gamblers met the criteria for problem gambling in accordance with the Problem Gambling Severity Index, 29% met the criteria for risky gambling and 32.7% of gamblers met the criteria for problem gambling at a low level. Other studies also confirm greater exacerbation of problem gambling among online than offline gamblers [16,19,20], which is, according to some, even three to five times greater [21]. In Austrian studies, 31% of online gamblers showed symptoms of problem gambling, while 18% of offline gamblers displayed such symptoms in accordance with Lie-Bet questionnaire results [54].

The last aspect we analysed included sociodemographic variables coexisting with gambling addiction.

The first important factors differentiating gamblers at risk of a gambling disorder from non-problem gamblers were male gender and age from 40 to 49 years old. These results are surprising because Poles addicted to offline gambling are mainly younger people (18–24 years old) [53]. Nevertheless, the results obtained by us are consistent with the Austrian research of Yazdi and Katzian, in the light of which addicted online gamblers most often belong to the age range 30–49 years [54]. It seems that due to the relatively short period of online gambling being available in Poland, these games are mainly used by mature men who have longer experience with offline gambling, and are, therefore, consciously looking for a new offer of already known entertainment.

The level of education also differentiated problem and non-problem gamblers. Problem e-gamblers more often have primary education, which is also the case with offline gamblers in Poland.

The next important factor differentiating gamblers at risk of a gambling disorder from non-problem gamblers was the presence of children in the household. Gamblers at risk constituted a group that more often had children than representatives of the non-addicted group. This may be due to the higher age of problem e-gamblers. At this stage of study, we are still considering how to understand this relationship. It may be argued that people who are interested in gambling—and have children—have been more inclined to opt for online games which are more accessible due to time constraints. As studies confirm the stronger addictive potential of online gambling, this activity is, thus, more likely to turn into addiction. It can also be assumed that gamblers who do not have children gamble offline as well, but also opt for alternative, non-addictive offline entertainment, which is less accessible to those with children. Online gambling is more absorbing, allowing the gambler to play several games at once, as emphasised by both Cotte et al. and Gainsbury et al. [30,31]. The structural characteristics of online games—such as directness, accessibility, ease of betting, and the fact that they pose a particular risk of addiction—are also highlighted by Chóliz [24].

Accessibility factors are also revealed when linking residence to problem gambling. In light of the results, problem e-gamblers come, more often, from the countryside. Despite the fact that rural residents do not gamble online more often than urban residents, they develop problem e-gambling more often. It can be assumed that these people, with limited possibilities of enjoying other entertainment (including offline gambling), engage in e-gambling more intensively, which translates into an increased risk of developing addiction to these games.

Another factor significantly co-existing with the risk of gambling addiction was the type of game being played. In light of the results, gamblers at risk of addiction are more often involved in sports betting (including "fantasy sports"). These results correlate with McCormack's study, which showed that the risk of problem online gambling is significantly higher for, among others, online sports betting gamblers [23]. Given that sports betting is one of the most popular online gambling services in Poland, this is an important discovery. Problem e-gamblers are also more often involved in online scratch cards, which are one the most popular offline gambling game types in Poland [53].

Summarising the results of the study, it is worth once again referring to the Polish legal regulations on gambling. When the study was conducted, legitimate gambling, apart from sports betting, was in its early stages. It would be significant to monitor the development of Poles' involvement in online gambling as it becomes more widespread. Taking into account the relatively low involvement of Poles in online gambling, it may be assumed that the results obtained stem from the fact that these games were not yet very popular at the time the study was conducted. For instance, Chóliz [24] analysed the changes that occurred between 2012 (when online gambling was legalised in Spain) and the turn of 2014/2015, during which period the number of people who started treatment for pathological gambling quadrupled. Additionally, patients indicated online gambling as the main source of their problems nearly ten times more often in 2014/2015 than in 2012. With this in mind, it is extremely important to continue epidemiological studies on participation in online gambling and problem gambling to develop recommendations for legislators based on changes in the behaviour of gamblers resulting from the implementation of legal amendments. Legalisation of online gambling is a very important issue. Researchers note that the use of legitimate gambling sites causes less gambling-related harm than the use of illegal sites [40]. However, the legalisation of online gambling alone cannot be the only preventive factor. Its effects should be monitored and the next steps need to be adapted accordingly. It would be worthwhile to conduct future studies on the relationship between multi-gambling and gambling problems, especially as researchers have pointed out a research deficit in this area [23]. It would also be important to highlight the differences between "pure" online gamblers, "pure" offline gamblers, and "mixed-mode" gamblers. It is also significant to recognise the differences between the genders in terms of online gambling activities. As the online gambling market in Poland is constantly evolving, it is important to use the experience of Western countries when implementing responsible gambling policy. Internet gamblers should be informed by operators about the risks of gambling. In addition, it would be important for operators to monitor online gambler behaviour and identify at risk gamblers and direct messages to them about threats and the possibilities of seeking help. Gamblers should be able to exclude themselves from the site for a certain period of time, and this should also be offered to at risk gamblers. Some activities in this area are already being implemented; however, it is important to conduct research on the effectiveness of preventive measures taken, because cultural factors can modify it.

Limitations

Despite the pioneering character of this study in Poland, this study also has its limitations. The first one is the BBGS, the research tool used, which, despite its psychometric properties, only has a screening character and is used relatively rarely in epidemiological studies. Earlier studies on offline gambling in Poland employed a different scale (CPGI), so it is difficult to compare those results with the results of the present study. The BBGS was used due to the preliminary nature of this study, the continuation of which is being planned. Besides, the adjustment of BBGS to online gambling by rewording the questions, being our attempt to remedy to the lack of distinction between online and offline forms of gambling, is a very unusual technique, and it is uncertain how that step affected the results obtained. The next limitation was the restricted number of questions in the survey and the resulting failure to include more variables, including psychological ones. A more elaborate study is, however, currently underway. There were also no questions about offline gambling in the survey, which makes it impossible to determine whether the outspoken gamblers are "pure" online gamblers. In light of the study by Gainsbury, there are differences between pure online and offline gamblers and "mixed-mode" gamblers [18]. Another limitation of research is the fact that it was conducted in the same month in which the online gambling market was expanded. The result of this may have been that the study only captured gamblers very advanced in using new technologies who were the first to reach games in a new form. This confirms the connection between the use of online gambling games and the intensity of Internet involvement. Another hypothesis may be that the research revealed players looking for new types of gambling. This hypothesis, however, is partly undermined by the results of studies in the light of which most Poles practiced Lottery of Sports Totalizator and online sports betting. Lotteries are the most popular offline games in Poland; they are widely recognized and their publicity is allowed, which translates into their high availability, and therefore—greater involvement of Poles in them. On the other hand, online sports betting has been available in Poland since 2012, which is why it is not a "new" type of game. Research should certainly be continued to learn more about the specifics of Poles' involvement in online gambling.

5. Conclusions

This study provided a characterisation of Poles' involvement in online gambling. This is all the more relevant because in December 2018 new types of online gambling services were introduced. We thus managed to capture the 'initial' state—that is, the very beginning of the new reality of online gambling in Poland. As a result, it is possible to observe changes arising from the introduction of new legal regulations. Studies have shown that 4.1% of Poles made an online bet in the 12-monthnperiod prior to the survey. Lotteries, sports and e-sports betting proved to be the most popular online gambling games. Online gambling was more popular among younger men, with incomes lower than the national average salary, who were highly engaged Internet users. Among all gamblers, 26.8% were reported to be at risk of gambling addiction based on the results of the BBGS screening questionnaire. Addicted online gamblers more often had children and preferred sports betting.

Author Contributions: Conceptualization, B.L.-K. and R.P.B.; methodology, B.L.-K., R.P.B., M.W., and J.C.; validation, B.L.-K. and R.P.B.; formal analysis, R.P.B. and M.W.; investigation, B.L.-K., J.C., M.W., and R.P.B.; resources, B.L.-K., J.C., and R.P.B.; data curation, R.P.B. and M.W.; writing—original draft preparation, B.L.-K., M.W., R.P.B.; writing—review and editing, B.L.-K., R.P.B., J.C., M.W., and I.N.; visualization, M.W.; supervision, I.N.; project administration, B.L.-K.; funding acquisition, J.C. and B.L.-K. All authors have read and agreed to the published version of the manuscript.

References

1.   Gaboury, A.; Ladouceur, R.; Bussières, O. Structures des loteries et comportements des joueurs. [Structure of lotteries and behaviour of players]. *Rev. Psychol. Appliquée* **1989**, *39*, 197–207.
2.   Ladouceur, R.; Mayrand, M. Depressive behaviors and gambling. *Psychol. Rep.* **1987**, *60*, 1019–1022. [CrossRef] [PubMed]
3.   American Psychiatric Association. *Diagnostic and Statistical Manual of Mental Disorders [DSM-5]*, 5th ed.; American Psychiatric Association: Washington, DC, USA, 2013.
4.   World Health Organization. International Classification of Diseases for Mortality and Morbidity Statistics (11th Revision). Available online: https://icd.who.int/en (accessed on 16 December 2019).
5.   Freimuth, M.; Moniz, S.; Kim, S.R. Clarifying exercise addiction: Differential diagnosis, co-occurring disorders, and phases of addiction. *Int. J. Environ. Res. Public Health* **2011**, *8*, 4069–4081. [CrossRef] [PubMed]
6.   Lesieur, H.R.; Rosenthal, R.J. Pathological gambling: A review of the literature (prepared for the American Psychiatric Association Task Force on DSM-IV Committee on Disorders of Impulse Control Not Elsewhere Classified). *J. Gambl. Stud.* **1991**, *7*, 5–39. [CrossRef]
7.   Thompson, W.N.; Gazel, R.; Rickman, D. Social and legal costs of compulsive gambling. *Gaming Law Rev.* **1997**, *1*, 81–89. [CrossRef]
8.   Bischof, A.; Meyer, C.; Bischof, G.; John, U.; Wurst, F.M.; Thon, N.; Lucht, M.; Grabe, H.J.; Rumpf, H.-J. Suicidal events among pathological gamblers: The role of comorbidity of axis I and axis II disorders. *Psychiatry Res.* **2015**, *225*, 413–419. [CrossRef]
9.   Bischof, A.; Meyer, C.; Bischof, G.; John, U.; Wurst, F.M.; Thon, N.; Lucht, M.; Grabe, H.-J.; Rumpf, H.-J. Type of gambling as an independent risk factor for suicidal events in pathological gamblers. *Psychol. Addict. Behav.* **2016**, *30*, 263–269. [CrossRef]
10. Walker, D.M.; Barnett, A.H. The social costs of gambling: An economic perspective. *J. Gambl. Stud.* **1999**, *15*, 181–212. [CrossRef]
11. McBride, J.; Derevensky, J. Internet gambling behavior in a sample of online gamblers. *Int. J. Ment. Health Addict.* **2008**, *7*, 149–167. [CrossRef]
12. Griffiths, M.; Parke, A.; Wood, R.; Parke, J. Internet gambling: An overview of psychosocial impacts. *UNLV Gaming Res. Rev. J.* **2005**, *10*, 27–39.

13. LaBrie, R.A.; LaPlante, D.A.; Nelson, S.E.; Schumann, A.; Shaffer, H.J. Assessing the playing field: A prospective longitudinal study of internet sports gambling behavior. *J. Gambl. Stud.* **2007**, *23*, 347–362. [CrossRef] [PubMed]

14. Meyer, G.; Fiebig, M.; Häfeli, J.; Mörsen, C. Development of an assessment tool to evaluate the risk potential of different gambling types. *Int. Gambl. Stud.* **2011**, *11*, 221–236. [CrossRef]

15. Monaghan, S. Internet gambling—Not just a fad. *Int. Gambl. Stud.* **2009**, *9*, 1–4. [CrossRef]

16. Williams, R.J.; Wood, R.T.; Parke, J. *Routledge International Handbook of Internet Gambling*; Routledge: London, UK, 2012.

17. Philander, K.S.; MacKay, T.L. Online gambling participation and problem gambling severity: Is there a causal relationship? *Int. Gambl. Stud.* **2014**, *14*, 214–227. [CrossRef]

18. Gainsbury, S.M. Online gambling addiction: The relationship between internet gambling and disordered gambling. *Curr. Addict. Rep.* **2015**, *2*, 185–193. [CrossRef] [PubMed]

19. Williams, R.J.; Wood, R.T. The proportion of Ontario gambling revenue derived from problem gamblers. *Can. Public Policy* **2007**, *33*, 367–388. [CrossRef]

20. Wood, R.T.; Williams, R.J. *Internet Gambling: Prevalence, Patterns, Problems, and Policy Options*; Ontario Problem Gambling Research Centre: Guelph, ON, Canada, 2009.

21. Canale, N.; Griffiths, M.D.; Vieno, A.; Siciliano, V.; Molinaro, S. Impact of internet gambling on problem gambling among adolescents in Italy: Findings from a large-scale nationally representative survey. *Comput. Hum. Behav.* **2016**, *57*, 99–106. [CrossRef]

22. Effertz, T.; Bischof, A.; Rumpf, H.J.; Meyer, C.; John, U. The effect of online gambling on gambling problems and resulting economic health costs in Germany. *Eur. J. Health Econ.* **2018**, *19*, 967–978. [CrossRef]

23. McCormack, A.; Shorter, G.W.; Griffiths, M.D. An examination of participation in online gambling activities and the relationship with problem gambling. *J. Behav. Addict.* **2013**, *2*, 31–41. [CrossRef]

24. Chóliz, M. The challenge of online gambling: The effect of legalization on the increase in online gambling addiction. *J. Gambl. Stud.* **2016**, *32*, 749–756. [CrossRef]

25. Storer, J.; Abbott, M.; Stubbs, J. Access or adaptation? A meta-analysis of surveys of problem gambling prevalence in Australia and New Zealand with respect to concentration of electronic gaming machines. *Int. Gambl. Stud.* **2009**, *9*, 225–244. [CrossRef]

26. Welte, J.W.; Barnes, G.M.; Wieczorek, W.F.; Tidwell, M.C.O.; Hoffman, J.H. Type of gambling and availability as risk factors for problem gambling: A tobit regression analysis by age and gender. *Int. Gambl. Stud.* **2007**, *7*, 183–198. [CrossRef]

27. Hing, N.; Haw, J. The development of a Multi-dimensional Gambling Accessibility Scale. *J. Gambl. Stud.* **2009**, *25*, 569–581. [CrossRef] [PubMed]

28. Thomas, A.C.; Sullivan, G.B.; Allen, F.C.L. A theoretical model of EGM problem gambling: More than a cognitive escape. *Int. J. Ment. Health Addict.* **2009**, *7*, 97–107. [CrossRef]

29. Chóliz, M. Experimental analysis of the game in pathological gamblers: Effect of the immediacy of the reward in slot machines. *J. Gambl. Stud.* **2010**, *26*, 249–256. [CrossRef]

30. Cotte, J.; Latour, K.A. Blackjack in the kitchen: Understanding online versus casino gambling. *J. Consum. Res.* **2009**, *35*, 742–758. [CrossRef]

31. Gainsbury, S.; Wood, R.; Russell, A.; Hing, N.; Blaszczynski, A. A digital revolution: Comparison of demographic profiles, attitudes and gambling behavior of Internet and non-Internet gamblers. *Comput. Hum. Behav.* **2012**, *28*, 1388–1398. [CrossRef]

32. Hing, N.; Russell, A.M.T.; Gainsbury, S.M.; Nuske, E. The public stigma of problem gambling: Its nature and relative intensity compared to other health conditions. *J. Gambl. Stud.* **2016**, *32*, 847–864. [CrossRef]

33. Barrault, S.; Varescon, I. Online and live regular poker players: Do they differ in impulsive sensation seeking and gambling practice? *J. Behav. Addict.* **2016**, *5*, 41–50. [CrossRef]

34. LaPlante, D.A.; Nelson, S.E.; Gray, H.M. Breadth and depth involvement: Understanding internet gambling involvement and its relationship to gambling problems. *Psychol. Addict. Behav.* **2014**, *28*, 396–403. [CrossRef]

35. Gainsbury, S.M.; Russell, A.; Blaszczynski, A.; Hing, N. Greater involvement and diversity of Internet gambling as a risk factor for problem gambling. *Eur. J. Public Health* **2015**, *25*, 723–728. [CrossRef] [PubMed]

36. Wardle, H.; Moody, A.; Spence, S.; Orford, J.; Volberg, R.; Jotangia, D.; Griffiths, M.; Hussey, D.; Dobbie, F. *British Gambling Prevalence Survey 2010*; National Centre for Social Research: London, UK, 2011.

37. Columb, D.; O'Gara, C. A national survey of online gambling behaviours. *Ir. J. Psychol. Med.* **2017**, *35*, 311–319. [CrossRef] [PubMed]

38. Gainsbury, S.; Wood, R. Internet gambling policy in critical comparative perspective: The effectiveness of existing regulatory frameworks. *Int. Gambl. Stud.* **2011**, *11*, 309–323. [CrossRef]

39. Fiedler, I. Regulation of online gambling. *Econ. Bus. Lett.* **2018**, *7*, 162–168. [CrossRef]

40. Costes, J.M.; Kairouz, S.; Eroukmanoff, V.; Monson, E. Gambling patterns and problems of gamblers on licensed and unlicensed sites in France. *J. Gambl. Stud.* **2016**, *32*, 79–91. [CrossRef]

41. Planzer, S.; Gray, H.M.; Shaffer, H.J. Associations between national gambling policies and disordered gambling prevalence rates within Europe. *Int. J. Law Psychiatry* **2014**, *37*, 217–229. [CrossRef]

42. *Ustawa z Dnia 15 Grudnia 2016 o Zmianie Ustawy o Grach Hazardowych oraz Niektórych Innych Ustaw [Act of 15 December 2016 on the Amendment of the Gambling Activities Act and Certain Other Acts]*; Chancellery of the Sejm of the Republic of Poland: Warsaw, Poland, 2016; pp. 1–22. Available online: http://prawo.sejm.gov.pl/isap.nsf/DocDetails.xsp?id=WDU20170000088 (accessed on 12 November 2019).

43. United Nations Global Compact. *Przeciwdziałanie Szarej Strefie w Polsce [Counteracting the Gray Area in Poland]*; Global Compact Poland: Warsaw, Poland, 2016.

44. Lelonek, B. *Psychospołeczne Korelaty Uzależnień od Gier Hazardowych [Psychosocial Correlates of Gambling Addiction]*; Towarzystwo Naukowe Katolickiego Uniwersytetu Lubelskiego: Lublin, Poland, 2012.

45. Gebauer, L.; LaBrie, R.; Shaffer, H.J. Optimizing DSM-IV-TR classification accuracy: A brief biosocial screen for detecting current gambling disorders among gamblers in the general household population. *Can. J. Psychiatry* **2010**, *55*, 82–90. [CrossRef]

46. Niewiadomska, I.; Augustynowicz, W.; Palacz-Chrisidis, A.; Bartczuk, R.P.; Wiechetek, M.; Chwaszcz, J. *Bateria Metod Służących Do Oceny Ryzyka Zaburzeń Związanych z Hazardem [A Battery of Methods to Assess the Risk of Gambling-Related Disorders]*; Instytut Psychoprofilaktyki i Psychoterapii: Stowarzyszenie Natanaelum: Lublin, Poland, 2014.

47. Brett, E.I.; Weinstock, J.; Burton, S.; Wenzel, K.R.; Weber, S.; Moran, S. Do the DSM-5 diagnostic revisions affect the psychometric properties of the Brief Biosocial Gambling Screen? *Int. Gambl. Stud.* **2014**, *14*, 447–456. [CrossRef]

48. Hing, N.; Russell, A.M.; Browne, M. Risk factors for gambling problems on online electronic gaming machines, race betting and sports betting. *Front. Psychol.* **2017**, *8*, 779. [CrossRef]

49. IBM Corporation. *IBM SPSS Statistics for Windows*; IBM Corporation: Armonk, NY, USA, 2016.

50. Badora, B.; Gwiazda, M.; Herrmann, M.; Kalka, J.; Moskalewicz, J. *Oszacowanie Rozpowszechnienia oraz Identyfikacja Czynników Ryzyka i Czynników Chroniących w Odniesieniu do Hazardu, w Tym Hazardu Problemowego (Patologicznego) oraz Innych Uzależnień Behawioralnych [Estimation of Prevalence and Identification of Risk and Protective Factors in Relation to Gambling, Including Problem (Pathological) Gambling and Other Behavioural Addictions]*; Centrum Badania Opinii Społecznej: Warsaw, Poland, 2012.

51. Costes, J.M.; Eroukmanoff, V. Les pratiques de jeux d'argent sur Internet en France en 2017 [Internet gambling practices in France in 2017]. *Notes L'Observatoire Jeux* **2018**, *9*, 1–8.

52. Rémond, J.J.; Romo, L. Analysis of gambling in the media related to screens: Immersion as a predictor of excessive use? *Int. J. Environ. Res. Public Health* **2018**, *15*, 58. [CrossRef] [PubMed]

53. Moskalewicz, M.; Badora, B.; Feliksiak, M.; Głowacki, A.; Gwiazda, M.; Herrmann, M.; Kawalec, I.; Roguska, B. *Oszacowanie Rozpowszechnienia oraz Identyfikacja Czynników Ryzyka i Czynników Chroniących Hazardu i Innych Uzależnień Behawioralnych—Edycja 2018/2019 [Estimation of Prevalence and Identification of Risk and Protective Factors for Gambling and Other Behavioural Addictions—2018/2019 Edition]*; Centrum Badania Opinii Społecznej: Warsaw, Poland, 2019.

54. Yazdi, K.; Katzian, C. Addictive potential of online-gambling. A prevalence study from Austria. *Psychiatr. Danub.* **2017**, *29*, 376–378. [CrossRef] [PubMed]

7

Empirical Relationships between Problematic Alcohol Use and a Problematic Use of Video Games, Social Media and the Internet and their Associations to Mental Health in Adolescence

Lutz Wartberg [1] and Rudolf Kammerl [2,*]

[1] Department Psychology, Faculty of Life Sciences, MSH Medical School Hamburg, 20457 Hamburg, Germany; lutz.wartberg@medicalschool-hamburg.de

[2] Department of Education, Chair for Pedagogy with a Focus on Media Education, Friedrich-Alexander-University Erlangen-Nuremberg, 90478 Nuremberg, Germany

* Correspondence: rudolf.kammerl@fau.de

Abstract: Adolescents frequently show risky behavior, and these problematic behavior patterns often do not occur in isolation, but together. Problematic alcohol use is widespread among youth, as is problematic use of the Internet and of specific online applications (video games or social media). However, there is still a lack of findings for minors regarding the relations between these behavioral patterns (particularly between problematic alcohol use and problematic gaming or problematic social media use). Standardized instruments were used to survey problematic alcohol use, problematic gaming, problematic social media use, problematic Internet use and mental health among 633 adolescents (mean age: 15.79 years). Bivariate correlation and multivariable linear regression analyses were conducted. The correlation analyses showed statistically significant positive bivariate relationships between all four behavioral patterns each. Antisocial behavior was related to all problematic behavioral patterns. Whereas, emotional distress, self-esteem problems and hyperactivity/inattention were associated with substance-unrelated problematic behavior patterns only. Anger control problems were related to problematic alcohol use and problematic gaming. In adolescence, the findings revealed small effect sizes between substance-related and substance-unrelated problematic behavior patterns, but moderate to large effect sizes within substance-unrelated behavioral patterns. Similarities and differences were found in the relations between the behavioral patterns and mental health.

Keywords: Internet addiction; pathological Internet use; Internet gaming disorder; gaming disorder; social networking site addiction; social media addiction; Facebook addiction; problem drinking; alcohol; adolescent

1. Introduction

In adolescence, new developmental tasks can pose great challenges and psychological stress for minors [1]. In addition to effective problem-solving strategies, dysfunctional stress management strategies (e.g., use of psychotropic substances) are often used to cope with these developmental tasks [1], which can also serve the striving for independence (e.g., from parents) or the search for identity [2]. According to the Problem-Behavior Theory of Jessor [3], these dysfunctional stress management strategies or problematic behavior patterns often do not occur in isolation, but together. Problematic alcohol use (often referred to as problem drinking) is explicitly mentioned by Jessor [3] (p. 602). The extensive technological changes in recent years and decades call for the concept of Problem-Behavior Theory to be expanded in content. Some authors (e.g., De Leo & Wulfert [4]) now also include a problematic use of the Internet or its applications in this context. Considering the widespread occurrence of substance-related problematic behavior patterns and problematic use of digital media in adolescence, it seems quite relevant to examine whether there are empirical relationships. Initial studies (e.g., [5]) have conducted a combined investigation of substance-related problem behavior (e.g., problematic alcohol use) and problem behavior unrelated to substance use (e.g., problematic Internet use or problematic use of specific online applications). Another important approach specifically to explain Internet-use disorders is the Interaction of Person-Affect-Cognition-Execution (I-PACE) model by Brand et al. [6]. In the I-PACE model specific Internet-use disorders "... are considered to be the consequence of interactions between predisposing factors" (e.g., biopsychological constitution, psychopathology, personality, social cognitions and specific motives for using), "... coping styles and Internet-related cognitive biases. . . " and "... affective and cognitive responses to situational triggers in combination with reduced executive functioning" (p. 252).

The increasing relevance of problem behavior unrelated to substance use was demonstrated by the American Psychiatric Association (APA) with the inclusion of "Internet Gaming Disorder" in the appendix of the DSM-5 [7] (as a condition for which further studies are required), and by the World Health Organization (WHO) with the inclusion of "Gaming Disorder" in the ICD-11 [8]. In addition to use of video games (in the following referred to as gaming), the use of social media is often mentioned as another Internet application with potential for problematic use by adolescents (e.g., [9]). The collective term "social media" includes the use of websites of social networks and messengers as well as blogs, etc. [10]. In addition, an increasing number of studies is examining problematic use of the Internet on a more general level [11]. According to available empirical findings, it seems appropriate to differentiate between general problematic Internet use and the use of specific applications (such as online gaming, in cross-section: (e.g., [12]), in longitudinal section: [13]).

As an important substance-related behavior pattern, problematic consumption of alcohol and its consequences in adolescence have been a relevant aspect of public health efforts and scientific research for a long time (in Germany, for example, an increase in the age of first alcohol use from 14.1 years in 2004 to 15.0 years in 2018 has been observed [14]). Indeed, alcohol use among adolescents remains widespread in many countries. Following the European School Survey Project on Alcohol and Other Drugs (ESPAD) risky patterns of alcohol consumption are still highly prevalent in youth. In 1995, in the first ESPAD study, 36% of the examined European students reported heavy episodic drinking. In 2015, in the last ESPAD investigation, the observed prevalence for heavy episodic drinking was 35% [15]. Besides, a substantial percentage of youth already shows a problematic alcohol use. In Germany (where the present study was conducted), the one-year prevalence estimation for problematic alcohol use in a representative sample of adolescents was 5.0% [16].

In addition to substance-related problem behavior (especially alcohol consumption), the relevance of problem behavior unrelated to substance use (such as problematic Internet use, problematic gaming, and problematic social media use) has often been discussed and empirically investigated especially in adolescence. Surveys of representative samples of youth show high prevalence values for problematic Internet use, problematic gaming, and problematic social media use. Based on latent profile and latent class analyses in representative samples, prevalence estimates between 3.2% and 4.7% were observed for problematic Internet use in German minors [17–19]. For problematic gaming, in representative samples prevalence values of 2.6% among Slovenian students and 3.5% in German adolescents were reported [20,21]. Bányai et al. [22], investigated a representative sample of Hungarian students, conducted a latent profile analysis and obtained a prevalence estimate of 4.5% for problematic social media use. At present, it is still largely unclear how often problematic alcohol use and problematic use of the Internet use or specific online applications occur combined in adolescence.

According to the Problem-Behavior Theory of Jessor [3], associations between problematic alcohol and problematic use of the Internet or specific online applications seem not unlikely, but relatively few empirical findings on these relations have been published. Relationships between problematic Internet use and general substance use in adolescents have been investigated more frequently (see for example the systematic review of Lanthier-Labonté et al. [23]). However, it is important to distinguish between general alcohol consumption (which in Germany occurs among a majority of minors) and problematic alcohol use in adolescence (which only affects a minority, but which clearly can have serious consequences, see for instance the review of McCambridge et al. [24]).

In the few available studies, relations between problematic alcohol use and problematic Internet use in adolescence were usually examined in cross-sectional surveys. Pallanti et al. [25] observed a statistically significant positive correlation (0.38) between problematic alcohol use and problematic Internet use among Italian youth (average age: 16.67 years). In the study by Ha et al. [26], problematic alcohol use in South Korean adolescents (mean age: 15.8 years) did not occur more frequently in youth with problematic Internet use than among those without problematic Internet use. In contrast, Ko et al. [5] reported that problematic alcohol use occurred more often in Taiwanese adolescents with problematic Internet use than without problematic Internet use (average age of the sample was 16.26 years). Golpe et al. [27] found a statistically significant positive correlation (0.36) between problematic alcohol use and problematic Internet use among Spanish youth (mean age: 14.52 years). Rial et al. [28] obtained more problematic alcohol use among Spanish minors (average age: 14.41 years) with problematic Internet use than among adolescents without problematic Internet use. In addition, in a longitudinal study Gámez-Guadix et al. [29] showed that negative consequences of problematic Internet use predicted an increase in problematic alcohol use in Spanish minors (mean age: 14.92 years) six months later.

For relations between problematic alcohol use and problematic gaming there are so far only findings from studies with adults. Na et al. [30] observed relatively often (in 165 of the 1819 surveyed 20- to 49-year olds) a comorbid occurrence of problematic alcohol use and problematic gaming in South Korea and this comorbidity group showed more severe psychopathological impairments compared to the adults affected by only one of the two problem behavioral patterns. In contrast, the survey by Erevik et al. [31] showed a negative association between "high-level gaming" and problematic alcohol use among Norwegian university students (average age: 25.8 years). Problematic gaming was a protective factor against problematic alcohol use in this investigation. For relations between problematic alcohol use and problematic social media use only one result (also in adults) has been published so far [32]. Lyvers et al. [32] obtained a statistically significant positive correlation (0.42) between problematic alcohol use and problematic social media use in Australian adults (mean age: 26.1 years).

Furthermore, in both the I-PACE model ("psychopathology") [6] and the Problem-Behavior Theory (e.g., "low self-esteem") [3] associations to mental health were also mentioned. Problematic alcohol use (e.g., [33]), problematic gaming (e.g., [9]), problematic social media use (e.g., [9]) and problematic Internet use (e.g., [12]) are each associated with a higher psychopathological burden, but there are very few studies that have examined several of these patterns and their links to mental health in one sample (e.g., [33]).

To sum up, empirical evidence predominantly suggests relations between problematic alcohol use and problematic Internet use in adolescence [5,25,27–29]. Whether such associations exist between problematic alcohol use and problematic gaming or problematic social media use is currently unclear for youth. Accordingly, the present study is the first to investigate empirically associations between problematic alcohol use and problematic gaming and problematic social media use in adolescence. Furthermore, we wanted to explore and compare associations between problematic alcohol use, problematic gaming, problematic social media use, problematic Internet use and different aspects of mental health.

2. Materials and Methods

2.1. Research Questions

In the present study the following research questions (RQs) were examined:

RQ1 What is the relationship between problematic alcohol use and problematic gaming in adolescents?

RQ2 What is the relationship between problematic alcohol use and problematic social media use in adolescents?

RQ3 What is the relationship between problematic alcohol use and problematic Internet use in adolescents?

RQ4 What are the relationships between problematic alcohol use, problematic gaming, problematic social media use, problematic Internet use and different aspects of mental health?

2.2. Procedure

Data collection was conducted in Germany within the framework of the VEIF project in accordance with the Declaration of Helsinki. The Ethics Committee of the German Educational Research Association (Deutsche Gesellschaft für Erziehungswissenschaft, DGfE) approved the proceedings (approval number: 01/2018/DGfE). Informed consent was obtained both from the surveyed adolescents and from one of their parents. The findings reported below are based on nation-wide data collected in the first quarter of 2019 by a market research institute. The VEIF project is a longitudinal study in which data had previously been collected at annual intervals in the first quarter 2016, in the first quarter 2017 and in the first quarter 2018. At the time of the first data collection (2016), youth were aged between 12 and 14, and in 2019 between 14 and 17. As formulated in the research questions, relations between problematic alcohol use and problematic use of the Internet and specific online applications should be investigated. For the first time in the 2019 data collection, due to the increased age of the sample, a substantial and sufficient number of adolescents (n = 57) reported problematic alcohol use. The data collection was carried out in 2019 by 134 interviewers directly at the families' homes. Using computer-assisted personal interviewing (CAPI), one adolescent and one parent (dyad) were surveyed each. For the dyads, the parent was examined first and afterwards the adolescent. In the VEIF project, a sample with an increased risk of problematic use of digital media compared to the general population is examined. For this purpose, an oversampling of youth with an increased risk of problematic use of digital media was carried out before the first data collection in 2016 (a more detailed description of the study design and the recruitment process conducted at the beginning of the VEIF project can be found at Wartberg et al. [34]).

2.3. Measures

Problematic alcohol use in the last 12 months was measured with the Alcohol Use Disorders Identification Test-Consumption (AUDIT-C, Bush et al. [35]). We used the German version by Lampert and Kuntz [36]. The screening questionnaire comprises three items. In the first AUDIT-C question, the adolescents were surveyed how often they have a drink containing alcohol (five-step response format: 0 = "never", 1 = "monthly or less", 2 = "2–4 times a month", 3 = "2–3 times a week", 4 = "4 or more times a week"). In the second AUDIT-C question, the youth should rate how many drinks containing alcohol they consume on a typical day when they are drinking (five-step response format: 0 = "1–2", 1 = "3–4", 2 = "5–6", 3 = "7–9", 4 = "10 or more"). In the third AUDIT-C question, the adolescents were asked how often they consume six or more drinks on one occasion (five-step response format: 0 = "never", 1 = "less than monthly", 2 = "monthly", 3 = "weekly", 4 = "daily or almost daily"). An AUDIT-C sum value is formed by adding up the answers to all three questions and a higher sum value indicates a more pronounced problematic alcohol use. The reliability of the AUDIT-C was 0.72 in the investigated sample.

Problematic gaming in the past 12 months was assessed with the Internet Gaming Disorder Scale (IGDS, Lemmens et al. [37], we used the German version by Wartberg et al. [38]). The IGDS consists of nine questions with a binary answer format (0 = "no", 1 = "yes"). An IGDS total value is calculated from the nine items. A higher total figure indicates a more pronounced problematic gaming. The reliability of the IGDS was 0.82 in the examined sample.

Problematic social media use in the last 12 months was measured with the Social Media Disorder Scale (SMDS, van den Eijnden et al. [10]). The SMDS also comprises nine items with a binary response format (0 = "no", 1 = "yes"). An SMDS sum value can be calculated from the answers to the nine questions and a higher value indicates a more pronounced problematic social media use. The reliability of the SMDS was 0.83 in the surveyed sample.

To assess problematic Internet use, we utilized the Young Diagnostic Questionnaire (YDQ, Young [39], validation of the German version: Wartberg et al. [40]). The YDQ consists of eight items with a binary answer format (0 = "no", 1 = "yes") from which a sum value can be formed. A higher figure indicates a more pronounced problematic Internet use. The reliability of the YDQ was 0.70 in the investigated sample.

To assess adolescent mental health within the last six months, we applied the German adaption of the Reynolds Adolescent Adjustment Screening Inventory [41]: Screening psychischer Störungen im Jugendalter-II (SPS-J-II) [42]. The SPS-J-II consists of 32 questions (3-level response format: 0 = "never or almost never", 1 = "sometimes", 2 = "nearly all the time"). The questionnaire is divided into four scales assessing the frequency of adolescent antisocial behavior, anger control problems, emotional distress (combined measure of anxiety and depressiveness), and self-esteem problems. In each of the four scales, a higher sum value indicates a greater degree of adolescent psychopathological burden. We observed the following reliability coefficients (Cronbach's α): antisocial behavior: $\alpha = 0.77$, anger control problems: $\alpha = 0.79$, emotional distress: $\alpha = 0.88$ and self-esteem problems: $\alpha = 0.68$.

To collect a parental rating of adolescent hyperactivity/inattention over the last six months, we utilized the scale hyperactivity/inattention of the well-established Strengths and Difficulties Questionnaire (SDQ) [43]. This SDQ subscale comprises five questions with a 3-level response format (0 = "not true", 1 = "somewhat true", 2 = "certainly true"). A higher total value in this scale indicates a higher level of adolescent hyperactivity/inattention. In our sample, the reliability coefficient of the SDQ scale was $\alpha = 0.75$. Furthermore, socio-demographic characteristics (e.g., gender of the adolescent and age at the time of the survey) were collected.

2.4. Statistical Analyses

Overall, 319 adolescents had stated in the first question of the AUDIT-C [35] that they had never consumed alcohol in the last year. All these 319 cases did not have to answer the following two questions of the AUDIT-C and their AUDIT-C sum value was set to "0". Similarly, 40 minors had reported that they had never played video games in the last twelve months. These 40 cases did not have to answer the IGDS questions [37] and their IGDS total value was set to "0". Frequencies, mean values, standard deviations, reliability coefficients, correlations as well as multivariable linear regression analyses were calculated with SPSS version 25 (IBM, 2017, New York, NY, USA). First, bivariate correlation analyses were calculated. Subsequently, multivariable linear regression analyses were conducted (whereby all explanatory variables were simultaneously included in the regression models). In the four multivariable linear regression analyses problematic alcohol use, problematic gaming, problematic social media use, problematic Internet use were the dependent variable in one regression model each. In addition to gender, the different aspects of mental health (antisocial behavior, anger control problems, emotional distress, self-esteem problems, and hyperactivity/inattention) were utilized as explanatory variables.

3. Results

3.1. Descriptive Statistics

The sociodemographic characteristics of the total sample ($n = 633$) are presented in Table 1. In line with expectations (given the age of the sample and compulsory schooling in Germany), most of the adolescents interviewed were still attending school (93.5% of the total sample or 592 cases). For those youth who were still attending school, parents were asked to provide a prognosis for their future school leaving certificate (forecast). A total of 40 minors had already finished school (eight adolescents had achieved a graduation on a medium education level and another 32 adolescents on a high education level) and one girl did not go to school anymore (at the time of the survey she had no school leaving certificate).

Table 1. Sociodemographic characteristics of the sample.

Variable	Total Sample (n = 633) % or M (SD)
Gender	
Female	47.2%
Male	52.8%
Age [a]	15.79 (0.96)
Achieved or prospective level of graduation [b]	
Low-educational level	9.3%
Medium educational level	46.1%
High-educational level	44.5%

Note. [a] In years. [b] Prospective level: Forecast for all adolescents still attending school.

3.2. Bivariate Correlation Analyses

Answers to RQ1, RQ2 and RQ3: In the bivariate correlation analyses, we observed statistically significant positive associations between problematic alcohol use and problematic gaming behavior, problematic social media use and problematic Internet use (see Table 2). Furthermore, statistically significant positive relations between problematic gaming behavior, problematic social media use and problematic Internet use were found (see Table 2).

Table 2. Bivariate correlation analyses regarding the relationships of problematic alcohol use, problematic gaming behavior, problematic social media use and problematic Internet use in adolescents.

Variable	1	2	3	4
(1) Problematic alcohol use [a]	–			
(2) Internet gaming disorder [b]	0.12 **	–		
(3) Problematic social media use [c]	0.14 ***	0.45 ***	–	
(4) Problematic Internet use [d]	0.13 **	0.57 ***	0.63 ***	–

Note. [a] AUDIT-C sum value. [b] IGDS sum value. [c] SMDS sum value. [d] YDQ sum value; ** $p < 0.01$; *** $p < 0.001$.

3.3. Multiple Linear Regression Models

Answer to RQ4: In the multiple linear regression models problematic alcohol was associated with stronger antisocial behavior and lower anger control problems (see Table 3). Problematic gaming behavior was related to male gender and increased burden in all mental health aspects (antisocial behavior, anger control problems, emotional distress, self-esteem problems and hyperactivity/inattention) investigated. Problematic social media use was associated with female gender and higher levels of antisocial behavior, emotional distress, self-esteem problems and hyperactivity/inattention. Problematic Internet use was related to stronger antisocial behavior, higher emotional distress and more pronounced hyperactivity/inattention.

Table 3. Multiple linear regression models regarding the associations between mental health aspects and problematic alcohol use, problematic gaming behavior, problematic social media use and problematic Internet use in adolescents.

Mental Health Aspects	Problematic Alcohol Use	Internet Gaming Disorder	Problematic Social Media Use	Problematic Internet Use
	Standardized Beta Coefficients (95% CI)	Standardized Beta Coefficients (95% CI)	Standardized Beta Coefficients (95% CI)	Standardized Beta Coefficients (95% CI)
Gender [a]	−0.01 (−0.08; 0.07)	−0.33 *** (−0.39; −0.27)	0.18 *** (0.12; 0.24)	−0.02 (−0.08; 0.05)
Antisocial behavior	0.52 *** (0.42; 0.62)	0.18 *** (0.11; 0.26)	0.26 *** (0.17; 0.34)	0.19 *** (0.10; 0.27)
Anger control problems	−0.15 ** (−0.25; −0.04)	0.13 *** (0.04; 0.21)	0.08 (−0.01; 0.17)	0.02 (−0.08; 0.11)
Emotional distress	−0.06 (−0.15; 0.03)	0.09 * (0.01; 0.16)	0.13 ** (0.05; 0.20)	0.28 *** (0.20; 0.36)
Self-esteem problems	0.02 (−0.06; 0.10)	0.10 ** (0.03; 0.16)	0.12 ** (0.05; 0.18)	0.06 (−0.01; 0.13)
Hyperactivity/inattention	0.01 (−0.09; 0.10)	0.22 *** (0.15; 0.29)	0.26 *** (0.19; 0.34)	0.26 *** (0.19; 0.33)

Note. [a] Coding: 0 = male, 1 = female. * $p < 0.05$; ** $p < 0.01$; *** $p < 0.001$.

4. Discussion

In the present study, we investigated associations between problematic alcohol use and problematic use of the Internet and its specific applications (video games and social media) in adolescents. The first published findings already suggested relations between problematic alcohol use and problematic Internet use in adolescence [5,25,27–29]. We also found relationships between problematic alcohol use (operationalized via the established screening instrument AUDIT-C, which is recommended for use in adolescents, for example by Rumpf et al. [44]) and problematic Internet use (operationalized via the internationally frequently used YDQ [39]) in our sample of adolescents. Accordingly, our findings complement and confirm the international state of research on problematic alcohol use and problematic Internet use in adolescence.

Going beyond the current state of research, this study was the first to show empirically associations between problematic alcohol use and problematic gaming or problematic social media use in adolescence (a few findings have been reported from samples of adults). According to published empirical results (cross-sectional: e.g., Rosenkranz et al. [12], longitudinal: Wartberg et al. [13]), it does not seem advisable to transfer findings for a general problematic Internet use to a problematic use of specific online applications without further examination. In the context of the present study, it also seems helpful to distinguish between general problematic Internet use (in the cognitive-behavioral model of Davis [45] that would correspond to a "generalized pathological Internet use") and the problematic use of specific applications (such as video games or social media, in Davis' model [45] that could be a "specific pathological Internet use" each).

Regarding the associations between problematic alcohol use and problematic gaming, there have so far been only two results in adults [30,31]. However, these studies revealed heterogeneous findings. While the study by Na et al. [30] showed a positive relation between problematic alcohol use and problematic gaming, Erevik et al. [31] observed a negative association. The present survey could not confirm Erevik et al.'s finding [31] that problematic gaming in adults functioned as a protective factor against problematic alcohol use. This result of the present investigation indicates a positive relationship between problematic alcohol use and problematic gaming in adolescence, but naturally requires verification in further empirical surveys. Concerning the relation between problematic alcohol use and problematic social media use, only one study in adults [32] is available. Lyvers et al. [32] reported a positive correlation between both problematic behavioral patterns, which we observed in the present study also for adolescents. Again, this finding needs to be verified in future studies.

According to Jessors Problem-Behavior Theory [3], problematic behavior in adolescence often does not occur in isolation but in combination (this applies not only to problematic alcohol use but also to the examined three problematic patterns of Internet use or its applications). However, a combined survey of substance-unrelated problematic behavioral patterns has so far only been carried out very rarely. Estévez et al. [46] investigated the importance of emotion regulation in a mixed sample of adolescents and young adults in Spain for various problematic behaviors related and unrelated to substance use. In the correlation table of all constructs studied, positive statistically significant correlations were found for alcohol abuse with both problematic Internet use (0.28) and video game addiction (0.13) and between problematic Internet use and video game addiction (0.35) [46]. In our sample of adolescents, we also observed statistically significant correlations between problematic alcohol use and problematic gaming ($r = 0.12$), problematic social media use ($r = 0.14$) and problematic Internet use ($r = 0.13$, see Table 2). However, it should be noted that, according to the classification of Cohen [47], these correlations were small, while the correlation between problematic gaming and problematic social media use was moderate ($r = 0.45$). There were large correlations between problematic Internet use and problematic gaming ($r = 0.57$) as well as between problematic Internet use and problematic social media use ($r = 0.63$). Correspondingly, the associations between problem behaviors without substance relations were much more pronounced than to the substance-related problem behavior. Large correlation coefficients between problematic Internet use and problematic gaming in adolescents have been reported before by Király et al. [48] with 0.59 (p. 752) and by van Rooij et al. [49] with 0.63 (p. 509).

With regard to the associations between the problematic behaviors and mental health aspects (as described previously in the Problem-Behavior Theory [3] and the I-PACE model [6]), we observed both similarities and differences. More pronounced antisocial behavior was related to problematic alcohol use, problematic gaming behavior, problematic social media use and problematic Internet use and therefore seems to be consistently relevant for all four problematic behavioral patterns. Whereas, emotional distress, self-esteem problems and hyperactivity/inattention were associated with substance-unrelated problematic behavior patterns, but not with problematic alcohol use. This finding is a further contribution to the question of whether problematic alcohol consumption is related to depressiveness, where the published empirical findings are still heterogeneous (e.g., [50]). More anger control problems were associated with problematic gaming, but surprisingly less pronounced anger control problems with problematic alcohol use. The finding that problematic alcohol use is associated with fewer anger control problems and more pronounced antisocial behavior is novel and needs further investigation. Whereas the relationship between a problematic alcohol use and more externalizing problems (e.g., conduct problems or antisocial behavior) is considered empirically well established.

The present survey has various limitations. The VEIF project does not examine a representative sample, because a higher percentage of youth with a higher risk of problematic use of digital media was included than in the general population (oversampling). This may limit the transferability of the results to the general population as well as to other age groups (e.g., adults). Findings of a cross-sectional analysis were reported. Therefore, no cause-effect relationships or conclusions that one behavior leads to another can be deduced between the characteristics examined (this would require a longitudinal design). In addition to the investigated behavior patterns, further problematic behavior patterns unrelated to substance use are conceivable (e.g., problematic gambling), which could also be relevant for problematic alcohol use in adolescence, but were not considered in the study design of the VEIF project. Therefore, we cannot provide a complete model to explain adolescent problematic alcohol use (too many relevant variables, such as substance use of the peers, were not collected).

5. Conclusions

Despite the limitations mentioned above, the present investigation revealed some interesting new findings. The empirical associations between problematic alcohol use and a problematic gaming and a problematic social media use among adolescents extended existing research. With regard to a common etiology and for the development of comprehensive prevention programs (e.g., life skills trainings), it seems quite promising to examine several problematic behavior patterns and their associations to mental health together. Therefore, the findings of the present survey can be used to develop or revise preventive measures. Furthermore, if there are indications of problem behaviors in youth related or unrelated to substance use, they should be screened for further substance-related or non-substance-related problematic behavior patterns as part of a comprehensive diagnostic procedure (e.g., before the start of an intervention measure in an outpatient or inpatient setting) in order to exclude or take them into account as comorbidities in treatment.

Author Contributions: Conceptualization, R.K. and L.W.; methodology, L.W.; software, L.W.; validation, R.K. and L.W.; formal analysis, L.W.; investigation, R.K. and L.W.; resources, R.K. and L.W.; data curation, L.W.; writing—original draft preparation, L.W.; writing—review and editing, R.K.; visualization, L.W.; supervision, R.K.; project administration, R.K.; funding acquisition, R.K. and L.W. All authors have read and agreed to the published version of the manuscript.

Acknowledgments: We thank all adolescents and parents who participated in the study.

References

1. Faltermaier, T. *Gesundheitspsychologie [Health Psychology]*; Kohlhammer: Stuttgart, Germany, 2017.
2. Scheithauer, H.; Hayer, T.; Niebank, K. *Problemverhalten und Gewalt im Jugendalter: Erscheinungsformen, Entstehungsbedingungen, Prävention und Intervention*; Kohlhammer: Stuttgart, Germany, 2008.
3. Jessor, R. Risk behavior in adolescence: A psychosocial framework for understanding and action. *J. Adolesc. Health* **1991**, *12*, 597–605. [CrossRef]
4. De Leo, J.A.; Wulfert, E. Problematic Internet use and other risky behaviors in college students: An application of problem-behavior theory. *Psychol. Addict. Behav.* **2013**, *27*, 133–141. [CrossRef]
5. Ko, C.H.; Yen, J.Y.; Yen, C.F.; Chen, C.S.; Weng, C.C.; Chen, C.C. The Association between Internet Addiction and Problematic Alcohol Use in Adolescents: The Problem Behavior Model. *Cyberpsychol. Behav.* **2008**, *11*, 571–576. [CrossRef] [PubMed]
6. Brand, M.; Young, K.S.; Laier, C.; Wölfling, K.; Potenza, M.N. Integrating psychological and neurobiological considerations regarding the development and maintenance of specific Internet-use disorders: An Interaction of Person-Affect-Cognition-Execution (I-PACE) model. *Neurosci. Biobehav. Rev.* **2016**, *71*, 252–266. [CrossRef] [PubMed]
7. American Psychiatric Association. *Diagnostic and Statistical Manual of Mental Disorders, DSM-5*, 5th ed.; American Psychiatric Publishing: Washington, DC, USA, 2013; ISBN 978-0890425558.
8. WHO. Gaming Disorder. 2018. Available online: who.int/news-room/q-a-detail/gaming-disorder (accessed on 25 May 2020).
9. Mérelle, S.M.Y.; Kleiboer, A.M.; Schotanus, M.; Cluitmans, T.L.M.; Waardenburg, C.M.; Kramer, D.; van de Mheen, D.; van Rooij, T. Which health-related problems are associated with problematic video-gaming or social media use in adolescents? A large-scale cross-sectional public health study. *Clin. Neuropsychiatry* **2017**, *14*, 11–19.
10. Van den Eijnden, R.J.; Lemmens, J.S.; Valkenburg, P.M. The social media disorder scale. *Comput. Hum. Behav.* **2016**, *61*, 478–487. [CrossRef]
11. Lopez-Fernandez, O. Generalised Versus Specific Internet Use-Related Addiction Problems: A Mixed Methods Study on Internet, Gaming, and Social Networking Behaviours. *Int. J. Environ. Res. Public Health* **2018**, *15*, 2913. [CrossRef]
12. Rosenkranz, T.; Müller, K.W.; Dreier, M.; Beutel, M.E.; Wölfling, K. Addictive potential of internet applications and differential correlates of problematic use in internet gamers versus generalized internet users in a representative sample of adolescents. *Eur. Addict. Res.* **2017**, *23*, 148–156. [CrossRef]
13. Wartberg, L.; Zieglmeier, M.; Kammerl, R. An Empirical Exploration of Longitudinal Predictors for Problematic Internet Use and Problematic Gaming Behavior. *Psychol. Rep.* **2020**. [CrossRef]
14. Orth, B.; Merkel, C. *Der Alkoholkonsum Jugendlicher und Junger Erwachsener in Deutschland. Ergebnisse des Alkoholsurveys 2018 und Trends*; BZgA-Forschungsbericht: Köln, Germany, 2019. [CrossRef]
15. EMCDDA and ESPAD. *ESPAD Report 2015—Results from the European School Survey Project on Alcohol and Other Drugs*; Publications Office of the European Union: Luxembourg, 2016.
16. Wartberg, L.; Kriston, L.; Thomasius, R. Prevalence of problem drinking and associated factors in a representative German sample of adolescents and young adults. *J. Public Health* **2019**, *41*, 543–549. [CrossRef]
17. Wartberg, L.; Kriston, L.; Kammerl, R.; Petersen, K.-U.; Thomasius, R. Prevalence of pathological Internet use in a representative German sample of adolescents: Results of a latent profile analysis. *Psychopathology* **2015**, *48*, 25–30. [CrossRef] [PubMed]

18. Rumpf, H.-J.; Vermulst, A.A.; Bischof, A.; Kastirke, N.; Gürtler, D.; Bischof, G.; Meerkerk, G.-J.; John, U.; Meyer, C. Occurence of internet addiction in a general population sample: A latent class analysis. *Eur. Addict. Res.* **2014**, *20*, 159–166. [CrossRef]

19. Wartberg, L.; Kriston, L.; Bröning, S.; Kegel, K.; Thomasius, R. Adolescent problematic Internet use: Is a parental rating suitable to estimate prevalence and identify familial correlates? *Comput. Hum. Behav.* **2017**, *67*, 233–239. [CrossRef]

20. Pontes, H.M.; Macur, M.; Griffiths, M.D. Internet Gaming Disorder among Slovenian primary schoolchildren: Findings from a nationally representative sample of adolescents. *J. Behav. Addict.* **2016**, *5*, 304–310. [CrossRef] [PubMed]

21. Wartberg, L.; Kriston, L.; Thomasius, R. Internet gaming disorder and problematic social media use in a representative sample of German adolescents: Prevalence estimates, comorbid depressive symptoms and related psychosocial aspects. *Comput. Hum. Behav.* **2020**, *103*, 31–36. [CrossRef]

22. Bányai, F.; Zsila, Á.; Király, O.; Maraz, A.; Elekes, Z.; Griffiths, M.D.; Andreassen, C.S.; Demetrovics, Z. Problematic social media use: Results from a large-scale nationally representative adolescent sample. *PLoS ONE* **2017**, *12*, e0169839. [CrossRef]

23. Lanthier-Labonté, S.; Dufour, M.; Milot, D.M.; Loslier, J. Is problematic Internet use associated with alcohol and cannabis use among youth? A systematic review. *Addict. Behav.* **2020**, *106*, 106331. [CrossRef]

24. McCambridge, J.; McAlaney, J.; Rowe, R. Adult consequences of late adolescent alcohol consumption: A systematic review of cohort studies. *PLoS Med.* **2011**, *8*, e1000413. [CrossRef]

25. Pallanti, S.; Bernardi, S.; Quercioli, L. The Shorter PROMIS Questionnaire and the Internet Addiction Scale in the assessment of multiple addictions in a high-school population: Prevalence and related disability. *CNS Spectr.* **2006**, *11*, 966–974. [CrossRef]

26. Ha, J.H.; Kim, S.Y.; Bae, S.C.; Bae, S.; Kim, H.; Sim, M.; Lyoo, I.K.; Cho, S.C. Depression and Internet addiction in adolescents. *Psychopathology* **2007**, *40*, 424–430. [CrossRef]

27. Golpe, S.; Gómez, P.; Braña, T.; Varela, J.; Rial, A. The relationship between consumption of alcohol and other drugs and problematic Internet use among adolescents. *Adicciones* **2017**, *29*, 268–277. [CrossRef] [PubMed]

28. Rial, A.; Golpe, S.; Isorna, M.; Braña, T.; Gómez, P. Minors and problematic Internet use: Evidence for better prevention. *Comput. Hum. Behav.* **2018**, *87*, 140–145. [CrossRef]

29. Gámez-Guadix, M.; Calvete, E.; Orue, I.; Las-Hayas, C. Problematic Internet use and problematic alcohol use from the cognitive–behavioral model: A longitudinal study among adolescents. *Addict. Behav.* **2015**, *40*, 109–114. [CrossRef] [PubMed]

30. Na, E.; Lee, H.; Choi, I.; Kim, D.J. Comorbidity of Internet gaming disorder and alcohol use disorder: A focus on clinical characteristics and gaming patterns. *Am. J. Addict.* **2017**, *26*, 326–334. [CrossRef]

31. Erevik, E.K.; Torsheim, T.; Andreassen, C.S.; Krossbakken, E.; Vedaa, Ø.; Pallesen, S. The associations between low-level gaming, high-level gaming and problematic alcohol use. *Addict. Behav. Rep.* **2019**, *10*, 100186. [CrossRef]

32. Lyvers, M.; Narayanan, S.S.; Thorberg, F.A. Disordered social media use and risky drinking in young adults: Differential associations with addiction-linked traits. *Aust. J. Psychol.* **2019**, *71*, 223–231. [CrossRef]

33. Wartberg, L.; Brunner, R.; Kriston, L.; Durkee, T.; Parzer, P.; Fischer-Waldschmidt, G.; Resch, F.; Sarchiapone, M.; Wasserman, C.; Hoven, C.W.; et al. Psychopathological factors associated with problematic alcohol and problematic Internet use in a sample of adolescents in Germany. *Psychiatry Res.* **2016**, *240*, 272–277. [CrossRef]

34. Wartberg, L.; Kriston, L.; Kammerl, R. Associations of social support, friends only known through the Internet, and health-related quality of life with Internet Gaming Disorder in adolescence. *Cyberpsychol. Behav. Soc. Netw.* **2017**, *20*, 436–441. [CrossRef]

35. Bush, K.; Kivlahan, D.R.; McDonell, M.B.; Fihn, S.D.; Bradley, K.A. The AUDIT alcohol consumption questions (AUDIT-C): An effective brief screening test for problem drinking. *Arch. Intern. Med.* **1998**, *158*, 1789–1795. [CrossRef]

36. Lampert, T.; Kuntz, B. Tabak- und Alkoholkonsum bei 11- bis 17-jährigen Jugendlichen. Ergebnisse der KiGGS-Studie—Erste Folgebefragung (KiGGS Welle 1). *Bundesgesundheitsblatt Gesundh. Gesundh.* **2014**, *57*, 830–839. [CrossRef]

37. Lemmens, J.S.; Valkenburg, P.M.; Gentile, D.A. The Internet Gaming Disorder Scale. *Psychol. Assess.* **2015**, *27*, 567–582. [CrossRef] [PubMed]

38. Wartberg, L.; Kriston, L.; Thomasius, R. The Prevalence and Psychosocial Correlates of Internet Gaming Disorder. *Dtsch. Arztebl. Int.* **2017**, *114*, 419–424. [CrossRef] [PubMed]

39. Young, K.S. Internet Addiction: The Emergence of a New Clinical Disorder. *Cyberpsychol. Behav.* **1998**, *1*, 237–244. [CrossRef]

40. Wartberg, L.; Durkee, T.; Kriston, L.; Parzer, P.; Fischer-Waldschmidt, G.; Resch, F.; Sarchiapone, M.; Wasserman, C.; Hoven, C.W.; Carli, V.; et al. Psychometric Properties of a German Version of the Young Diagnostic Questionnaire (YDQ) in two Independent Samples of Adolescents. *Int. J. Ment. Health Addict.* **2017**, *15*, 182–190. [CrossRef]

41. Reynolds, W.M. *Reynolds Adolescent Adjustment Screening Inventory™ (RAASI™): Professional Manual*; Psychological Assessment Resources: Lutz, Germany, 2001.

42. Hampel, P.; Petermann, F. Screening psychischer Störungen im Jugendalter-II (SPS-J-II). In *Deutschsprachige Adaptation des Reynolds Adolescent Adjustment Screening Inventory (RAASI) von William M. Reynolds (2. erweiterte Auflage)*, 2nd ed.; Huber: Bern, Switzerland, 2012.

43. Goodman, R. The Strengths and Difficulties Questionnaire: A research note. *J. Child Psychol. Psychiatry* **1997**, *38*, 581–586. [CrossRef]

44. Rumpf, H.J.; Wohlert, T.; Freyer-Adam, J.; Grothues, J.; Bischof, G. Screening Questionnaires for Problem Drinking in Adolescents: Performance of AUDIT, AUDIT-C, CRAFFT and POSIT. *Eur. Addict. Res.* **2013**, *19*, 121–127. [CrossRef]

45. Davis, R.A. A cognitive-behavioral model of pathological Internet use. *Comput. Hum. Behav.* **2001**, *17*, 187–195. [CrossRef]

46. Estévez, A.; Jauregui, P.; Sanchez-Marcos, I.; Lopez-Gonzalez, H.; Griffiths, M.D. Attachment and emotion regulation in substance addictions and behavioral addictions. *J. Behav. Addict.* **2017**, *6*, 534–544. [CrossRef]

47. Cohen, J. *Statistical Power Analysis for the Behavioral Sciences*; Lawrence Erlbaum Associates: Hillsdale, MI, USA, 1988.

48. Király, O.; Griffiths, M.D.; Urbán, R.; Farkas, J.; Kökönyei, G.; Elekes, Z.; Tamás, D.; Demetrovics, Z. Problematic Internet use and problematic online gaming are not the same: Findings from a large nationally representative adolescent sample. *Cyberpsychol. Behav. Soc. Netw.* **2014**, *17*, 749–754. [CrossRef]

49. van Rooij, A.J.; Schoenmakers, T.M.; Van den Eijnden, R.J.J.M.; Vermulst, A.A.; van de Mheen, D. Video game addiction test: Validity and psychometric characteristics. *Cyberpsychol. Behav. Soc. Netw.* **2012**, *15*, 507–511. [CrossRef]

50. Pesola, F.; Shelton, K.H.; Heron, J.; Munafò, M.; Hickman, M.; van den Bree, M.B. The developmental relationship between depressive symptoms in adolescence and harmful drinking in emerging adulthood: The role of peers and parents. *J. Youth Adolesc.* **2015**, *44*, 1752–1766. [CrossRef] [PubMed]

8

Psychological Characteristics and Addiction Propensity According to Content Type of Smartphone Use

Jinhee Lee [1,2], Joung-Sook Ahn [1,2], Seongho Min [1] and Min-Hyuk Kim [1,*]

[1] Department of Psychiatry, Yonsei University Wonju College of Medicine, 20 Ilsan-ro, Gangwon-do, Wonju 26426, Korea; jinh.lee95@yonsei.ac.kr (J.L.); jsahn@yonsei.kr (J-S.A.); mchorock@yonsei.ac.kr (S.M.)

[2] Division of Child and Adolescent Psychiatry, Yonsei University Wonju College of Medicine, 20 Ilsan-ro, Gangwon-do, Wonju 26426, Korea

* Correspondence: mhkim09@yonsei.kr

Abstract: The aim of this study was to evaluate the association between content type of smartphone use and psychological characteristics and addiction propensity, including the average time of smartphone use and problematic smartphone use. Data were obtained from the 2017 Korea Youth Risk Behavior Web-Based Survey, a nationally representative survey of middle- and high-school students ($n = 62{,}276$). The content type of smartphone use was divided into four categories: (1) Study, (2) Social-Networking Services (SNS), (3) Game, and (4) Entertainment. The association of depressive mood and suicidal ideation with content type of smartphone use was analyzed, using multiple and binary logistic regression analyses, respectively. The relationship between content type of smartphone use and time spent on smartphone use and problematic smartphone use was analyzed by using multiple logistic regression, adjusted for related covariables. The results of this study revealed that depressive mood and suicidal ideation were significantly associated with the SNS smartphone use group, compared with the other groups. Our results also indicate that the SNS group showed higher addiction propensity, such as overuse and experiencing adverse consequences of smartphone use.

Keywords: suicide; suicide attempts; intervention; case management; smartphone use; addiction

1. Introduction

Smartphones are perceived as indispensable information and communication tools in daily life for many people and are now the most frequently used technology worldwide [1]. For adolescents, in particular, who are sensitive to new technology and media use, smartphones have become an important part of their life. Recent studies estimate that 84% of adolescents in Japan [2] and 97% of adolescents in Switzerland [3] have their own smartphone. Furthermore, similar to substance or other types of behavioral addictions, adolescents are known to be vulnerable to smartphone addiction. A prior study reported that 60% of adolescents in the UK are highly addicted to their smartphones [2], and the rate of smartphone addiction among adolescents was double for adults in South Korea [2]. Prior studies have suggested some neurobiological evidences of the vulnerability toward smartphone addiction among adolescents, such as the dual processing model and an imbalance between the go and stop networks [4,5].

Smartphones are useful for multiple purposes, including study, information searching, social communication, and entertainment [6]. Compared with the traditional forms of computer and internet use, the portability and connectivity of smartphones give users easier access to information and entertainment content—nearly anytime and anywhere. These characteristics can also make people more vulnerable to behavioral addiction [7] in the form of habitual checking or excessive use of smartphones. Previous studies have reported that excessive smartphone use in adolescents is associated with psychopathologies (i.e., depression, anxiety, high-stress levels, and low mood) and behavioral problems [8,9], because adolescents are easily affected by external stimulus, interpersonal issues, and emotional changes. Another study on young adults suggested that excessive smartphone use is related to high stress, and it is also inversely related to academic performance, as well as life satisfaction [10].

Previous studies have used the smartphone addiction scale, smartphone usage time, or the frequency of use to clarify the relationship between addictive smartphone use and adverse effects on physical and mental health. However, despite the possible associations between the purpose of smartphone use and the risk of addictive behaviors, little is known regarding the relative impact of the content type of smartphone use on addiction and adverse consequences of smartphone use, including adolescent mental health. Andreassen and her colleagues have suggested that addictive online behaviors, including both addictive social networking and video gaming, are associated with underlying psychiatric disorders, such as ADHD, OCD, anxiety, and depression [11]; however, the differences in specific associations according to the purpose of its use have not been clarified. Another study has indicated that social-networking addiction and internet-gaming disorder can augment the symptoms of each other and simultaneously contribute to deterioration of overall psychological health in a similar fashion [12]. Some evidence shows that internet addiction comprises strongly directed internet activities, such as excessive online-video-game playing, excessive use of online pornography, or online shopping, and there are indeed different forms of internet addiction [13–15].

Thus, we aim to investigate the association between content type of smartphone use and adolescent mental health, with the hypothesis that psychological characteristics and addiction propensity are related with content type of smartphone use. This study examines the average time of smartphone use and problematic smartphone use, using a school-based, nationally representative dataset of the Korean adolescent population.

2. Materials and Methods

2.1. Methods

Study Population and Source of Data

Data on the study population were obtained from the 13th Korea Youth Risk Behavior Web-Based Survey (KYRBS), which was administered in 2017 by the Korean Ministry of Education, Science and Technology; the Ministry of Health and Welfare; and the Korea Centers for Disease Control and Prevention. KYRBS is a self-reported anonymous online survey of a nationally representative sample of Korean adolescents (aged 12–18 years) [16]. The sample design of this survey used a stratified multistage cluster strategy with 123 questions divided into 15 sections inquiring about health-related behaviors and mental and physical health. In the 13th KYRBS, 64,991 students from 800 middle and high schools were randomly selected, and 62,276 (31,636 boys and 30,640 girls) students (95.8% response rate) from 799 schools responded to the survey [17]. Participants were provided with identification numbers and were guaranteed anonymity, and written informed consent was obtained from each participant after the survey had been fully explained. All data used in this study were fully anonymized before we accessed them. This consent procedure was approved by the Institutional Review Board of the Korea Centers for Disease Control and Prevention (2014-06EXP-02-P-A).

2.2. Measures

2.2.1. Content Type of Smartphone Use

The exposure variable, content type of smartphone use, was assessed by the question "In the last 30 days, please select only one service that you used mainly, when using your smartphone", and the answers were classified into four categories: (1) Study; (2) Social-Networking Services (SNS) (e.g., messaging and chat, communities, and social networks); (3) Game; and (4) Entertainment (e.g., watching movies, reading comics and fiction, listening to music, creating User-Created Content and videos).

2.2.2. Sociodemographic and General Characteristics

The sociodemographic characteristics reported included age, sex, residential area, and family economic status of the participant. Respondents who lived in the country or rural areas were categorized as "Rural"; those who lived in small, middle-sized or large cities were categorized as "Urban". Family economic status was assessed by the question "What is your family economic status?" The five possible response categories, very high/high/middle/low/very low, were grouped into three categories, for the purpose of our analysis: high (very high or high), middle (middle), and low (very low or low) [18]. Sleep hours were divided into two categories: under 6 h; and 6 or more hours. Physical activity was divided into two categories, Yes/No, from the question "In the last 7 days, did you have physical activity with higher heart rate than usual?"

2.2.3. Psychological Characteristics

Subjective stress was measured by the question "How much stress do you usually feel?" The five possible response categories of very high//high/middle/low/very low were grouped into three categories: high (very high or high), middle (middle), and low (very low or low). Current alcohol consumption was assessed by the question "How many days during the past 30 days did you drink more than one cup of alcohol? (None/1–2 days/3–5 days/6–9 days/10–19 days/20–29 days/Every day)" Respondents who responded "None" were classified as not current alcohol drinkers, and those who responded between "1–2 days" and "Every day" were classified as current alcohol drinkers. The current cigarette smoking was assessed by using the following question: "How many days during the past 30 days did you smoke a cigarette? (None/1–2 days/3–5 days/6–9 days/10–19 days/20–29 days/Every day)". Respondents who responded "No" to the question were classified as not current cigarette smokers, and those who responded between "1–2 days" and "Every day" were classified as current cigarette smokers.

Depressed mood among the subjects was assessed by the question "In the past year, have you ever felt so sad or despaired that your feelings disturbed everyday life for two whole weeks?" Subjects responded with the following: (1) "No, I never felt it" or (2) "Yes, I have felt it". We also examined whether the subjects had suicidal ideations with the question "In the past year, did you ever seriously consider attempting suicide?" Subjects responded with the following: (1) "No, I never thought of it" or (2) "Yes, I have thought of it".

2.2.4. Addiction-Propensity-Related Factors

The average time spent using a smartphone was assessed by the question "On an average school day, how many hours do you use a smartphone?" According to the results of the previous study [3], the use of a smartphone over 5 h a day was defined as "smartphone overuse". Participants were also asked the following: "In the last 30 days, have you experienced severe conflicts with family due to your smartphone usage?" and "In the last 30 days, have you experienced severe conflicts with friends due to your smartphone usage?", (Yes/No), which would suggest a tolerance that is one of the important factors of smartphone addiction. They were also asked whether they had experienced poor academic performance due to smartphone use (Yes/No), by the question "In the last 30 days, were there any difficulties in your academic performance due to your smartphone usage?", which would suggest a daily disturbance due to smartphone addiction [1].

2.2.5. Statistical Analyses

The participants' general characteristics according to each content type of smartphone use were summarized by using either a one-way analysis of variance for continuous variables or a chi-squared test with Bonferroni correction for categorical variables. The relationships of the four different groups with psychological factors and problematic smartphone use were analyzed by using Pearson's chi-square. Subsequently, a multiple logistic regression analysis was performed to identify the associations between content type of smartphone use with depressed mood, suicidal ideation, and overuse of smartphones. General characteristics that showed a significant difference in the chi-square test were mutually adjusted for the analysis. Two-tailed analyses were conducted, and p-values lower than 0.05 were considered significant. Adjusted odds ratios (AORs) and 95% confidence intervals (CIs) were calculated. All statistical analyses were performed by using SPSS software (version 23.0, IBM Corp., Armonk, NY, USA).

3. Results

The descriptive characteristics according to the content type of smartphone use are presented in Table 1. Results of chi-square analysis revealed that there were significant differences depending on age, sex, residential area, family economic status, sleep hours, and physical activity by content type of smartphone use. The "Study" group was more likely to be older, live in large cities, and have a higher family economic status. The "SNS" group had a higher prevalence of female respondents and a lower prevalence of physical activity. The "Game" group was more likely to be younger, boys, living in rural areas, sleeping less than 6 h, and less physically active. The "Entertainment" group had a higher prevalence of low family economic status compared to other groups (all $p < 0.001$).

Table 1. General characteristics of participants, according to content type of smartphone use.

General Characteristics		Study (n = 4202, 10.7%)	SNS (n = 10,192, 25.9%)	Game (n = 7282, 18.5%)	Entertainment (n = 17,642, 44.9%)	p
Age (years)	Mean (SD)	15.58 ± 1.78	14.92 ± 1.66	14.31 ± 1.71	15.07 ± 1.76	< 0.001
Sex (%)						< 0.001
	Boys	62.9	28.9	87.9	50.8	
	Girls	37.1	71.1	12.1	49.2	
Region (%)						< 0.001
	Rural Area	7.3	7.2	8.5	7.8	
	Small City	45.6	47.3	50.3	47.3	
	Large City	47.1	45.5	41.2	44.9	
Family Economic Status (%)						< 0.001
	High	47.2	39.0	40.4	37.0	
	Middle	40.3	46.8	46.2	47.1	
	Low	12.5	14.2	13.4	15.9	
Sleep Hours (%)						< 0.001
	<6hrs	33.2	38.6	62.4	42.9	
	≥6hrs	66.8	61.4	37.6	57.1	
Physical Activity (%)						< 0.001
	No	34.2	38.9	32.0	36.5	
	Yes	65.8	61.1	68.0	64.0	

SNS: Social-Networking Services.

The psychological characteristics of participants according to content type of smartphone use are presented in Table 2. The "SNS" group had a higher prevalence of high subjective stress level, current cigarette smoking, and current alcohol drinking. The "SNS" group also had significantly higher prevalence of depressive mood and suicidal ideation compared to other groups. The "Game" group had the lowest proportion of depressive mood and suicidal ideation among groups (all $p < 0.001$).

The average amount of time spent using a smartphone was greater in the "SNS" group (322.17 ± 228.90 min/day) than in other groups and lower in the "Study" group (176.97 ± 173.06 min/day). The proportion of adverse consequences of smartphone use, including conflicts with family, conflicts with friends, and poor academic performance due to smartphone use, were higher in the "SNS" group (59.2%, 27.6%, and 58.4% respectively), whereas the "Study" group had a lower prevalence of adverse consequences (41.8%, 20.1%, and 43.0% respectively) (Table 3).

Table 2. Psychological characteristics of participants, according to content type of smartphone use.

Psychological Characteristics		Study (n = 4202, 10.7%)	SNS (n = 10,192, 25.9%)	Game (n = 7282, 18.5%)	Entertainment (n = 17,642, 44.9%)	p
Subjective Stress						< 0.001
	High	37.1	41.1	30.3	38.0	
	Middle	40.9	42.0	43.2	42.1	
	Low	22.0	16.6	26.5	19.8	
Current Cigarette Smoking						0.694
	No	93.4	93.2	93.6	93.3	
	Yes	6.6	6.8	6.4	6.7	
Current Alcohol Drinking						< 0.001
	No	77.7	74.7	77.4	75.5	
	Yes	22.3	25.3	22.6	24.5	
Depressive Mood						< 0.001
	No	76.2	71.1	82.5	76.2	
	Yes	23.8	28.9	17.5	23.8	
Suicidal Ideation						< 0.001
	No	89.5	85.3	90.6	87.7	
	Yes	10.5	14.7	9.4	12.3	

SNS: Social-Networking Services.

Table 3. Adverse consequences of smartphone use, according to content type of smartphone use.

Adverse Consequences		Study (n = 4202, 10.7%)	SNS (n = 10,192, 25.9%)	Game (n = 7282, 18.5%)	Entertainment (n = 17,642, 44.9%)	p
Average Spent Time Using a Smartphone (min/day)						< 0.001
	Mean (SD)	176.97 ± 173.06	322.17 ± 228.90	243.87 ± 191.73	255.10 ± 137.00	
Conflict with Family Members due to Smartphone Use (%)						< 0.001
	No	58.2	40.8	41.5	45.8	
	Yes	41.8	59.2	58.5	54.2	
Conflict with Friends due to Smartphone Use (%)						< 0.001
	No	79.9	72.4	74.1	78.4	
	Yes	20.1	27.6	25.9	21.6	
Poor Academic Performance due to Smartphone Use (%)						< 0.001
	No	57.0	41.6	51.9	47.4	
	Yes	43.0	58.4	48.1	52.6	

SNS: Social-Networking Services.

Compared to the "Study" group, the "SNS" group was significantly more likely to report a depressive mood (AOR 1.36; 95% CI 1.24–1.49) and suicidal ideation (AOR 1.49; 95% CI 1.32–1.69). The "Entertainment" group also showed a positive association with suicidal ideation (AOR 1.20; 95% CI 1.06–1.35), and the "Game" group showed a negative association with depressive mood (AOR 0.77; 95% CI 0.69–0.85) (Table 4).

Table 4. Multivariable logistic regression analysis of content type of smartphone use, for depressive mood and suicidal ideation.

Content Type	Depressive Mood		Suicidal Ideation	
	Crude OR	Adjusted OR *	Crude OR	Adjusted OR *
	OR (95% CI)	OR (95% CI)	OR (95% CI)	OR (95% CI)
Study	Ref.	Ref.	Ref.	Ref.
SNS	1.30 (1.20–1.41)	1.36 (1.24–1.49)	1.46 (1.31–1.64)	1.49 (1.32–1.69)
Game	0.68 (0.62–0.74)	0.77 (0.69–0.85)	0.87 (0.77–0.99)	0.95 (0.82–1.09)
Entertainment	1.00 (0.92–1.08)	1.02 (0.94–1.12)	1.19 (1.07–1.32)	1.20 (1.06–1.35)

* Adjustment for age, sex, region of residence, family economic status, sleep hours, and physical activity; SNS: Social-Network Services, OR: odds ratio.

The AORs for smartphone overuse (> 5 h per day) were 4.57 (95% CI, 4.20–4.98), 2.24 (95% CI, 2.05–2.45) and 2.60 (95% CI, 2.40–2.81) in the "SNS" group, "Game" group, and "Entertainment" group, respectively (Table 5).

Table 5. Multivariable logistic regression analysis of content type of smartphone use, for smartphone overuse (more than 5 h per day).

Content Type	Crude OR	Adjusted OR
	OR (95% CI)	OR (95% CI)
Study	Ref.	Ref.
SNS	4.67 (4.32–5.05)	4.57 (4.20–4.98)
Game	2.22 (2.04–2.40)	2.24 (2.05–2.45)
Entertainment	2.68 (2.49–2.88)	2.60 (2.40–2.81)

* Adjustment for age, sex, region of residence, family economic status, sleep hours, and physical activity; SNS: Social-Networking Services, OR: odds ratio

4. Discussion

This study examined the association of psychological characteristics and addiction propensity with content type of smartphone use, within a relatively large convenience sample of adolescents in Korea. The results of this study revealed that depressive mood and suicidal ideation are significantly associated with higher SNS use, compared with smartphone use for games, study, and entertainment. Our results also suggested that the "SNS" group showed higher addiction propensity, including overuse and adverse consequences of smartphone use.

The results of this study expanded upon and shared similarities with previous findings on the relationship between mental health and SNS use. A prior systematic review by Frost et al. reported associations between SNS use (i.e., Facebook) and mental-health outcomes, such as alcohol use, addiction, anxiety, and depression [19]. Several studies have indicated that the prolonged use of SNS may be related to signs and symptoms of depression, and some authors have indicated that certain SNS activities might be associated with low self-esteem, especially in children and adolescents [20–23]. On the other hand, our results were contrary to a previous study that reported that the use of non-social smartphone features (i.e., news consumption, entertainment, and relaxation) were most related to depression and problematic smartphone use [24]. Furthermore, a prior study by our research group reported a potential protective effect from moderate use (1–2 h) of smartphones for social purposes (i.e., SNS and messaging) in regard to suicide attempts [1]. In these contexts, we should also consider the positive psychological effects of SNS use. In this study, we did not simply divide content type of smartphone use as social and non-social, but instead we compared detailed non-social uses: study, game, entertainment, and SNS. According to our results, content type of smartphone use should not be classified simply as social and non-social use but should also take into account the detailed characteristics of SNS use and various other tasks, including differences in the effects of mental health on adolescents.

There has been wide discussion on the potential causes for depressive mood resulting from increased time on SNS. The most commonly used mediator to explain the association between SNS use and depression is self-esteem. It is an important factor in developing and maintaining mental health and overall quality of life, and low self-esteem is associated with numerous mental illnesses, including depression and addiction [25,26]. Some authors have presented that individuals higher in narcissism and lower in self-esteem also showed more online activity, including self-promotional content such as SNS [27]. On the other hand, there is the that hypothesis feelings of depression can be predicted indirectly by SNS addiction [21]. Authors have indicated that SNS allows the user to get virtual community gratification and gain gratification from creating a self-image online. Based on the uses and gratifications theory, SNS use can lead to SNS addiction, as the functions available to the users allow them to gain instant gratification from using the service, which in turn could lead to excessive use.

Contrary to previous research that indicated a negative association between online-game use and adolescent mental health [28,29], the current study did not find that smartphone-game use was associated with depressive mood and suicidal ideation. The results might reflect the characteristics of categorization and reference group of study. The "Game" group of this study included those who enjoyed "gaming" more than other contents of the smartphone, but it does not mean that they had a "gaming addiction". Specifically, if a person performs gaming in a regular pattern, the person may relieve his/her stress. However, if a person overly performs gaming, he or she may have increased psychological problems, as shown in the literature. On the other hand, because of the statistically low number of "non-smartphone users", we used "Study" as a reference group. Studying does not mean the person cannot be addicted to it, and using "Study" as the reference can create some biases. For example, a person who is over-studying may have increased distress. Therefore, we cannot capture whether gaming is related to increased distress if studying is associated with high distress.

Furthermore, smartphone-game use predicted problematic smartphone use compared to the "Study" group, but showed a weak association compared to the "SNS" or "Entertainment" groups. Smartphone games are somewhat different from computer-based online games, allowing users to access them anywhere, anytime, but there is a limit to the use of tools for the games. There have been a number of studies on problematic game use, and recently, a WHO ICD-11 proposal for a new category named "Gaming Disorder" [30]. However, most of the studies so far have been limited to computer-based online games [31–33]. Furthermore, considering the recent trend that the use of entertainment, such as the use of YouTube, is particularly popular among adolescents and has become dominant in the media market worldwide [34,35], the results of the current study indicated the necessity for further studies about game and entertainment on the smartphone. Smartphones, which are relatively simple tools compared to conventional computers, may be better suited for simple functions, such as watching videos, than for more complex tasks, such as playing games, which may result in adolescents indulging in media instead.

The present study has a number of limitations that should be considered when interpreting the findings. First, due to the cross-sectional nature of national surveys, the present findings have limitations in explaining the causal inferences between content type of smartphone use and psychological characteristics. Further studies with sufficient time for investigation are needed to develop a clear understanding about the association of psychological characteristics and addiction propensity with content type of smartphone use. Second, the psychological characteristics and internet use were measured through the ad hoc questions rather than mental-health experts' assessment or validated scales, because the data were collected through the participants' self-reports, and therefore, some reporting bias could have occurred. Moreover, because the group was divided only for one main purpose of smartphone use, we could not distinguish those who performed two or more content types. Third, in our study, the addictive propensity was estimated only by time spent using a smartphone, not by the scales for smartphone addiction. In addition, most variables in the study, including conflicts with family/friends, and poor academic performance due to smartphone use, were surveyed on the basis of a self-reported questionnaire, which has inherent limitations regarding the validity of the data and the recall bias. However, in the previous study, excessive smartphone use was validated as the most powerful independent predictor of smartphone addiction [8], and we can use this to estimate the propensity to addiction. Fourth, our data lacked information regarding the familiarity or personological profile of the participants that might affect individuals with mood disorder and/or addiction. Despite the limitations of this cross-sectional survey, the present study has some strengths. We used a multilevel multinomial logistic modeling approach based on a nationally representative sample of Korean adolescents, who have the highest smartphone ownership rate in the world. Moreover, the response rate to the survey was very high. To the best of our knowledge, this study is the first to report on the association of psychological characteristics and addiction propensity with the content type of smartphone use in adolescents.

5. Conclusions

In the present nationally representative sample of Korean adolescents aged 12–18 years, the significant and specific association between content type of smartphone use and the prevalence of depressed mood, suicidal ideation, and addiction propensity has been confirmed. Our findings indicate that SNS use was not only a stronger predictor of smartphone addiction than other content types, but also had stronger associations with negative psychological characteristics, including depressive mood and suicidal ideation. The results of this study suggest that careful consideration should be given to improving screening for the risk of smartphone addiction and mental health problems in adolescents, with a focus on SNS use. Further research is needed to understand the longitudinal impact of specific content type of smartphone use on the addictive behavior of adolescents, allowing for the development of effective prevention strategies and to help strengthen the current smartphone-use guidelines.

Author Contributions: Conceptualization, J.L. and M.-H.K.; methodology, J.L.; validation, J.-S.A. and S.M..; formal analysis, J.L.; investigation, J.L.; writing—original draft preparation, J.L.; writing—review and editing, M.-H.K.; supervision, J.-S.A. and S.M. All authors have read and agreed to the published version of the manuscript.

References

1. Kim, M.H.; Min, S.; Ahn, J.S.; An, C.; Lee, J. Association between high adolescent smartphone use and academic impairment, conflicts with family members or friends, and suicide attempts. *PLoS ONE* **2019**, *14*, e0219831. [CrossRef] [PubMed]

2. Davey, S.; Davey, A. Assessment of smartphone addiction in Indian adolescents: A mixed method study by systematic-review and meta-analysis approach. *Int. J. Prev. Med.* **2014**, *5*, 1500–1511. [PubMed]

3. Haug, S.; Castro, R.P.; Kwon, M.; Filler, A.; Kowatsch, T.; Schaub, M.P. Smartphone use and smartphone addiction among young people in Switzerland. *J. Behav. Addict.* **2015**, *4*, 299–307. [CrossRef] [PubMed]

4. Adisetiyo, V.; Gray, K.M. Neuroimaging the neural correlates of increased risk for substance use disorders in attention-deficit/hyperactivity disorder—A systematic review. *Am. J. Addict.* **2017**, *26*, 99–111. [CrossRef] [PubMed]

5. Sussman, C.J.; Harper, J.M.; Stahl, J.L.; Weigle, P. Internet and video game addictions: Diagnosis, epidemiology, and neurobiology. *Child Adolesc. Psychiatr. Clin.* **2018**, *27*, 307–326. [CrossRef]

6. Van Deursen, A.J.; Bolle, C.L.; Hegner, S.M.; Kommers, P.A. Modeling habitual and addictive smartphone behavior: The role of smartphone usage types, emotional intelligence, social stress, self-regulation, age, and gender. *Comput. Hum. Behav.* **2015**, *45*, 411–420. [CrossRef]

7. Demirci, K.; Orhan, H.; Demirdas, A.; Akpinar, A.; Sert, H. Validity and reliability of the Turkish Version of the Smartphone Addiction Scale in a younger population. *Klin. Psikofarmakol. Bülteni-Bull. Clin. Psychopharmacol.* **2014**, *24*, 226–234. [CrossRef]

8. Matar Boumosleh, J.; Jaalouk, D. Depression, anxiety, and smartphone addiction in university students-A cross sectional study. *PLoS ONE* **2017**, *12*, e0182239. [CrossRef]

9. Cerniglia, L.; Griffiths, M.D.; Cimino, S.; De Palo, V.; Monacis, L.; Sinatra, M.; Tambelli, R. A latent profile approach for the study of internet gaming disorder, social media addiction, and psychopathology in a normative sample of adolescents. *Psychol. Res. Behav. Manag.* **2019**, *12*, 651–659. [CrossRef]

10. Samaha, M.; Hawi, N.S. Relationships among smartphone addiction, stress, academic performance, and satisfaction with life. *Comput. Hum. Behav.* **2016**, *57*, 321–325. [CrossRef]

11. Andreassen, C.S.; Billieux, J.; Griffiths, M.D.; Kuss, D.J.; Demetrovics, Z.; Mazzoni, E.; Pallesen, S. The relationship between addictive use of social media and video games and symptoms of psychiatric disorders: A large-scale cross-sectional study. *Psychol. Addict. Behav.* **2016**, *30*, 252–262. [CrossRef] [PubMed]

12. Pontes, H.M. Investigating the differential effects of social networking site addiction and Internet gaming disorder on psychological health. *J. Behav. Addict.* **2017**, *6*, 601–610. [CrossRef] [PubMed]

13. Montag, C.; Bey, K.; Sha, P.; Li, M.; Chen, Y.F.; Liu, W.Y.; Zhu, Y.K.; Li, C.B.; Markett, S.; Keiper, J. Is it meaningful to distinguish between generalized and specific Internet addiction? Evidence from a cross-cultural study from Germany, Sweden, Taiwan and China. *Asia-Pac. Psychiatry* **2015**, *7*, 20–26. [CrossRef] [PubMed]

14. Davis, R.A. A cognitive-behavioral model of pathological Internet use. *Comput. Hum. Behav.* **2001**, *17*, 187–195. [CrossRef]

15. Wong, H.Y.; Mo, H.Y.; Potenza, M.N.; Chan, M.N.M.; Lau, W.M.; Chui, T.K.; Pakpour, A.H.; Lin, C.-Y. Relationships between Severity of Internet Gaming Disorder, Severity of Problematic Social Media Use, Sleep Quality and Psychological Distress. *Int. J. Environ. Res. Public Health* **2020**, *17*, 1879. [CrossRef]

16. Kim, Y.; Choi, S.; Chun, C.; Park, S.; Khang, Y.H.; Oh, K. Data Resource Profile: The Korea Youth Risk Behavior Web-based Survey (KYRBS). *Int. J. Epidemiol.* **2016**, *45*, 1076-1076e. [CrossRef]

17. Korea centers for disease control & prevention call center (KCDC). The 13th Korea Youth Risk Behavior Web-Based Survey. Available online: http://www.cdc.go.kr/yhs/home.jsp (accessed on 23 January 2020).

18. Lee, J.; Jang, H.; Kim, J.; Min, S. Development of a suicide index model in general adolescents using the South Korea 2012–2016 national representative survey data. *Sci. Rep.* **2019**, *9*, 1846. [CrossRef]

19. Frost, R.L.; Rickwood, D.J. A systematic review of the mental health outcomes associated with Facebook use. *Comput. Hum. Behav.* **2017**, *76*, 576–600. [CrossRef]

20. Pantic, I. Online social networking and mental health. *Cyberpsychol. Behav Soc. Netw.* **2014**, *17*, 652–657. [CrossRef]

21. Donnelly, E.; Kuss, D. Depression among users of social networking sites (SNSs): The role of SNS addiction and increased usage. *J. Addict. Prev. Med.* **2016**, *1*, 107. [CrossRef]

22. Jelenchick, L.A.; Eickhoff, J.C.; Moreno, M.A. "Facebook depression?" Social networking site use and depression in older adolescents. *J. Adolesc. Health* **2013**, *52*, 128–130. [CrossRef] [PubMed]

23. Cerniglia, L.; Guicciardi, M.; Sinatra, M.; Monacis, L.; Simonelli, A.; Cimino, S. The Use of Digital Technologies, Impulsivity and Psychopathological Symptoms in Adolescence. *Behav. Sci.* **2019**, *9*, 82. [CrossRef] [PubMed]

24. Elhai, J.D.; Levine, J.C.; Dvorak, R.D.; Hall, B.J. Non-social features of smartphone use are most related to depression, anxiety and problematic smartphone use. *Comput. Hum. Behav.* **2017**, *69*, 75–82. [CrossRef]

25. Mann, M.; Hosman, C.M.; Schaalma, H.P.; de Vries, N.K. Self-esteem in a broad-spectrum approach for mental health promotion. *Health Educ. Res.* **2004**, *19*, 357–372. [CrossRef]

26. J Kuss, D.; D Griffiths, M.; Karila, L.; Billieux, J. Internet addiction: A systematic review of epidemiological research for the last decade. *Curr. Pharm. Des.* **2014**, *20*, 4026–4052. [CrossRef]

27. Mehdizadeh, S. Self-presentation 2.0: Narcissism and self-esteem on Facebook. *Cyberpsychol. Behav. Soc. Netw.* **2010**, *13*, 357–364. [CrossRef]

28. Grüsser, S.M.; Thalemann, R.; Griffiths, M.D. Excessive computer game playing: Evidence for addiction and aggression? *Cyberpsychol. Behav.* **2006**, *10*, 290–292. [CrossRef]

29. Mentzoni, R.A.; Brunborg, G.S.; Molde, H.; Myrseth, H.; Skouverøe, K.J.M.; Hetland, J.; Pallesen, S. Problematic video game use: Estimated prevalence and associations with mental and physical health. *Cyberpsychol. Behav. Soc. Netw.* **2011**, *14*, 591–596. [CrossRef]

30. Aarseth, E.; Bean, A.M.; Boonen, H.; Colder Carras, M.; Coulson, M.; Das, D.; Deleuze, J.; Dunkels, E.; Edman, J.; Ferguson, C.J. Scholars' open debate paper on the World Health Organization ICD-11 Gaming Disorder proposal. *J. Behav. Addict.* **2017**, *6*, 267–270. [CrossRef]

31. Petry, N.M.; O'Brien, C.P. Internet gaming disorder and the DSM-5. *Addiction* **2013**, *108*, 1186–1187. [CrossRef]

32. Petry, N.M.; Rehbein, F.; Gentile, D.A.; Lemmens, J.S.; Rumpf, H.J.; Mößle, T.; Bischof, G.; Tao, R.; Fung, D.S.; Borges, G. An international consensus for assessing internet gaming disorder using the new DSM-5 approach. *Addiction* **2014**, *109*, 1399–1406. [CrossRef] [PubMed]

33. Ferguson, C.J. Do angry birds make for angry children? A meta-analysis of video game influences on children's and adolescents' aggression, mental health, prosocial behavior, and academic performance. *Perspect. Psychol. Sci.* **2015**, *10*, 646–666. [CrossRef] [PubMed]

34. Cranwell, J.; Murray, R.; Lewis, S.; Leonardi-Bee, J.; Dockrell, M.; Britton, J. Adolescents' exposure to tobacco and alcohol content in YouTube music videos. *Addiction* **2015**, *110*, 703–711. [CrossRef] [PubMed]

35. Chau, C. YouTube as a participatory culture. *New Dir. Youth Dev.* **2010**, *2010*, 65–74. [CrossRef]

9

Preventing Harmful Internet Use-Related Addiction Problems in Europe: A Literature Review and Policy Options

Olatz Lopez-Fernandez [1,*] and Daria J. Kuss [2]

[1] Monash Addiction Research Centre, Turning Point, Easter Health Clinical School, Monash University, Clayton, VIC 3800, Australia

[2] International Gaming Research Unit, Cyberpsychology Research Group, Psychology Department, Nottingham Trent University, Nottingham NG1 4FQ, UK; Daria.Kuss@ntu.ac.uk

[*] Correspondence: Olatz.Lopez-Fernandez@monash.edu or Lopez.Olatz@gmail.com

Abstract: Internet use-related addiction problems are increasingly being recognized on a European scale due to international health organizations considering gaming addiction. In April 2013, the American Psychiatric Association recognized Internet Gaming Disorder in the fifth Diagnostic and Statistical Manual of Mental Disorders, and in April 2018, the World Health Organization included Gaming Disorder in the eleventh International Classification of Diseases. However, findings on these problems within this period are lacking in Europe, and a preventive approach is missing globally. A detailed critical literature review was conducted using PsycINFO and Web of Science in this five-year period. A total of 19 studies were reviewed and problems identified were: generalized Internet addiction and online gaming and gambling addictions across seven European countries (i.e., Spain, Germany, France, Italy, Greece, The Netherlands, and Denmark). The individuals with problematic use were found to be educated adolescents, usually young males with comorbid disorders, and gaming and gambling disorders were implicated in the most severe cases. Cognitive behavioral therapy was the main treatment, sometimes combined with a systemic approach for adolescents. Prevalence, high-risk populations, and factors contributing to these addiction problems are discussed, and a set of policy options are developed for this region. The implications for early detection, diagnosis, treatment, and prevention in Europe are considered.

Keywords: Internet addiction; problematic Internet use; generalized Internet addiction; online gaming addiction; online gambling addiction; Europe; policy option; prevention; public health

1. Introduction

Contemporary use of the Internet has led to a number of benefits in the health field (e.g., digital health), but also negative impacts at an individual and psychological level (e.g., gaming addiction).

Excessive Internet use has been classed in the mid-nineties as Internet Addiction (IA) [1], Problematic Internet Use (PIU) [2], or as technological (behavioral) addiction [3]. This broad term, however, has evolved and at present encompasses many types of addiction problems related to generalized Internet addiction (GIA) and a set of specific addictive uses of the Internet [4]. These include online gambling, online gaming, social networking, and cybersex, which are the most prevalent ones that have evolved alongside gaming addiction [5]. These behavioral problems can be engaged in using any device as the Internet is ubiquitous. Accordingly, during the last decade, the Internet has facilitated the development of addiction problems through online technology in many ways, and is associated with health problems (e.g., distress, functional impairment, and comorbidity [6]).

During the last decade, international health bodies, which publish diagnostic manuals for mental health diseases, recognized two associated conditions as behavioral addictions, i.e., gambling and gaming disorders. First, the American Psychiatric Association (APA) proposed Internet Gaming Disorder (IGD) in its fifth Diagnostic and Statistical Manual of Mental Disorders (DSM-5) within its third appendix in April 2013 [7]. Subsequently, the World Health Organization (WHO) included Gaming Disorder (GD) in its first version of the eleventh International Classification of Diseases (ICD-11) in April 2018 [8]. This inclusion has produced the following consequences. Firstly, gambling and gaming disorders have been recognized in the mental health sciences and by health practitioners as behavioral or process addictions, leading to many debates [9,10]. Secondly, the mass media have alerted the general public regarding these emerging online addiction problems which usually affect young populations [11,12]. Thirdly, these addictions are now understood as international public health concern, and the preventive actions undertaken have had limited success and focused on English speaking countries (i.e., in American, European, and Australasian regions [13]), and Asian countries [14].

However, to the authors' knowledge, no literature review has been conducted focusing on the period when gaming addiction was officially recognized by global health organizations, within an intercultural continental region (i.e., Europe), to detect the main concerns, and to propose a set of policy options which are culturally and geographically based. For these reasons, the European Parliament's Scientific Foresight Unit (STOA) endeavored to perform a recent literature review to study the individual and psychological aspects of the harms associated with Internet use, including IA and related harms (e.g., gaming addiction) in the European Union (EU) [15].

To the authors' knowledge, only two reviews exist with similar characteristics, but both with an international scope rather than a regional focus performed in 2016 [6,16].

Kuss and Lopez-Fernandez [6] focused on clinical research on IA and reported characteristics of treatment seekers and online addiction treatments. First, treatment seeker characteristics from various continents included European clinical studies performed in Germany, The Netherlands, and Greece, and focused on both, GIA and gaming addiction problems (among other comorbidities). Second, psychopharmacotherapy was covered, which appeared to have positive effects in decreasing IA symptomatology and Internet gaming addiction problems through antidepressants and anxiolytics, and obsessive–compulsive disorders (OCD) and attention deficit hyperactivity disorder (ADHD) medications for comorbid problems. Third, psychological therapies usually with an individual approach (e.g., cognitive behavioral therapy (CBT)) were applied to outpatients, apart from a few group therapy approaches (e.g., multi-family group therapy (MFGT)). Fourth, combined treatments were researched, which included psychological treatment in combination with pharmacotherapy or electroacupuncture therapy.

Vondráčková and Gabrhelík's review [16] focused on IA prevention. First, they stated some target groups may benefit from prevention (e.g., children and adolescents) when it is indicated (e.g., focusing on psychopathological factors). Second, the need to improve specific skills with the help of professionals and other significant individuals (i.e., counsellors, parents) was emphasized. Third, program characteristics were deemed relevant (e.g., information-provision versus interactive interventions). Fourth, environmental interventions were indicated as being needed in some regions (e.g., in countries in which IA is a public health concern where regulation should be promoted, similar to the approach taken by the Chinese government [17]).

Apart from these reviews, a world-wide meta-analysis on IA performed by Chen and Li in 2014 [18] indicated that the global estimated prevalence rate was approximately 6%, with the lowest numbers found in Northern and Western Europe (2.6%). IA prevalence was inversely associated with self-perception of quality of life regarding subjective (e.g., life satisfaction) and objective indicators (e.g., environmental conditions). Furthermore, many cross-cultural studies on IA have emerged since 2012, especially in intercultural regions, such as Europe [19,20]. These studies were school based with adolescent samples and found between 1%–4% estimated prevalence of GIA (which was higher in males). There has been a continuing increase in the number of these studies in the field [21], including mostly cross-national intercontinental studies (covering Asia, America, and Europe), which have researched GIA and estimated its prevalence with psychometric scales, obtaining higher rates in Asian countries and in young male users.

Considering the above, the objective of the present paper was to present a timely critical review of the literature on Internet use-related addiction and associated problems published in Europe between April 2013 (i.e., when IGD was included in the DSM-5's III appendix) and April 2018 (i.e., when GD was first officially recognized in the ICD-11 beta test version). The aims were to critically analyze online harms by addressing: (i) the cross-cultural approach adopted within the EU, (ii) the users' characteristics based on community and clinical populations, (iii) Internet use-related addiction problems and the interventions to target the resultant harms in Europe, and (iv) its implications at a public health level with an eye towards prevention. Furthermore, we aim to provide the first set of policy options for harm minimization at the level of the individual in Europe.

2. Materials and Methods

A literature review was conducted using the databases PsycINFO and Web of Science between January and April 2018 at Nottingham Trent University (United Kingdom). The rationale to select these two scientific databases was to contain research in Psychology and related disciplines [15]. Initially, PubMed was also selected but the results almost duplicated all outcomes collected via the first two databases, and consequently this search was discarded. PsycINFO and Web of Science are also among the most relevant in the field of Internet addiction covering the majority of current scientific sources targeted in the present paper's aims. Moreover, they offered sufficient information to perform a timely, expeditious, and recent review, and are among the databases which are usually used in literature reviews published in this field from a disciplinary perspective (i.e., PsycINFO) and also using interdisciplinary approaches (i.e., Web of Science), which allowed us to study the individual and psychological aspects of the harms associated with IA.

The review comprised scientific papers published between April 2013 and April 2018 as this is the period between the official recognition of IGD and GD. The following search was undertaken using the following terms, clusters, and Boolean operators: ("Internet" OR "online" OR "game*" OR "gaming" OR "video gam*" OR "videogame*" OR "video-game*" OR "social network*" OR "social media") AND ("Addict*" OR "compuls*" OR "problem*" OR "disorder" OR "pathology*" OR "excess*") AND ("clinic*" OR "treat*" OR "therap*" OR "harm*" OR "risk factor" OR "prevent*"). The search was performed by paper titles as this was the only option available across both search engines.

The inclusion criteria were for studies to: (i) contain empirical data (i.e., data collected using quantitative, qualitative, and mixed methods approaches), (ii) assess online addictions in the EU, (iii) be published between 2013–2018, (iv) include community and clinical samples, (v) provide a full-text article, and (vi) be published in the languages the authors manage (i.e., English, Spanish, French, German, Polish, Italian, and Portuguese).

The literature review was performed as indicated in Figure 1 [22]. Over 390 sources resulted from the initial search. Of these, a great number were filtered out based on the following criteria: (i) duplicates, (ii) meeting and conference abstracts and non-empirical studies (e.g., case studies, anecdotal studies, reviews, editorials, letters, and commentaries), (iii) studies that did not assess IA and related harms in the EU, (iv) studies that were not published between April 2013 and April 2018 (both months included), (v) did not include the population groups targeted (i.e., community and clinical samples), (vi) did not provide a full text article, (vii) were not published in a language the authors manage. Thus, after removing duplicates ($n = 34$), articles in other languages ($n = 32$), conference abstracts ($n = 188$), non-empirical studies ($n = 81$) and non-EU papers ($n = 36$), 19 relevant sources were included in the final analysis.

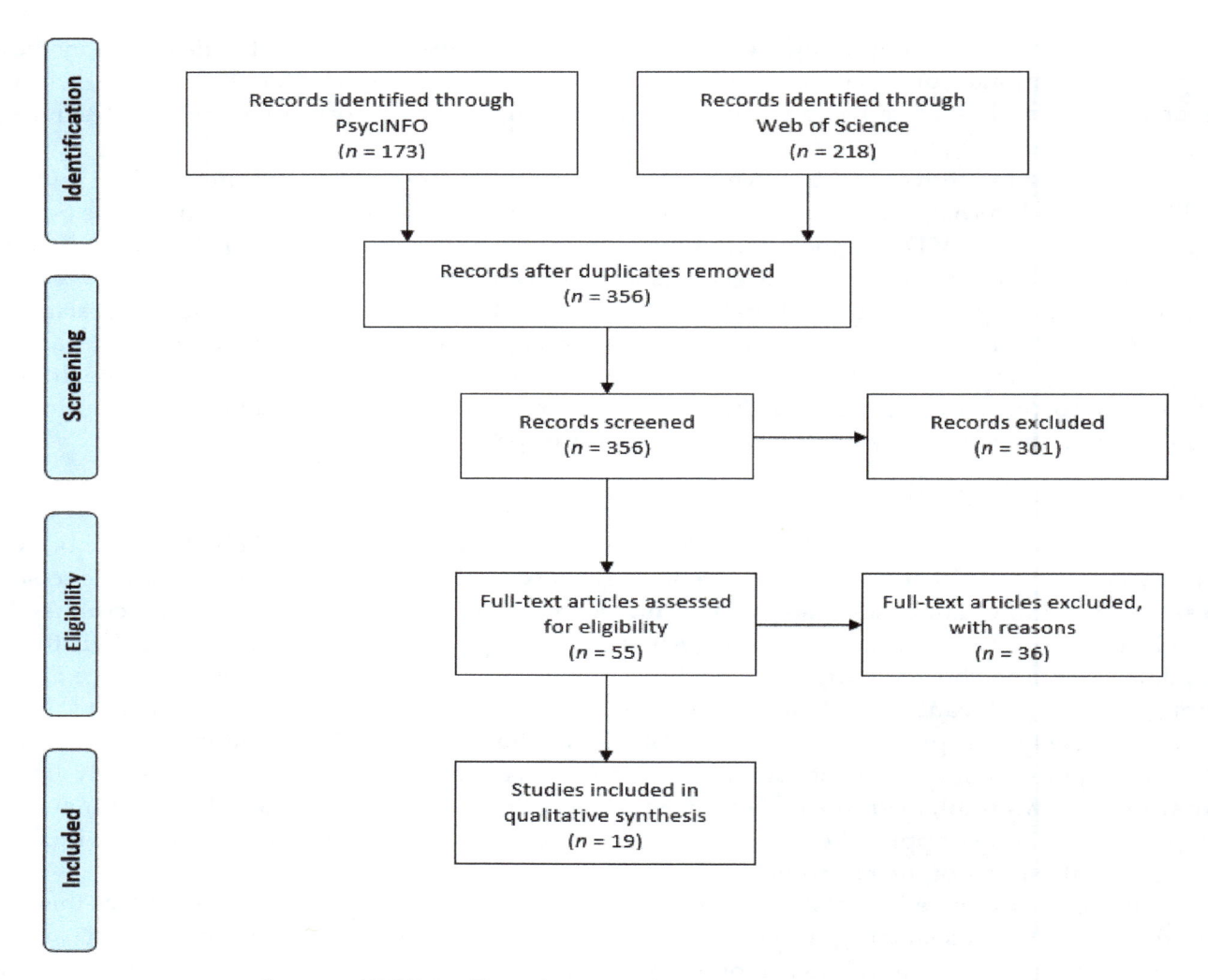

Figure 1. PRISMA Flow diagram of study selection processes.

Two rounds of searches were used: a first round (in January and February 2018) using PsycINFO and subsequently Web of Science, followed by a second round (in April 2018) to ensure all papers were consistently collected and no new paper was published within the specified period and in accordance with the inclusion and exclusion criteria. From the initial pool of 390 papers, after deleting duplicate papers, the remaining 324 results were manually scanned (i.e., title, abstract, key words, and, the paper) to identify the relevant outcomes. Thus, the literature search provided non-exclusive categories of Internet use-related addiction problems as follows: eight Internet addiction papers (i.e., seven by Internet addiction itself, and one including Internet addiction and gaming addiction), 11 online gaming addiction papers (i.e., eight with gaming addiction by itself, and two about gambling and gaming addictions together, and one including Internet addiction and gaming addiction), and three online gambling addiction papers (i.e., own with gambling addiction by itself, and two including gambling and gaming addictions together).

3. Results

Data were initially organized into four main categories which emerged in the qualitative analysis of the 19 European empirical papers undertaken by the two co-authors by categories (see Table 1).

Table 1. Papers selected for the review ($N = 19$).

Authors (Year) [Reference]	Country	Problem
Andrisano, Santoro, De Caro, Palmieri, Capunzo, Venuleo, & Boccia (2016) [23]	Italy	Internet addiction
Beranuy, Carbonell, & Griffiths (2013) [24]	Spain	Gaming addiction
Brand, Laier, & Young (2014) [25]	Germany	Internet addiction
Danet, & Miljkovitch (2016) [26]	France	Internet addiction
Floros, Siomos, Stogniannidou, Giouzepas, & Garyfallos (2014) [27]	Greece	Internet addiction
Frölich, Lehmkuhl, Orawa, BrombaWolf, & Görtz-Dorten (2016) [28]	Germany	Gaming addiction
González, & Orgaz (2014) [29]	Spain	Internet addiction
Holstein, Pedersen, Bendtsen, Madsen, Meilstrup, Nielsen, & Rasmussen (2014) [30]	Denmark	Gaming addiction
Jiménez-Murcia, Fernández-Aranda, Granero, Chóliz, La Verde, Aguglia, & del Pino-Gutiérrez (2014) [31]	Spain	Gambling & Gaming addictions
Lai, Altavilla, Mazza, Scappaticci, Tambelli, Aceto, & Tonioni (2017) [32]	Italy	Internet addiction
Luquiens, Tanguy, Lagadec, Benyamina, Aubin, & Reynaud (2016) [33]	France	Gambling addiction
Mallorquí-Bagué, Fernández-Aranda, Lozano-Madrid, Granero, Mestre-Bach, Baño, & Jiménez-Murcia (2017) [34]	Spain	Gambling & Gaming addictions
Marco, & Chóliz (2017) [35]	Spain	Gaming addiction
Martín-Fernández, Matalí, García-Sánchez, Pardo, Lleras, Castellano-Tejedor (2017) [36]	Spain	Gaming addiction
Müller, Beutel, & Wölfling (2014) [37]	Germany	Internet addiction
Taquet, & Hautekeete (2013) [38]	France	Gaming addiction
Torres-Rodríguez, Griffiths, Carbonell, Farriols-Hernando, & Torres-Jimenez (2017) [39]	Spain	Gaming addiction
Van Rooij, Schoenmaker, & van de Mheen (2017) [40]	The Netherlands	Gaming addiction
Wölfling, Beutel, Dreier, & Müller (2014) [41]	Germany	Internet addiction & Gaming addiction

Therefore, both authors independently first qualitatively analyzed the papers divided by categories (i.e., O.L.-F. performed the examination of gaming and gambling addiction articles [24,28,30,31,33–36, 38–40]; and D.J.K. evaluated Internet addiction articles [23,25–27,29,32,37,41]). Therefore, both authors reviewed the contents of the identified articles according to the following categories of analysis: title and journal, authors and country, sample, design, aim(s), measures, results, implications for policy options and prevention, and conclusions for harm minimization [15]. From this categorical analysis the authors proceeded to discuss the main preliminary results, and extracted the information based on the aims with the final purpose of creating a set of preliminary policy options and preventive actions for IA and related harms in Europe. This process included several rounds until theoretical saturation of the contents from all 19 papers was achieved, according to the aims.

The present qualitative and narrative analysis resulted in the division of identified research papers into four categories: (i) the characteristics of problem users (including community and clinical samples); (ii) GIA; (iii) specific IA problems (i.e., gaming, and gambling addictions); and (iv) policy options for preventing Internet use-related harm in Europe. The first category about users' characteristics is subdivided by Internet use-relate addiction problems (i.e., GIA and specific problems), as the literature shows there are differences in Internet users based on typology of disordered behaviour. Therefore, the categories related to GIA and specific problems were analyzed in detail covering both non-clinical and clinical studies, which were researched from a policy implications perspective. Lastly, the fourth category was divided into respective policy options to reduce Internet harm from an individual person perspective.

Regarding geographical location, half of the studies included in this review ($n = 10$; 53%) were from the Southern European region (countries are ordered from higher to lower frequency): Spain ($n = 7$), Italy ($n = 2$), and Greece ($n = 1$); and 42% ($n = 8$) were from the Western European region: Germany ($n = 4$), France ($n = 3$), and The Netherlands ($n = 1$). Finally, only one study (5%) was conducted in the Northern region (i.e., Denmark).

3.1. The Characteristics of Targeted Problem Internet Users

Almost all participants included in the studies were adolescents and young adults from high schools or universities, and the assessed studies dealt with GIA and gaming addiction. Only a few studies assessed online gambling addiction, with participants usually being middle-aged male adults.

3.1.1. Generalized Internet Addiction Users

The main characteristics extracted were:

- Sample sizes: variability depending on the method applied (all research methods were used);
- Age groups: majority of adolescents, and some adults;
- Gender: balanced in adolescent community samples, and more males in clinical samples;
- Regions: In Western and Southern Europe (i.e., Germany, France, Greece, Italy, and Spain).

Sample sizes included studies which varied in number depending on the research methods applied. For instance, samples ranged from 16 Italian Internet-addicted patients investigated through an experiment with a control group to assess the biological causes of IA [32] to a survey with 1,019 German adults to test a new model for GIA [25]. Regarding life stage, participants were usually adolescents and students in high schools [23,27,29], although a few studies included adults [25]. Regarding participant gender, studies on GIA tended to cover both genders in a balanced way. However, when participants were university students, there tended to be more females than males in the sample [25,26,29], and there were significantly more males in clinical samples [27,37]). No study analyzed potential differences between female and male problem Internet users.

3.1.2. Specific Internet Addiction Problem Users: Gamers and Gamblers

The main characteristics extracted from Internet-addicted gamers and gamblers were:

- Sample sizes ranged from one case study to group surveys including mixed methods studies;
- Age groups: majority of adolescents, and a few young adults who were gamers and only adult gamblers;
- Gender: more males, especially in clinical samples and gambling studies;
- Regions: all regions studied (i.e., Spain, France, Germany, The Netherlands, and Denmark).

Sample sizes included clinical case studies of one [38] and nine adolescent patients [24], and online surveys with gaming or gambling participants [30,31] used mixed methods studies combining interviews and surveys on Internet gambling [33,34]. Almost all studies about gaming addiction used adolescent samples [28,38–40], and the clinical studies were conducted with males who usually played Massively Multiplayer Online Role-Playing Games (MMORPGs [24,38,39]) and sometimes Multiplayer Online Battle Arena games (MOBA [39]) or First-Person Shooters (FPS [39]). Interestingly, these studies usually included family members (e.g., the mother, both parents, or a sibling [24,28,38,39]), type of family [41], or type of parenting style [28] to treat existing conflicts (e.g., loneliness and discussions with parents) and measured the impact of environmental factors and interventions [28,38–40].

However, studies on Internet gambling were conducted with patients within a pathological gambling unit [31,34] and explored factors related to IGD, and some participants were invited from an online gambling site (i.e., Winnimax [33]). These studies came from Spain [31,33–36,39], France [33,38], Germany [28,41], The Netherlands [40], and Denmark [30].

3.2. Generalised Internet Addiction Problems

Eight studies (42.1%) assessed GIA, and referred to non-specific Internet use (i.e., not reliant on the engagement with a particular online activity), and few considered prevention of IA [23]. The studies reviewed were from Germany [25,37], France [26], Greece [27], Italy [23,32], and Spain [29].

Findings suggested a wide range of problems could arise from overusing (e.g., difficulty cutting down, lack of sleep, fatigue, irritability, apathy, racing thoughts, declining grades or poor job performance, and neglecting other duties). Thus, the presence of addiction symptoms (e.g., tolerance), impairment in daily functioning, high comorbidity (i.e., anxiety, depression, and OCD), and risk factors (e.g., preoccupied and fearful attachment styles) were identified. Specifically, problem users tended to present psychological characteristics and co-occurring disorders (i.e., when two or more health problems occur at the same time, e.g., an addiction problem and a mental health disorder are present simultaneously). Usually, these other mental health disorders related to personality disorders, mood disorders, or anxiety disorders. For example, those who were affected by GIA also presented with poor coping strategies and low self-esteem [25], and attachment difficulties (e.g., preoccupied and fearful types [26]). Regarding co-occurring disorders, it seems at least half of the samples presented at least two problems [25,27]). The most prevalent associated problems were depression and anxiety disorder (e.g., the latter with the social subtype [25]). However, CBT emerged as effective in leading to significant changes in symptom experience.

The main characteristics of individuals with GIA in Europe were:

- Almost all studies used Young's psychometric tests, and their derivatives, whilst finding higher prevalence in clinical studies;
- Models in IA explain risk factors, which are diverse (cognitive, attachment styles, and comorbidity);
- Peer education programs when used as school interventions have good outcomes;
- Clinical interventions rely on cognitive and emotional components, including CBT approaches.

Prevalence rates were higher in clinical studies than in community studies. For instance, Müller et al. [37] estimated a prevalence of 71% of German treatment seekers with the clinical diagnosis of IA; while Andrisano and colleagues [23] found a prevalence rate of 4% of severe Internet-addicted Italian adolescent users among the community sample they studied, which was similar to the other community samples with young Spanish adults, where the prevalence was 10% according to Gonzalez and Orgaz [29]. The scale that most frequently used to measure IA [23,25,27] was the Internet Addiction Test (IAT [42]) and its short version (s-IAT [43]). However, other valid measures have also been used [27,29] (e.g., Online Cognitions Scale (OCS [44]); Index of Problematic Online Experiences (I-POE [45]), and the Assessment of Internet and Computer game Addiction—Scale (AICA-S [41])).

Brandt et al.'s [25] model on GIA explained 64% of GIA variance based on addiction symptoms, and included associated disorders and IA symptoms experience, suggesting users' cognitions (e.g., poor coping and cognitive expectations) increase the risk of IA. However, comorbidity can also mediate the relationship between symptomatology and factors which seem to act as a cause. Similarly, Danet and Miljkovitch [26] stated fearful and preoccupied attachments can be associated with IA, and Lai et al. [32] suggested a generalized impairment in emotional and cognitive processing abilities in those who suffer from IA, which can be linked to dissociative symptoms. Comorbidities in IA seem, therefore, to be diverse and present in half of Internet-addicted patients [25,27,37,41]. The identified comorbidities include depression, social anxiety, and associated symptoms experienced, such as low self-esteem, low self-efficacy, and high stress vulnerability. According to Müller et al. [27], the majority of treatment seekers present criteria sufficient to be diagnosed with IA, and half of them have comorbidities (i.e., depression, OCD, and dissociative symptoms) and stress. In general, comorbidities include Axis I diagnoses, such as:

- Anxiety Disorders (e.g., panic, social anxiety, and post-traumatic stress disorders);
- Mood Disorders (e.g., major depression, bipolar disorder);
- Eating Disorders (e.g., anorexia nervosa, bulimia nervosa);
- Psychotic Disorders;
- Dissociative Disorders;
- Substance Use Disorders (i.e., drug addictions).

Furthermore, it seems anxiety disorders are associated with the onset of GIA, and mood disorders can be precursors of or follow IA [27].

School interventions which have shown excellent outcomes are the peer education program evaluated by Andrisano and colleagues [23] in Italy, which included brainstorming and video co-creation. In Spain, potential Internet-addicted students [29] also presented with the problem, and this was associated with environmental factors (e.g., family, friends, online interactions, etc.). Both school-based studies came from Southern Europe, suggesting there is a need of educational policies to prevent GIA and related harms in this European region.

Clinical interventions usually aimed to validate tools and cut-off points to estimate the prevalence of GIA [37,41] (e.g., AICA-S [41]).

3.3. Specific Internet Addiction Problems: Gaming and Gambling

Twelve papers (63.2%) reported results on online gaming and gambling addictions, nine of which focused only on gaming (44.4%). Thus, these two problems together were more prevalent in comparison with GIA in the assessed samples of European studies.

3.3.1. Internet Gaming Addiction

The main characteristics of Internet gaming addiction in Europe were:

- All studies used different scales and methods (from qualitative to experiments) and addressed prevalence;
- A few models and risk factors emerged (i.e., cognitive, emotional, environmental, and comorbidity);
- Peer education programs used as school interventions have shown contradictory outcomes;
- Clinical studies relied on cognitive, emotional, and personality components and used CBT.

Studies that screened for gaming addiction in community samples were a minority in this section, and usually measured self-perceived problematic video gaming through different devices (e.g., computers and consoles) to assess both offline and online gaming through cross-sectional surveys in Denmark and Spain [30,35]. Regarding their commonalities, males and older adolescents were at a higher risk of gaming addiction problems, non-clinical measures were useful as preventive actions, and programs to reduce gaming were usually effective, and even more so if personality traits (such as impulsivity) were addressed in the interventions.

However, clinical studies were the most common in the samples that were included in the present review, coming from Spain [24,36,39], France [38], The Netherlands [40], and Germany [28]. Patients were brought to health centers by their families, usually by their mother or a sibling [24,38], and in general parent supervision was required [28]. The main factors associated with problematic MMORPG, MOBA and FPS behaviors were dissociation (i.e., a psychological mechanism of stepping out of oneself to be protected from external harm; e.g., bullying or the loss of a loved one), entertainment (e.g., enjoyment and escapism), and virtual friendship (e.g., social relationships in game without any need to personally know one's fellow gamers; the 'clan' or the 'guild') [24]. Therefore, there was a need to assess present motivations [38]: to change (e.g., if you continue gaming like this during a decade, what will happen to you?), and to work therapeutically (e.g., playing time was double the usual adult working time per week). Simultaneously, functional analyses were performed (e.g., to support the patient to treat themselves regarding the co-occurring disorders associated with gaming), treating the gaming behaviour (i.e., psychological gaming experience), while addressing alternative pastime opportunities, and improving other relationships.

In CBT interventions, the emotional component was as relevant as the cognitive component; e.g., using techniques related to empathy, self-esteem, self-control, assertiveness, communication skills, or insight [39]. One of the main aspects in the therapeutic intervention was relapse prevention [24,38,39]. Furthermore, one study [28,38–40] showed that nonspecific psychiatric disorders pose an increased risk for gaming addiction. This supports the argument that Internet gaming addiction might be a discrete psychiatric entity usually combined with emotional and social problems [24,38]. It can be related to ADHD, Asperger's, Autism, and other disorders, such as anxiety and depression, social phobia, pervasive developmental disorders, among other comorbid conditions and problems (e.g., parent–child relationship problems, school relationship problems, obesity, cannabis use, and anhedonia). The prognosis is generally positive at three or six months of treatment [24,36,38] for those patients with an externalized profile (i.e., disruptive behaviour disorder, ADHD, and adaptive disorder) or an internalized profile (i.e., anxiety, mood and personality disorders, social relationship problems, previous mental disorders family histories, and individuals who use gaming to escape discomfort experienced in their daily lives [39]). Furthermore, clinicians have stated that increasing numbers of patients sought help through families in the recent years in European public hospitals and health centers [34,36].

Thus, gaming addiction in Europe during the last decade has required both, the development of new short non-clinical measures to screen for it in young adolescents (e.g., using the computer gaming index, console gaming index, or the Internet use index [30]), while clinical studies usually were case studies and used mixed methods dealing with interventions through tailored CBT, including for instance the 'Individualized Psychotherapeutic Program for the Addiction to the Information and Communication Technologies' (PIPATIC [39]), and new psychometric tools (e.g., Clinical Video game Addiction test second version(C-VAT 2.0 [40]), or Assessment of Internet and Computer Game Addiction (AICA-S [41])). Related to prevalence, according to Martin-Fernandez et al. [36], 69% of Spanish adolescent patients met the DSM-5 criteria for IGD, and 91% of young Dutch patients met the IGD criteria through the C-VAT 0.2 [40]. However, only 37% of gamblers also experienced video game addiction as co-occurring disorder.

Furthermore, the effectiveness of impulsivity techniques to prevent gaming addiction has been demonstrated [35]. The most studied gaming problem is related to using MMORPGs [24,38,39], which has been researched through qualitative and mixed methods approaches to create a theoretical model [24] or to test CBT interventions [38,39]. The MMORPG online gaming addiction phenomenon has been described by Beranuy et al. [24], including use motivations (e.g., entertainment, escapism or disassociation, and virtual friendship) and factors associated with it, its symptomatology, and consequences (e.g., game context, conflict, and loss of control, respectively). Taquet and Hautekeete [38] and Torres-Rodriguez et al. [39] also highlighted good knowledge of the world of video games by the therapist and a balance between emotional and cognitive components in the intervention are positive factors to ensure therapeutic alliance and successful treatment outcome.

The scales used to measure gaming addiction in this European review were diverse and validated in different languages. These instruments include the AICA-S [41], Assessment of Pathological Computer Gaming (CSV-S [46]), Problem Video Game Playing Scale (PVP [47]), and the Video game dependency test (TDV [35]). Consequently, only a few of the assessed studies measured IGD, as stated by the APA [36,39,40] (e.g., the C-VAT 2.0 [40], the Internet Gaming Disorder test with 20 items (IGD-20 [48])).

School interventions have also been studied [30,35], usually to develop non-clinical measures for problematic gaming and Internet use, screen time, and other problems. The study from Denmark [30] did not find any problems regarding GIA or specific Internet uses in their population of study. On the other hand, a similar Spanish study [35] used an intervention for adolescents to prevent video gaming addiction and to treat two intervention groups with a program to prevent addiction to technologies (i.e., "PrevTec 3.1"). In one group, impulsivity management techniques were added to intensify the positive outcomes of the preventive program, in addition to a waitlist control group. They found the preventive program significantly reduced perceived dependence on video games, and the group who received instructions on impulsivity techniques maintained the successful results in the follow-up better than those who did not receive these techniques in the program. Accordingly, personality traits, such as impulsivity, appear to play a role in prevention on a long-term basis.

Ten lessons have been extracted regarding the problem gamer profile in Europe:

1. It appears they are high-school students,
2. Usually males,
3. Who usually play MMORPGs,
4. Spend considerable time at home alone and game for many hours daily,
5. Treatment is usually sought by parents,
6. These patients present distinct addiction symptomatology,
7. With specific comorbidities (internalized versus externalized profiles),
8. Together with problems with social relationships (e.g., social phobia),
9. CBT has positive results after three and six months, which are maintained after six months,
10. Prognosis improves if family support the treatment.

These studies also highlighted that preventative programs are effective over time in reducing gaming. However, in clinical settings, time spent gaming, age and gender, type of games (e.g., MMORPGs), and type of comorbidities were associated with gaming addiction (e.g., individuals with externalizing profiles have the best prognosis after three months and both profiles have a good prognosis at six months of treatment [36]). Moreover, lack of external parental control should be considered as important risk factor. However, one study did not find any specific psychiatric disorder as a risk factor for this addiction problem [28]. Thus, gaming addiction appears to be a unique clinical entity that can be treated by CBT (e.g., with a treatment length of three to six months). Follow-up studies are required to verify its benefits across groups and cultures.

3.3.2. Internet Gambling Addiction

The main characteristics of Internet gambling addiction in Europe were:

- All studies used different measures for gambling addiction;
- Risk factors emerged, especially when related to gaming addiction;
- Severe comorbidity exists when both Internet gambling and gaming problems were present;
- Clinical studies rely on self-seeking treatment and tailored interventions.

Three studies (15.8%) addressed mainly Internet Gambling Disorder in clinical samples, suggesting it is a different clinical entity in comparison to IGD, although both share some sociodemographic characteristics (e.g., both usually affect males) and psychological features (e.g., type of emotional distress, higher harm avoidance, and reward dependence traits).

The measures used to assess gambling addiction can be considered traditional (i.e., Stinchfield's Diagnostic Questionnaire for Pathological Gambling [49], and the Problem Gambling Severity Index (PGSI [50])).

In addition, when gambling was the main addiction and the patient played videogames, the comorbidity was more severe than for Internet gaming addiction itself [31,34,36], specifically if gaming addiction was identified together with gambling addiction (in which case paranoid ideation, distress, OCD, and interpersonal sensitivity were also present [31]). However, inversely, comorbidity did not appear in gamblers who were not gaming addicts, although the reviewed research indicated that gambling addiction appeared to be the more severe behavioral addiction. In other words, both disorders appear to be independent of each other, which is supported by evidence regarding their different clinical profiles [24]. Internet gambling had a higher mean age of disordered onset, disorder severity, somatization and depression symptoms, among other personality traits (i.e., novelty seeking and persistence) and associations with substance use (e.g., tobacco use). Furthermore, patients with both problems are younger, present more dysfunctional personality traits (e.g., lower self-directedness and higher persistence), and general psychopathology (e.g., depression, anxiety, and social phobia), higher body mass index (BMI) and food addiction (FA). In summary, although both addictive online behaviors share some emotional distress and personality traits, gambling disorder appeared to be more severe in the included studies.

Moreover, online interventions seem only to be effective when the gambler seeks treatment, and a commitment with a health professional is made, even if it is short-lived; inversely, if there is no help-seeking the efficacy of any intervention is counter-productive or may have an aversive effect [33]; therefore, 'more is not always better' in terms of prevention. Lastly, CBT should also be personalized to the type of gambling activity (e.g., online poker), which again requires knowledge from the therapist, as highlighted in the case of gaming [38].

3.4. European Policy Options to Prevent Internet Addiction Problems

From the present European literature review encompassing the period between 2013 and 2018, the following four policy options have been developed based on the included 19 studies (see Figure 2).

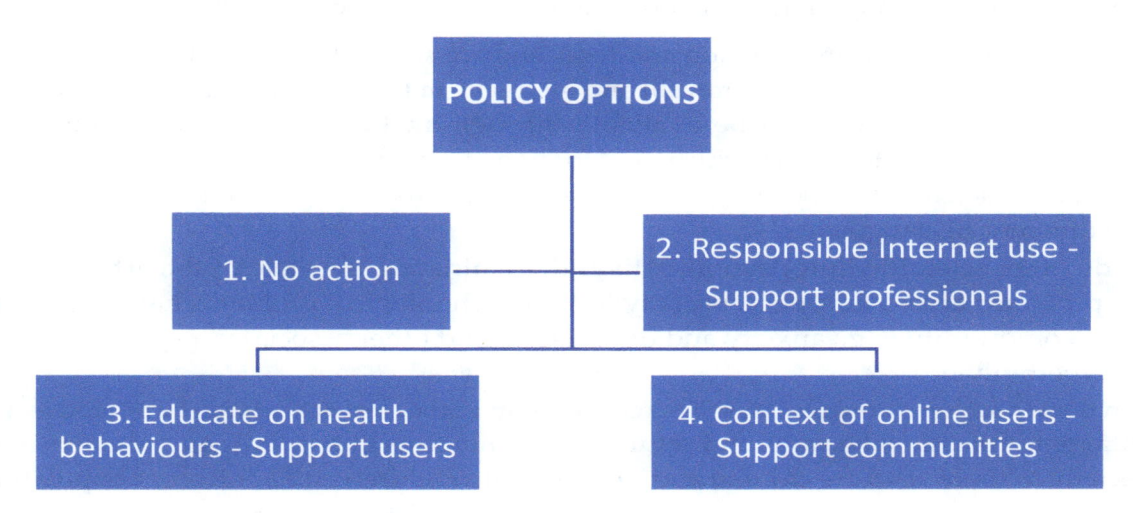

Figure 2. Policy options derived from the present literature review.

3.4.1. No Action

The first policy option concerns all stakeholders involved and should be considered with caution. In a few studies, contradictory findings have emerged which have highlighted it is not worth taking action if treatment is not sought [33] or if the problem does not emerge [30]. Thus, the first policy option is related to the following preventive actions:

- Internet addiction, Internet gaming, and gambling addictions can be hazardous (e.g., they can appear temporarily and last less than a year and then disappear). These respective problems are associated with a variety of internal and individual factors and are not always associated with the same comorbidity or associated symptom experiences. Environmental factors may also contribute to the emergence of different online addictions. Thus, Internet use-related addiction problems can appear temporarily and disappear spontaneously before they can be considered a disorder.
- This option should probably be considered when the period of the problem affecting users is less than a year, with no comorbidity or other associated severe symptoms and problems. However, if there is a suspicion of chronification (e.g., with a length of at least six months), preventive measures should be taken to avoid the development of the disorder and future disorder diagnosis.
- At present, this option seems to be unsustainable because the public health concern is growing and health practitioners are reporting increasing numbers of cases (e.g., more clinical papers than non-clinical) and interventions.

This option refers to natural recovery, which seems to exist but has not been studied much. However, due to the precautionary principle (i.e., which encourages policies that protect human health and the environment in the face of uncertain risks) it may jeopardize Europe's ability to prevent Internet use-related problems from emerging in the first place, and to take advantage of the instruments, therapeutic, and of preventive opportunities that the scientific literature on generalized and specific Internet addiction problems has recently provided.

3.4.2. Promote and Disseminate Applied Research on Responsible Internet Use and Prevention

The second policy option mainly addresses support organizations, professionals, and practitioners. Applied research is present in almost all reviewed studies, as research seeks to find solutions to the problems in European community and clinical settings. Only a couple of studies described models of GIA [25] and Internet gaming addiction [24] to provide an understanding about which factors contribute to the problems, their phenomenology, and therapy components to clinically address them. Moreover, providing information and interventions seem to be the key public health strategies to prevent and address the problem in all settings. Early preventive actions can:

- Promote evidence-based information and tools and are supported by applied research outcomes for professionals who can help to prevent and intervene in Internet use-related addiction problems. For instance, information can be available through an EU webpage with public resources (e.g., containing validated scales which exist for non-clinical measures), contact details for support organizations across the respective European countries, a list of experts, and information provided in the different EU languages.
- Include other scientific European initiatives disseminating the state of the art of research into these problems across Europe, especially if these technological problems have associated risks, such as comorbidity (e.g., anxiety and depression) and other associated psychosocial problems (e.g., cyberbullying).
- When these problems are present, self-screen tools and other test actions can be offered as a package to different professional groups and settings (e.g., clinicians in hospitals and teachers in schools), especially to those who are close to and/or work with children and adolescent populations.

There is a need to improve this research field to diversify the methodologies used and translate them to the professional sector, and to promote joint clinical and educational research. It is also crucial for standardized measures to assess problems and compare them in order to support diagnosis and treatment success (e.g., cross-culturally and trans-diagnostically). These preventive actions can provide support for decision-makers to better understand the problems from a European public health perspective, and to promote responsible Internet use and media literacy.

3.4.3. Promote Education on Offline and Online Health Behaviors in Young Populations

The third policy option addresses all Internet users, especially those who have appeared as more at risk for developing Internet use-related addiction problems. All reviewed studies have highlighted common aspects related to promoting healthy Internet use, especially in adolescents and young adults, as some gaming genres are very demanding regarding competition and social involvement (e.g., MMORPGs). The following options are preventive actions which can be introduced:

- To encourage alternative motivations, engagement in alternative entertainment behaviors (also those including Internet use), new coping skills, cognitive and emotional skills, healthy attachment styles to reduce the risk of Internet use-related problems and to reduce Internet usage, if needed (e.g., through alerts and notifications) and to provide alternative options of relaxation (e.g., reading, meeting people, and engaging in physical activities).
- To detect the risk of experiencing other comorbidities or problems and address them with professional support and the support of significant others (e.g., caregivers in the case of adolescents), and to embrace systemic approaches.
- If a problem with Internet usage is present, all Internet use-related addictions should be simultaneously assessed, as many of the reviewed studies were clinical studies on gaming addiction, which together with gambling in young adults seemed to indicate the worst-case scenario regarding these problems.

In the EU, there is a need for programs and campaigns addressing children and youth to promote awareness of the risks of online behaviors at an individual person's level. Studies have shown school interventions are usually effective, even more so if they include a psychological component (e.g., impulsivity management techniques when gaming). Young individuals should be engaged in conversations and activities concerning offline and online health, potential positive and negative implications of excessive online behaviors, and provided with information on alternative pastime activities and alternative coping strategies not involving Internet use.

The usual problem user is an adolescent who increasingly spends time gaming alone at home, usually plays MMORPGs, and experiences co-occurring problems and negative impacts in their daily life. Thus, problem cases should be treated on a case-by-case basis when detected with tailored psychological and educational interventions, including CBT, whilst ensuring treatment encompasses interventions for comorbidities. The young user should be able to determine which functions the maladaptive Internet use fulfils in his or her life, and which other options are available to him or her with professional support. These actions can be supported by other initiatives in educational and health settings, which require resources and action plans (e.g., providing funding and resources).

3.4.4. Support Communities and Significant Others of Problematic Internet Users

In addition to supporting professionals (i.e., the second policy option) and users (i.e., the third policy option), communities (i.e., the fourth policy option) also need attention. The preventive actions for this group are the following:

- Enhanced family, partner, and peer communication and caretaking (e.g., through parents, siblings, partners or friends) can prevent the problems from emerging when risk indicators appear and develop progressively (e.g., excessive time spent playing online games, lack of sleep due to constant online connection, irritability and mood changes when disconnecting, neglecting school or relationships). Thus, 'keeping an eye' on time spent and having conversations about online uses can be the first measure of prevention in families and friendship groups.

- Information should also be available for users' environments (e.g., for families, schools and communities) about the risks of habitually engaging in online role-playing games or online gambling applications which can be out of control and cause negative health consequences (i.e., functional impairment and distress) or financial problems (i.e., online gambling).

These problems usually affect families, education or workplace organizations, and communities. Thus, basic information, education, social, and clinical support can help individuals in the immediate context of problem users with community support. The EU should consider facilitating information provision to healthcare providers to support general practitioners when taking care of communities in health settings. Moreover, the implementation of actions, programs, and services for information, early detection, and facilitation of support and treatment routes for future problem users and their significant others are options to develop. For instance, at a school and community level, actions to promote prevention can be provided together with those for other related problems (e.g., substance use disorders and cyberbullying).

4. Discussion

This timely European literature review provides an overview of the currently available research on Internet use-related addiction problems in this region in the period between gaming addiction recognition by the APA and the WHO (i.e., April 2013–April 2018). It has used a public health approach and a preventative perspective to offer a set of policy options and preventive actions. The aims, therefore, were to use a cross-cultural approach across the EU to identify the problematic users' profiles for risk management in community and clinical settings; to ascertain how Internet addiction problems have been researched in Europe within the period when gaming disorder was officially recognized by health organizations; to understand the scope of their harm implications; and, at a public health level, which preventive actions can be extracted and policy options proposed.

An update of these problems at an individual level in the EU has been provided as Internet use-related addiction problems seem to have increased world-wide in the past two decades [6,18,19], with an estimated global prevalence of 6% [18]. Low rates have generally been reported in European regions in school community sample studies (e.g., via meta-analyses and cross-cultural studies) published between 2012 and 2015 (with an average of a 2.5% prevalence [18–21]). However, this review has highlighted the prevalence is growing, as GIA in similar adolescent and young community samples is now approximately 4%–10% [23,29]. Indeed, a recent cross-cultural study has indicated that the prevalence of PIU in Europe is relatively higher than previously indicated, although this observation is based on an adult community sample (i.e., where prevalence rates ranged from 14% to 55% [51]). However, caution is needed to be considered a cause for concern in the present general population due to the highlighted conceptual and methodological issues in the respective studies of these addiction problems.

On the other hand, another indicator that requires attention and has appeared in this review is the higher rates of GIA and online gaming addiction in European clinical samples [36,37,40] compared with community samples [23,29], which range between 69%–91% for both addiction problems. This is in line with Carbonell et al.'s [52] and Lopez-Fernandez's [53] bibliometric studies of IA and other specific online addiction problems published in the last two decades. It seems increasing world-wide Internet use is accompanied by an increasing number of publications on Internet addiction problems. However, it also seems clear gaming addiction has surpassed IA, probably due to IGD recognition by the APA [5] within the period studied, which was the starting point for this review and attracted the attention of clinicians and researchers who deal with these health problems and have published their findings since. The fact that the number of publications on gaming disorders in Europe, and internationally, is increasing may be due to the official recognition of gaming addiction as a disorder, which is indicated by the number of recent reviews [54–59]. Furthermore, neurological functions have commonalities and differences across these two behavioral addictions [54].

The number of studies included in this literature review, however, is scarce compared to other previous international reviews on GIA and IGD [5,6,16,21,54–58]. One explanation is that these health concerns are less prevalent in Europe relative to Asian regions, which is supported by the scientific literature. However, this does not mean that the precautionary principle cannot be applied [10], and almost no reviews have analyzed papers cross-culturally using different languages [6]. In the reviewed European samples, no study from Eastern Europe has been identified, and the regions that have seen more publications are both Southern and Western Europe for GIA, and Northern regions for gaming addiction. This is consistent with a previous cross-cultural study on dependent mobile phone use [60]. In that case, the Northern and Southern regions were the ones with heaviest online mobile use (the Northern countries especially for gaming), and the Eastern regions had lower rates. France appeared as one of the countries with the highest problematic mobile phone use, although Spain has seen a larger number of publications on Internet use-related addiction problems in the period studied.

The European scientific evidence reviewed here published between April 2013–April 2018 identified three potential problems: GIA, online gaming, and gambling disorders at community and clinical levels, which usually affected adolescents and young male adults, except for online gambling (middle-aged adults). This distribution corresponds to previous literature [5,6,16,54–57], specifically as gambling requires financial resources. However, recent empirical European and international studies on IA and gaming addiction show that females are increasingly affected, although they have not been the main study group yet [51,61]. To the best of the authors' knowledge, no review on these problems at an individual person level in the EU has been published yet, and the main findings correspond to the results presented in two previous international reviews on clinical issues related to IA [6,55].

Furthermore, comorbidity seems to be the norm [6,59], and usually includes depression, social anxiety disorder, social phobia, OCD, ADHD, hostility, substance use disorders (e.g., gambling, alcohol, marihuana, nicotine, and cocaine use), eating disorders (e.g., binge eating disorder, bulimia, and obesity), and certain personality traits and personality disorders (e.g., impulsivity, borderline, avoidant personality, or antisocial disorders) [6,55]. However, the present review showed different comorbidities depending on the type of Internet use-related addiction problems, a novel finding which reinforces the independent identities of GIA and gaming addiction [5,24,38,53–59]. In GIA, half of the investigated samples present with comorbid Axis I disorders, which is consistent with previous research [25,27,62]. This suggests a complete psychiatric evaluation is needed for these types of problems. Nevertheless, this review also highlights the need of a psychological evaluation as other emotional, cognitive, and behavioral features have emerged, such as the role of self-esteem [25,32,39], attachment or defense styles [26,60], cognitive coping and disassociation [25,32], and other personality traits and mental disorders [6,25,27,37,41,59] in specific developmental stages (i.e., adolescence [58]). In gaming addiction, however, the spectrum of comorbid disorders is more diverse and severe, especially if gambling is one of the co-occurring disorders, including internalizing and externalizing profiles which need to be considered regarding recovery length [24,35,36,38,39,59]. A European gamer profile has also emerged where environmental factors appear for the etiology, development, and recovery of these problems (e.g., CBT with a systemic approach for adolescent gamers).

At present, research has moved the field forward considerably, resulting in clinicians and researchers recognizing Internet use-related addiction problems across different devices [30,53,60,62] as more scientific research is emerging [5,6,52], and so is the demand for diagnosis and treatment [24,34,36,38,39,41]. The present literature is slightly contradictory, as it has been suggested that the device used to engage in gaming can be associated with the occurrence, course, and prognosis of IGD [62], and it has also been stated that the device does not influence gaming addiction problems [30]. The most alarming studies on gaming addiction and the role of gaming devices come from Asia, and those studies which contradict the findings related to the role of gaming devices in gaming addiction were mainly conducted in Europe.

On the other hand, other contradictions regarding gaming addiction, such as comorbidity or associated symptom experience identified, are the reasons why, together with the low number of prevention research studies in the field [13,16,57,59,63], it seems essential to start addressing possible preventive actions regarding IA and related harms at all levels (i.e., by regions and globally). Simultaneously, qualitative work is needed to address the uniqueness of the phenomenological expression of these types of behavioral addiction problems [64] facilitated through the Internet.

Regarding the policy options, the first one (i.e., no action) has also been put forward in similar preventive studies on substance use disorders. This action is based on the available knowledge on natural recovery, which is considered in the context of IGD as well [65]. However, as almost no follow-up studies have produced evidence on long-term relapse and the natural recovery rates, caution must be applied for this first policy option. The second policy option will aid informing and training professionals and practitioners and is aligned with the few international reviews on IA and prevention. For instance, according to Vondráčková and Gabrhelík [16], the improvement of skills in specific professions (i.e., for researchers, counsellors, and teachers) can support preventive action and better intervention plans or, as Kiraly et al. [57] stated, measures are taken to make health services available to gamers who experience problems. The third policy option, related to users, also highlights the need to pay attention to those who are among the highest risk groups, individuals of particular age (e.g., children and youth, especially MMORPG gamers), gender (males), engaged in a general or specific Internet activity, and who experience comorbidity [6,15,16,55,57–59]. The fourth policy option is aimed at supporting communities, including signposting families, schools, institutions, and governments [13,16,57,63,66,67].

Nevertheless, as King et al. [13] highlighted, in Western cultures including Europe, at the moment community-based support derives from non-profit organizations and the private sector; although a few countries are starting to provide support through their national health systems, such as Germany [10]. However, not all measures that have been put into place to prevent Internet and gaming addiction have obtained effective results [13,57], and there is a bias regarding what is known through the current literature, which is dominated by English language publications from English and Asian regions [13,57]. Thus, the current scientific literature base may not sufficiently reflect what other non-English speaking countries are already doing regarding prevention at all levels (e.g., Switzerland [10]).

This review also has its limitations, including the strategy applied to identify the included studies. For instance, the period of five years selected, and the number of databases used can be considered short and small, but both decisions have a rationale (i.e., recognition of gaming addiction, and disciplinary and interdisciplinary scientific search engines associated with the aims, respectively). Preliminary findings are relevant as they have shown, for example, the emergence of clinical research in online addiction problems in Europe with its specificities (e.g., gamer profile and specific comorbidity depending on internet use-related problems). However, in this emergent field, other literature reviews have also been undertaken with even shorter periods of analysis for relevant reasons and with a larger or smaller number of databases (e.g., internet use-related to self-harm and suicidal behaviour using Medline, Cochrane, and PsychINFO, and covering four years [68], or the utility of magnetic resonance imaging to study IA using Scopus, which covered a three year period [69]). The keywords applied did not take into consideration other possible Internet addiction problems which are currently being researched in Europe (e.g., cybersex). However, the identified limited number of studies produced preliminary findings to achieve the present aims to obtain an overview of the status quo in Europe regarding these problems from a cross-cultural and preventive perspectives, with a qualitative analysis using the lens of harm minimization to develop a set of policy options with preventive actions. Future research should first extend a similar procedure to non-European countries and also collect grey literature with non-English language publications to produce a holistic perspective of the policy options and prevention actions and consequences of what kinds of initiatives are already taken in several countries, which can be useful at local and global levels. Thus, this review offers a brief and timely snapshot of scientific studies in the recent period where gaming addiction has been officially recognized. Indeed, it is the first review on these problems at a European level using a preventive approach. However, methodological improvements can aid more robust future research, which should apply methods and procedures to compute other quantitative inter-rater reliability measures to complement the qualitative inter-rated reliability obtained through sharing and comparing coding agreements in iterative rounds until arriving at a consensus and theoretical saturation of findings (e.g., the Cohen's Kappa coefficient [70]), and complementary quality checks of the procedure (e.g., the Critical Appraisal Skills Programme (CASP) [71]). The included studies' findings have been synthesized and analyzed in detail in the present literature review to provide an overview regarding these emerging addiction problems in Europe, which can be used with caution as the present literature review constitutes a qualitative narrative synthesis, for international comparisons, and to translate some of the identified policy options into preventive actions.

5. Conclusions

In summary, the most prevalent Internet addiction problems appeared to be generalized Internet addiction and online gaming addiction in the EU between April 2013 and April 2018, both of which tend to present with specific comorbid disorders. More clinical studies compared to non-clinical studies were identified and analyzed which shows the emergence of and need for action, public health, and prevention. Gaming and gambling addictions were usually more severe problems compared to generalized Internet addiction. In addition, gambling appears to be more severe than gaming. However, the current scientific literature base does not report much prevention work in Europe (and internationally). A set of preventive recommendations and policy options have been formulated, which can support future harm minimization actions.

Author Contributions: Conceptualization, O.L.-F.; methodology, O.L.-F. and D.J.K.; formal analysis, O.L.-F. and D.J.K.; investigation, O.L.-F. and D.J.K.; resources, O.L.-F.; data curation, O.L.-F. and D.J.K.; writing—original draft preparation, O.L.-F.; writing—review and editing, O.L.-F. and D.J.K.; visualization, O.L.-F.; supervision, O.L.-F. and D.J.K.; project administration, O.L.-F.; funding acquisition, O.L.-F. and D.J.K. All authors have read and agreed to the published version of the manuscript.

Acknowledgments: We would like to acknowledge the contribution of the European Parliament through the Science and Technology Options Assessment (STOA) Panel and thank them for their invitation to develop this research project: Gianluca Quaglio, Damir Plese, and Emilia Bandeira Morais. To Nottingham Trent University for facilitating the development of the project, which included a research assistant in the data collection: Bailey Foster.

References

1. Young, K.S. Psychology of computer use: XL. Addictive use of the Internet: A case that breaks the stereotype. *Psychol. Rep.* **1996**, *79*, 899–902. [CrossRef]
2. Shapira, N.A.; Goldsmith, T.D.; Keck, P.E., Jr.; Khosla, U.M.; McElroy, S.L. Psychiatric features of individuals with problematic internet use. *J. Affect. Disord.* **2000**, *57*, 267–272. [CrossRef]
3. Griffiths, M. Technological addictions. *Clin. Psych. For.* **1995**, *76*, 14–19.
4. Davis, R.A. A cognitive–behavioral model of pathological Internet use. *Comput. Hum. Behav.* **2001**, *17*, 187–195. [CrossRef]
5. Lopez-Fernandez, O. How has internet addiction research evolved since the advent of internet gaming disorder? An overview of cyberaddictions from a psychological perspective. *Curr. Addict. Rep.* **2015**, *2*, 263–271. [CrossRef]
6. Kuss, D.J.; Lopez-Fernandez, O. Internet addiction and problematic Internet use: A systematic review of clinical research. *World J. Psychiatry* **2016**, *6*, 143–176. [CrossRef]
7. American Psychiatric Association (APA). *Diagnostic and Statistical Manual of Mental Disorders 5th Edition (DSM-5)*; American Psychiatric Association Publishing: Washington, DC, USA, 2013.
8. World Health Organization (WHO). ICD-11 Beta Draft—Mortality and Morbidity. StatisticsMental, Behavioural or Neurodevelopmental Disorders. 2018. Available online: https://icd.who.int/dev11/l-m/en# /http://id.who.int/icd/entity/1448597234 (accessed on 29 February 2020).
9. Van Rooij, A.J.; Ferguson, C.J.; Carras, M.C.; Kardefelt-Winther, D.; Shi, J.; Brus, A.; Coulson, M.; Deleuze, J.; Dullur, P.; Dunkels, E.; et al. A weak scientific basis for gaming disorder: Let us err on the side of caution. *J. Behav. Addict.* **2018**, *7*, 1–9. [CrossRef]
10. Rumpf, H.J.; Achab, S.; Billieux, J.; Bowden-Jones, H.; Carragher, N.; Demetrovics, Z.; Higuchi, S.; King, D.L.; Mann, K.; Potenza, M.; et al. Including gaming disorder in the ICD-11: The need to do so from a clinical and public health perspective. *J. Behav. Addict.* **2018**, *7*, 556–561. [CrossRef]
11. NY Times. Video Game Addiction Tries to Move from Basement to Doctor's Office. Available online: https://www.nytimes.com/2018/06/17/business/video-game-addiction.html (accessed on 29 February 2020).
12. Time. 'Gaming Disorder' is Now an Official Medical Condition, According to the WHO. Available online: https://time.com/5597258/gaming-disorder-icd-11-who/ (accessed on 29 February 2020).
13. King, D.L.; Delfabbro, P.H.; Doh, Y.Y.; Wu, A.M.; Kuss, D.J.; Pallesen, S.; Mentzoni, R.; Carragher, N.; Sakuma, H. Policy and prevention approaches for disordered and hazardous gaming and Internet use: An international perspective. *Prev. Sci.* **2018**, *19*, 233–249. [CrossRef]
14. Choi, J.; Cho, H.; Lee, S.; Kim, J.; Park, E.C. Effect of the online game shutdown policy on Internet use, Internet addiction, and sleeping hours in Korean adolescents. *J. Adolesc. Health* **2018**, *62*, 548–555. [CrossRef]
15. Lopez-Fernandez, O.; Kuss, D. *Internet addiction—PartI: Internet addiction and problematic internet use*—Report Scientific Foresight Unit—Panel for the Future of Science and Technology, Science and Technology Options Assessment (STOA). In Proceedings of the Directorate for Impact Assessment and European Added Value, Directorate-General for Parliamentary Research Services, European Parliament, Brussels, Belgium, 31 January 2019; pp. 1–80. Available online: https://www.europarl.europa.eu/stoa/en/document/EPRS_STU(2019)624249 (accessed on 29 February 2020).
16. Vondráčková, P.; Gabrhelík, R. Prevention of Internet addiction: A systematic review. *J. Behav. Addict.* **2016**, *5*, 568–579. [CrossRef]
17. Kuss, D.J. Policy, prevention and regulation for Internet Gaming Disorder: A commentary on Király et al. (2017). *J. Behav. Addict.* **2018**, *7*, 553–555. [CrossRef]

18. Cheng, C.; Li, A.Y. Internet addiction prevalence and quality of (real) life: A meta-analysis of 31 nations across seven world regions. *Cyberpsychol. Behav. Soc. Netw.* **2014**, *17*, 755–760. [CrossRef]

19. Durkee, T.; Kaess, M.; Carli, V.; Parzer, P.; Wasserman, C.; Floderus, B.; Apter, A.; Balazs, J.; Barzilay, S.; Bobes, J.; et al. Prevalence of pathological internet use among adolescents in Europe: Demographic and social factors. *Addiction* **2012**, *107*, 2210–2222. [CrossRef]

20. Tsitsika, A.; Janikian, M.; Schoenmakers, T.M.; Tzavela, E.C.; Ólafsson, K.; Wojcik, S.; Macarie, G.F.; Tzavara, C.; Richardson, C. Internet addictive behavior in adolescence: A cross-sectional study in seven European countries. *Cyberpsychol. Behav. Soc. Netw.* **2014**, *17*, 528–535. [CrossRef]

21. Lopez-Fernandez, O. Cross-cultural research on Internet addiction: A systematic review. *I Arch. Addict. Res. Med.* **2015**, *1*, 1–5.

22. Moher, D.; Liberati, A.; Tetzlaff, J.; Altman, D.G.; The PRISMA Group. Preferred Reporting Items for Systematic Reviews and Meta-Analyses: The PRISMA Statement. *PLoS Med.* **2009**, *6*, e1000097. [CrossRef]

23. Andrisano, R.; Santoro, E.; De Caro, F.; Palmieri, L.; Capunzo, M.; Venuleo, C.; Boccia, G. Internet Addiction: A prevention action-research intervention. *Epidem. Biostat Public Health* **2016**, *13*, e11817-1. [CrossRef]

24. Beranuy, M.; Carbonell, X.; Griffiths, M.D. A qualitative analysis of online gaming addicts in treatment. *Int. J. Ment Health Addict.* **2013**, *11*, 149–161. [CrossRef]

25. Brand, M.; Laier, C.; Young, K.S. Internet addiction: Coping styles, expectancies, and treatment implications. *Front. Psychol.* **2014**, *5*, 1256. [CrossRef]

26. Danet, M.; Miljkovitch, R. Etre soi-même sur le net: Un facteur de risque à l'usage problématique d'Internet chez les personnes insécures. *L'Encéphale* **2016**, *42*, 506–510. [CrossRef] [PubMed]

27. Floros, G.; Siomos, K.; Stogiannidou, A.; Giouzepas, I.; Garyfallos, G. Comorbidity of psychiatric disorders with Internet addiction in a clinical sample: The effect of personality, defense style and psychopathology. *Addict. Behav.* **2014**, *39*, 1839–1845. [CrossRef] [PubMed]

28. Frölich, J.; Lehmkuhl, G.; Orawa, H.; Bromba, M.; Wolf, K.; Görtz-Dorten, A. Computer game misuse and addiction of adolescents in a clinically referred study sample. *Comput. Hum. Behav.* **2016**, *55*, 9–15. [CrossRef]

29. González, E.; Orgaz, B. Problematic online experiences among Spanish college students: Associations with Internet use characteristics and clinical symptoms. *Comput. Hum. Behav.* **2014**, *31*, 151–158. [CrossRef]

30. Holstein, B.E.; Pedersen, T.P.; Bendtsen, P.; Madsen, K.R.; Meilstrup, C.R.; Nielsen, L.; Rasmussen, M. Perceived problems with computer gaming and internet use among adolescents: Measurement tool for non-clinical survey studies. *BMC Pubic Health* **2014**, *14*, 361. [CrossRef]

31. Jiménez-Murcia, S.; Fernández-Aranda, F.; Granero, R.; Chóliz, M.; Verde, M.L.; Aguglia, E.; Signorelli, M.S.; Sá, G.M.; Aymamí, N.; Gómez-Peña, M.; et al. Video game addiction in gambling disorder: Clinical, psychopathological, and personality correlates. *BioMed Res. Int.* **2014**, *315062*, 1–11. [CrossRef]

32. Lai, C.; Altavilla, D.; Mazza, M.; Scappaticci, S.; Tambelli, R.; Aceto, P.; Luciani, M.; Corvino, S.; Martinelli, D.; Alimonti, F.; et al. Neural correlate of Internet use in patients undergoing psychological treatment for Internet addiction. *J. Ment. Health* **2017**, *26*, 276–282. [CrossRef]

33. Luquiens, A.; Tanguy, M.; Lagadec, M.; Benyamina, A.; Aubin, H.J.; Reynaud, M. The efficacy of three modalities of Internet-based psychotherapy for non-treatment-seeking online problem gamblers: A randomized controlled trial. *J. Med. Internet Res.* **2016**, *18*, e36. [CrossRef]

34. Mallorquí-Bagué, N.; Fernández-Aranda, F.; Lozano-Madrid, M.; Granero, R.; Mestre-Bach, G.; Baño, M.; Jiménez-Murcia, S. Internet Gaming Disorder and Online Gambling Disorder: Clinical and personality correlates. *J. Behav. Addict.* **2017**, *6*, 669–677. [CrossRef]

35. Marco, C.; Chóliz, M. Eficacia de las técnicas de control de la impulsividad en la prevención de la adicción a videojuegos. *Ter. Psicológica* **2017**, *35*, 57–69. [CrossRef]

36. Martín-Fernández, M.; Matalí, J.L.; García-Sánchez, S.; Pardo, M.; Lleras, M.; Castellano-Tejedor, C. Adolescents with Internet Gaming Disorder (IGD): Profiles and treatment response. Adolescentes con Trastorno por juego en Internet (IGD): Perfiles y respuesta al tratamiento. *Adicciones* **2017**, *29*, 125–133. [CrossRef]

37. Müller, K.; Beutel, M.E.; Wölfling, K. A contribution to the clinical characterization of Internet addiction in a sample of treatment seekers: Validity of assessment, severity of psychopathology and type of co-morbidity. *Compr. Psychiatry* **2014**, *55*, 770–777. [CrossRef] [PubMed]

38. Taquet, P.; Hautekeete, M. Prise en charge TCC d'une addiction aux jeux vidéo: L'expérience de jeu contribue à la thérapie. *J. Thérapie Comport. Cogn.* **2013**, *23*, 102–112. [CrossRef]

39. Torres-Rodríguez, A.; Griffiths, M.D.; Carbonell, X. The treatment of internet gaming disorder: A brief overview of the pipatic program. *Int. J. Ment. Health Addict.* **2018**, *16*, 1000–1015. [CrossRef] [PubMed]

40. van Rooij, A.J.; Schoenmakers, T.M.; van de Mheen, D. Clinical validation of the C-VAT 2.0 assessment tool for Gaming Disorder: A sensitivity analysis of the proposed DSM-5 criteria and the clinical characteristics of young patients with 'video game addiction'. *Addict. Behav.* **2017**, *64*, 269–274. [CrossRef] [PubMed]

41. Wölfling, K.; Beutel, M.E.; Dreier, M.; Müller, K.W. Treatment outcomes in patients with Internet addiction: A clinical pilot study on the effects of a cognitive-behavioral therapy program. *BioMed Res. Int.* **2014**, *2014*, 425924. [CrossRef]

42. Young, K.S. *Caught in the Net: How to Recognize the Signs of Internet Addiction–and a Winning Strategy for Recovery*; John Wiley & Sons: New York, NY, USA, 1998.

43. Pawlikowski, M.; Altstötter-Gleich, C.; Brand, M. Validation and psychometric properties of a short version of Young's Internet Addiction Test. *Comput. Hum. Behav.* **2013**, *29*, 1212–1223. [CrossRef]

44. Davis, R.A.; Flett, G.L.; Besser, A. Validation of a new scale for measuring problematic Internet use: Implications for pre-employment screening. *CyberPsychology Behav.* **2002**, *5*, 331–345. [CrossRef]

45. Mitchell, K.J.; Sabina, C.; Finkelhor, D.; Wells, M. Index of Problematic Online Experiences: Item characteristics and correlation with negative symptomatology. *CyberPsychology Behav.* **2009**, *12*, 707–711. [CrossRef]

46. Wölfling, K.; Müller, K.W.; Beutel, M. Reliability and validity of the Scale for the Assessment of Pathological Computer-Gaming (CSV-S). *Psychother. Psychosom. Med. Psychol.* **2011**, *61*, 216–224. [CrossRef]

47. Salguero, R.A.T.; Morán, R.M. Measuring problem video game playing in adolescents. *Addiction* **2002**, *97*, 1601–1606. [CrossRef] [PubMed]

48. Pontes, H.M.; Király, O.; Demetrovics, Z.; Griffiths, M.D. The conceptualisation and measurement of DSM-5 Internet Gaming Disorder: The development of the IGD-20 Test. *PLoS ONE* **2014**, *9*, e110137. [CrossRef] [PubMed]

49. Stinchfield, R. Reliability, validity and classification accuracy of a measure of DSM-IV diagnostic criteria for pathological gambling. *Am. J. Psychiatry* **2003**, *160*, 180–182. [CrossRef] [PubMed]

50. Holtgraves, T. Evaluating the problem gambling severity index. *J. Gambl. Stud.* **2009**, *25*, 105. [CrossRef] [PubMed]

51. Laconi, S.; Kaliszewska-Czeremska, K.; Gnisci, A.; Sergi, I.; Barke, A.; Jeromin, F.; Király, O. Cross-cultural study of Problematic Internet Use in nine European countries. *Comput. Hum. Behav.* **2018**, *4*, 430–440. [CrossRef]

52. Carbonell, X.; Guardiola, E.; Beranuy, M.; Bellés, A. A bibliometric analysis of the scientific literature on Internet, video games, and cell phone addiction. *J. Med. Libr. Assoc.* **2009**, *97*, 102–107. [CrossRef]

53. Lopez-Fernandez, O. Generalised Versus specific Internet use-related addiction problems: A mixed methods study on Internet, gaming, and social networking behaviours. *Int. J. Environ. Res. Pubic Health* **2018**, *15*, 2913. [CrossRef]

54. Kuss, D.J.; Griffiths, M.D. Internet and gaming addiction: A literature review of neuroimaging studies. *Brain Sci.* **2012**, *2*, 347–374. [CrossRef]

55. Ko, C.H.; Yen, J.Y.; Yen, C.F.; Chen, C.S.; Chen, C.C. The association between Internet addiction and psychiatric disorder: A review of the literature. *Eur. Psychiatry* **2012**, *27*, 1–8. [CrossRef]

56. Kuss, D.J.; Griffiths, D.M.; Karila, L.; Billieux, J. Internet addiction: A review of epidemiological research for the last decade. *Curr. Pharm. Des.* **2014**, *20*, 4026–4052. [CrossRef]

57. Kiraly, O.; Griffiths, M.D.; King, D.L.; Lee, H.K.; Lee, S.Y.; Banyai, F.; Zsila, Á.; Takacs, Z.K.; Demetrovics, Z. Policy responses to problematic video game use: A review of current measures and future possibilities. *J. Behav. Addict.* **2017**, *1*, 1–15. [CrossRef] [PubMed]

58. Paulus, F.W.; Ohmann, S.; Von Gontard, A.; Popow, C. Internet gaming disorder in children and adolescents: A systematic review. *Dev. Med. Child. Neurol.* **2018**, *60*, 645–659. [CrossRef] [PubMed]

59. González-Bueso, V.; Santamaría, J.J.; Fernández, D.; Merino, L.; Montero, E.; Ribas, J. Association between Internet Gaming Disorder or Pathological Video-Game Use and Comorbid Psychopathology: A Comprehensive Review. *Int. J. Environ. Res. Public Health* **2018**, *15*, 668. [CrossRef] [PubMed]

60. Lopez-Fernandez, O.; Kuss, D.J.; Pontes, H.M.; Griffiths, M.D.; Dawes, C.; Justice, L.V.; Männikkö, N.; Kääriäinen, M.; Rumpf, H.-J.; Bischof, A.; et al. Measurement invariance of the short version of the Problematic Mobile Phone Use Questionnaire (PMPUQ-SV) across eight languages. *Int. J. Environ. Res. Public Health* **2018**, *15*, 1213. [CrossRef] [PubMed]

61. Lopez-Fernandez, O.; Williams, A.J.; Kuss, D.J. Measuring female gaming: Gamer profile, predictors, prevalence, and characteristics from psychological and gender perspectives. *Front. Psychol.* **2019**, *10*, 898. [CrossRef]

62. Paik, S.-H.; Cho, H.; Chun, J.-W.; Jeong, J.-E.; Kim, D.-J. Gaming device usage patterns predict Internet Gaming Disorder: Comparison across different gaming device usage patterns. *Int. J. Environ. Res. Pubic Health* **2017**, *14*, 1512. [CrossRef]

63. Throuvala, M.A.; Griffiths, M.D.; Rennoldson, M.; Kuss, D.J. School-based prevention for adolescent Internet addiction: Prevention is the key. A literature review. *Curr. Neuropharmacol.* **2019**, *17*, 507–525. [CrossRef]

64. Billieux, J.; Rooij, A.J.; Heeren, A.; Schimmenti, A.; Maurage, P.; Edman, J.; Blaszczynski, A.; Khazaal, Y.; Kardefelt-Winther, D. Behavioural addiction open definition 2.0–using the Open Science Framework for collaborative and transparent theoretical development. *Addiction* **2017**, *112*, 1723–1724. [CrossRef]

65. Petry, N.M.; Rehbein, F.; Ko, C.H.; O'Brien, C.P. Internet gaming disorder in the DSM-5. *Curr. Psychiatry Rep.* **2015**, *17*, 72. [CrossRef]

66. Neverkovich, S.D.; Bubnova, I.S.; Kosarenko, N.N.; Sakhieva, R.G.; Sizova, Z.M.; Zakharova, V.L.; Sergeeva, M.G. Students' Internet addiction: Study and prevention. *Eurasia J. Math. Sci. Technol. Educ.* **2018**, *14*, 1483–1495.

67. Bağatarhan, T.; Siyez, D.M. Programs for preventing Internet addiction during adolescence: A review. *Addicta Turk. J. Addict.* **2017**, *4*, 243–265.

68. Marchant, A.; Hawton, K.; Stewart, A.; Montgomery, P.; Singaravelu, V.; Lloyd, K.; Purdy, N.; Daine, K.; John, A. A systematic review of the relationship between internet use, self-harm and suicidal behaviour in young people: The good, the bad and the unknown. *PLoS ONE* **2017**, *12*, e0181722. [CrossRef] [PubMed]

69. Sharifat, H.; Rashid, A.A.; Suppiah, S. Systematic review of the utility of functional MRI to investigate internet addiction disorder: Recent updates on resting state and task-based fMRI. *MJMHS* **2018**, *14*, 21–33.

70. Sun, S. Meta-analysis of Cohen's kappa. *Health Serv. Outcomes Res. Meth.* **2011**, *11*, 145–163. [CrossRef]

71. Critical Appraisal Skills Programme UK. Critical Appraisal Skills Programme Making Sense of Evidence. 2012. Available online: http://www.casp-uk.net (accessed on 14 May 2020).

10

Association between Internet Gaming Disorder or Pathological Video-Game Use and Comorbid Psychopathology

Vega González-Bueso [1,†], Juan José Santamaría [1,*,†], Daniel Fernández [2,3], Laura Merino [1], Elena Montero [1] and Joan Ribas [1]

[1] Atención e Investigación en Socioadicciones (AIS), Mental Health and Addictions Network, Generalitat de Catalunya (XHUB), C/Forn-7-9 Local, 08014 Barcelona, Spain; vgonzalez@ais-info.org (V.G.-B.); lmerino@ais-info.org (L.M.); emontero@ais-info.org (E.M.); 38039jrs@comb.cat (J.R.)

[2] Research and Development Unit, Parc Sanitari Sant Joan de Déu, Fundació Sant Joan de Déu, CIBERSAM, Dr. Antoni Pujadas, 42, Sant Boi de Llobregat, 08830 Barcelona, Spain; df.martinez@pssjd.org

[3] School of Mathematics and Statistics, Victoria University of Wellington, Wellington 6140, New Zealand

* Correspondence: jsantamaria@ais-info.org

† These authors contributed equally to this work.

Abstract: The addictive use of video games is recognized as a problem with clinical relevance and is included in international diagnostic manuals and classifications of diseases. The association between "Internet addiction" and mental health has been well documented across a range of investigations. However, a major drawback of these studies is that no controls have been placed on the type of Internet use investigated. The aim of this study is to review systematically the current literature in order to explore the association between Internet Gaming Disorder (IGD) and psychopathology. An electronic literature search was conducted using PubMed, PsychINFO, ScienceDirect, Web of Science and Google Scholar (r.n. CRD42018082398). The effect sizes for the observed correlations were identified or computed. Twenty-four articles met the eligibility criteria. The studies included comprised 21 cross-sectional and three prospective designs. Most of the research was conducted in Europe. The significant correlations reported comprised: 92% between IGD and anxiety, 89% with depression, 85% with symptoms of attention deficit hyperactivity disorder (ADHD), and 75% with social phobia/anxiety and obsessive-compulsive symptoms. Most of the studies reported higher rates of IGD in males. The lack of longitudinal studies and the contradictory results obtained prevent detection of the directionality of the associations and, furthermore, show the complex relationship between both phenomena.

Keywords: pathological video-game use; Internet Gaming Disorder; comorbid psychopathology; review

1. Introduction

The problematic use of video games is recognized by mental health professionals as an addictive behavior with clinical relevance. This is due to the negative consequences it may have for affected people in several functional areas such as relationship conflicts, sleep problems or occupational functioning [1,2]. However, in the current literature, the terms "Internet addiction" (IA) and "pathological Internet use" (PIU) have commonly been used to refer to all sorts of activities including, but not limited to, the use of video games. All these activities are derived from the excessive use of devices connected to the Internet (i.e., computers, smartphones and other devices to play on and navigate). This classification has frequently been criticized as being too broad and not distinguishing between problematic activities and the medium itself on which they take place [3,4], despite the fact that persons engaged in these activities have different sociodemographic characteristics and motivations [5]. For example, the Internet preference activities for males are those related to entertainment and leisure, whereas women tend to choose activities related to interpersonal communication and educational assistance; additionally, these differences may be mediated by age [6].

The non-inclusion of IA as a diagnosis, and the inclusion of "Internet Video-Game Disorder" (Internet Gaming Disorder, IGD) in Section III of the diagnostic manual DSM-5 [7] as a condition that requires further study, seems to support considering both disorders as different problems. Likewise, the most recent inclusion of Gaming Disorder in the beta version of the ICD-11 (International Classification of Diseases) of the World Health Organization [8] seems to confirm this trend. In this document, the problem is defined as "a pattern of persistent or recurrent gaming behavior ('digital gaming' or 'video-gaming'), which may be online (i.e., over the Internet) or offline, manifested by: (1) impaired control over gaming (e.g., onset, frequency, intensity, duration, termination, context); (2) increasing priority given to gaming to the extent that gaming takes precedence over other life interests and daily activities; and (3) continuation or escalation of gaming despite the occurrence of negative consequences. The behavior pattern is of sufficient severity to result in significant impairment in personal, family, social, educational, occupational or other important areas of functioning. The pattern of gaming behavior may be either continuous or, on the other hand, episodic and recurrent. The gaming behavior and other features are normally evident over a period of at least 12 months for a diagnosis to be assigned, although the required duration may be shortened if all diagnostic requirements are met and symptoms are severe".

The psychopathology associated with addictive behaviors, with or without substance, can result from a problem or, alternatively, lead to further issues [9,10]. If the association between two disorders is higher than expected by chance, it is likely that there are mechanisms contributing to that association. Four general models of increased comorbidity have been described [11–13]: common factor models, secondary substance-use disorder models, secondary psychiatric disorder models, and bidirectional models. In the first instance, both disorders share risk factors and the higher comorbidity is the result. In the second case, the addictive disorder contributes to other psychiatric disorders. In the third condition, the psychiatric disorder precipitates the addictive behavior. Finally, either disorder can increase vulnerability to the other disorder; in such cases the higher comorbidity reported may be due to inappropriate sampling, assessment, study design or other biases in the published studies.

In the case of behavioral addictions, the temporal linearity of that relationship remains unclear. Associations between IA or PIU and various psychiatric symptoms have been reported in the literature. Specifically, they have been related to depression, attention deficit hyperactivity disorder (ADHD), anxiety, obsessive-compulsive symptoms, and hostility or aggression [14]. Depression seems to be the most common comorbidity in all age groups (adolescents, adults and the general population). However, the designs used to explore these relationships are not sufficiently comprehensive or complex to confirm the hypothesis for the above models. It is possible that a specific psychiatric problem might have an influence on developing an IA, or that a person with an IA diagnosis, due to various negative consequences, will later develop a comorbid psychiatric disorder. It is also possible that both problems share biological, sociodemographic or psychological underlying mechanisms that make people vulnerable to both pathologies; these may thus become evident at the same time [15]. A major drawback of these studies is that, in most, the type of Internet use is not controlled or, alternatively, the results are not separated by use. In many studies, playing video games is the most common activity among people with IA [16–19]; still, the results have been analyzed without taking this aspect into account.

Therefore, some interesting questions remain. One is whether IGD has similar comorbidities to IA or, rather, the comorbidities are different. In the latter case, one may wonder if other Internet-based issues are affecting in some way the results of studies focused on IA in general. An additional question pertains to the directionality of both conditions (IGD and psychopathology).

The aim of this study is to review systematically the current literature to elicit epidemiological evidence supporting or refuting the association between Internet gaming addiction and psychopathology. An additional objective is to explore the relationship between these conditions. Such results can furnish clinicians with updated information and provide a direction for future investigative endeavors.

2. Materials and Methods

This systematic review was conducted in accordance with the Preferred Reporting Items for Systematic Reviews and Meta-Analyses-P 2015 statement for systematic review and meta-analysis protocols [20]. The databases reviewed between October and December 2017 were PubMed, PsychINFO, ScienceDirect, Web of Science, and Google Scholar, using the following search terms and logic: "(Internet OR online) gaming addiction AND (psychopathology OR comorbidity)". Without considering the results in Google Scholar, these database search parameters yielded a total of 688 results, including the following results in each database: PubMed (54 results), PsychINFO (354 results), and ScienceDirect (280 results). Due to the large number of results provided by Google Scholar (more than 17,500 results), we reviewed only the first 30 pages of results. Additional articles were identified through searching the citations in the literature selected.

The studies were systematically and independently reviewed by the authors (Vega González-Bueso and Juan José Santamaría); paying attention to the study type, study population, methodology, outcome measures, effect sizes and interpretation of results. In cases of discrepancies, these were resolved through consensus or referral to a third reviewer (Laura Merino). The inclusion criteria were: (i) the inclusion of empirically collected data; (ii) IGD assessed by standardized questionnaires or other proposed criteria based on international disease classifications; (iii) psychiatric comorbidity assessed by standardized questionnaires; (iv) availability of the full text; (v) published after the year 2010 (this allowed us to review the most recent research in a field where the subject of addiction evolves rapidly); (vi) written in English or in Spanish (the two languages known by the authors); and (vii) article published in a peer-reviewed journal.

Studies were also included if the object of research was IA, only if it was specified that the Internet was used to play video games, and/or the results were separated according to Internet use and whether video games were one of those activities.

The exclusion criteria were: (i) articles containing only anecdotal evidence on psychopathology associated with IGD; (ii) authors not providing a specific definition or criteria for IGD; (iii) case reports and case series; (iv) studies only reporting results on phenomenons such as motivation to play video games, decision-making, stress, lifestyle, impulsivity and sexual attitude, without reporting other psychiatric comorbidity.

A review protocol exists at the PROSPERO International prospective register of systematic reviews [21] registration number CRD42018082398.

In order to facilitate the comparisons with pathological Internet use, the reviewing method applied by Carli et al. in 2013 [14] was followed: the effect sizes of the associations between IGD and psychopathology were identified by the reviewed publications or calculated using the data provided by the authors, when available. In order to compare the different associations, the effect sizes d and R^2 were stated as small, moderate, or large, according to Cohen [22]; OR were converted into these groups according to Chinn [23]. The effect sizes were interpreted accordingly: small (d = 0.2, R^2 = 0.01, OR = 1.45), moderate (d = 0.5, R^2 = 0.06, OR = 2.50), and large (d = 0.8, R^2 = 0.14, OR = 4.25). Full association was considered when a correlation was found for both genders after multivariate analyses. If a correlation was identified for only one gender, it was classified as a partial association. The geographical distribution of studies was also mapped (Figure 1).

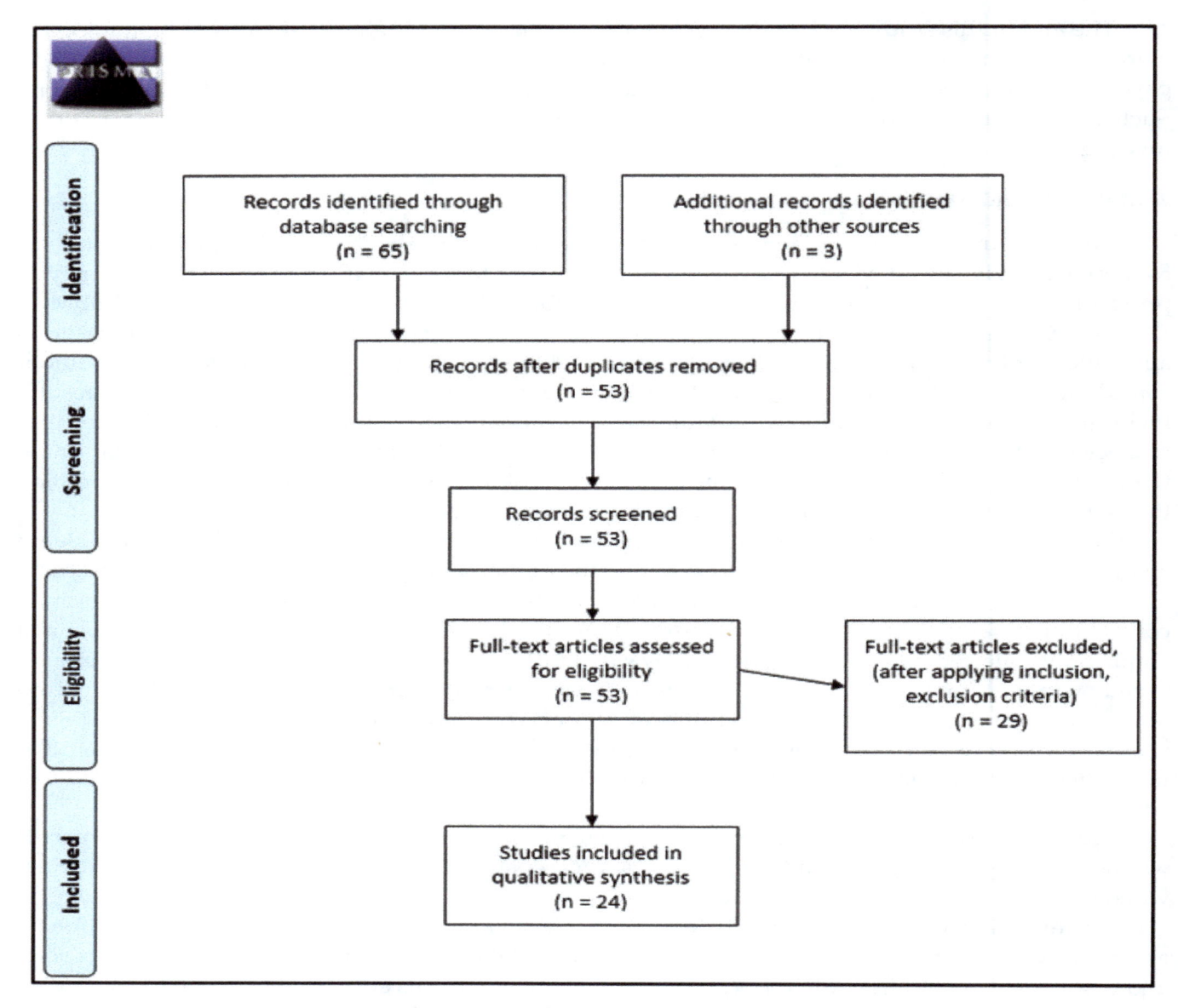

Figure 1. PRISMA 2009 protocols flow diagram.

3. Results

After deleting duplicate studies, a total of 68 articles were screened and identified through the present systematic search. After applying inclusion and exclusion criteria, a total of 24 studies were selected and included. Table 1 shows a summary of the main characteristics of the studies examining the relationship between IGD and comorbid psychopathology, including effect sizes.

Table 1. Studies examining the relationship between Internet Gaming Disorder (IGD) and comorbid psychopathology, including effect sizes.

Source	Study Type	N	Population Age [a]	Sex	Country	IGD Measures	Psychopathology Measures	Psychopathology Outcome	Association	Effect Size	95% CI of d
Baer et al., 2011 [24]	cross-sectional	102	adolescents 13.7 ± 1.9	M/F	Canada	Computer/Gaming-station Addiction Scale (CGAS)	Strengths and Difficulties Questionnaire	Emotional problems	full	$R^2 = 0.29$	–
								Hyperactivity	full	$R^2 = 0.18$	–
Cole & Hooley, 2013 [25]	cross-sectional	163	general population 27.3 ± 9.1	M/F	USA	Generalized Problematic Internet Use Scale (GPIUS)	State-Trait Anxiety Inventory (STAI)	Anxiety state	full	$d = 0.26$	−0.05–0.57
								Anxiety trait	full	$d = 1.07$	0.74–1.40
							Social Phobia Scale	Social phobia	full	$d = 1.17$	0.83–1.50
Jiménez-Murcia et al., 2014 [26]	cross-sectional	193	adults with GD 42.4 ± 13.4	M/F	Spain	Video-game Dependency Test (VDT)	Symptom Checklist 90-revision	Somatization	full	$d = 0.57$	0.16–0.983
								Obsessive-Compulsive	full	$d = 0.84$	0.424–1.257
								Interpersonal Sensitivity	full	$d = 0.76$	0.341–1.169
								Depression	full	$d = 0.58$	0.17–0.991
								Anxiety	full	$d = 0.64$	0.216–1.064
								Hostility	full	$d = 0.68$	0.255–1.106
								Phobic-Anxiety	full	$d = 0.55$	0.127–0.973
								Paranoid Ideation	full	$d = 0.83$	0.402–1.259
								Psychoticism	full	$d = 0.56$	0.137–0.983
Kim et al., 2016 [27]	cross-sectional	3041	adults 20–49	M/F	South Korea	IGD diagnostic criteria in DSM-5	Brief Symptom Inventory (BSI)	Somatization	full	$d = 1.59$	1.481–1.703
								Obsessive-Compulsive	full	$d = 1.67$	1.557–1.78
								Interpersonal Sensitivity	full	$d = 1.61$	1.499–1.721
								Depression	full	$d = 1.75$	1.642–1.867
								Anxiety	full	$d = 1.75$	1.642–1.866
								Hostility	full	$d = 1.72$	1.61–1.834
								Phobic-Anxiety	full	$d = 1.82$	1.705–1.928
								Paranoid Ideation	full	$d = 1.74$	1.623–1.847
								Psychoticism	full	$d = 1.76$	1.646–1.87
King et al., 2013 [28]	cross-sectional	1287	adolescents 12–18	M/F	Australia	Pathological Technology Use (PTU)	Revised Children's Anxiety and Depression Scale	Depression	none	–	

Table 1. *Cont.*

Source	Study Type	N	Population Age [a]	Sex	Country	IGD Measures	Psychopathology Measures	Psychopathology Outcome	Association	Effect Size	95% CI of d
								Obsessive-Compulsive Disorder (OCD)	none	–	
								Anxiety	none	–	
King & Delfabbro, 2016 [29]	cross-sectional	824	adolescents 14.1 ± 1.5	M/F	Australia	IGD Diagnostic criteria in DSM-5	Depression Anxiety Stress Scales, 21-item version	Depression	full *	d = 0.62	0.087–1.155
								Anxiety	full *	d = 0.50	−0.035–1.025
Laconi et al., 2017 [30]	cross-sectional	418	adults 21.9 ± 3	M/F	France	Internet Gaming Disorder Test-10 (IGDT-10)	Center for Epidemiologic Studies, Depression Scale-10	Depression	full	d = 2.687	1.969–3.405
Männikkö et al., 2015 [31]	cross-sectional	293	general population 18.7 ± 3.4	M/F	Finland	Gaming Addiction Scale (GAS)	School Health Promotion (SHP)	Depression	full	$R^2 = 0.17$	-
								Anxiety	full	$R^2 = 0.11$	-
Mentzoni, et al., 2011 [32]	cross-sectional	816	general population 15–40	M/F	Norway	Gaming Addiction Scale for Adolescents (GASA)	Hospital Anxiety and Depression Scale (HADS)	Depression	full	n/a	-
								Anxiety	full	n/a	-
Müller et al., 2015 [33]	cross-sectional	12,938	adolescents 15.8 ± 0.7	M/F	Germany	Assessment of Internet and Computer Game Addiction (AICGA)	Youth Self-Report	Anxious-Depression	full	d = 0.34	0.183–0.496
								Withdrawn-Depression	full	d = 0.35	0.347–0.507
Na et al., 2017 [34]	cross-sectional	1819	adults 20–49	M/F	South Korea	IGD diagnostic criteria in DSM-5	Symptom Checklist 90-revision	Depression	full	n/a	-
								Anxiety	full	n/a	-
Starcevic et al., 2011 [35]	cross-sectional	1945	general population over 14	M/F	Australia	Video-Game Use Questionnaire (VGUQ)	Symptom Checklist 90	Somatization	partial>	d = 1.02	0.854–1.187
								Obsessive-Compulsive	partial	d = 1.365	1.196–1.534
								Interpersonal Sensitivity	partial	d = 1.228	1.059–1.396
								Depression	partial	d = 1.264	1.096–1.433
								Anxiety	partial>	d = 1.149	0.981–1.317
								Hostility	partial>	d = 1.276	1.108–1.445

Table 1. *Cont.*

Source	Study Type	N	Population Age [a]	Sex	Country	IGD Measures	Psychopathology Measures	Psychopathology Outcome	Association	Effect Size	95% CI of d
								Phobic-Anxiety	partial>	d = 1.131	0.964–1.299
								Paranoid Ideation	partial>	d = 1.203	1.035–1.371
								Psychoticism	partial>	d = 1.368	1.199–1.537
Stetina et al., 2011 [36]	cross-sectional	468	general population 11–67	M/F	Austria	Problematic Internet use scale (ISS-20)	Questionnaire for depression diagnostics (FDD for DSM-IV)	Depression	none	-	-
Strittmatter et al., 2015 [37]	cross-sectional	9758	adolescents 15.0 ± 1.3	M/F	Germany	Young Diagnostic Questionnaire (YDQ)	Beck Depression Inventory II	Depression	full	d = 0.58	0.449–0.702
							Strengths and Difficulties Questionnaire (SDQ)	Hyperactivity	full	d = 0.53	0.399–0.652
Vadlin et al., 2016 [38]	cross-sectional	N1 (1868) N2 (242)	adolescents 12–18	M/F	Sweden	Gaming Addiction Identification (GAIT)	Depression Self-Rating Scale (DSRS-A)	Depression	full	OR 2.47 (1.44–4.25)	-
							Spence Children's Anxiety Scale (SCAS)	Anxiety	full	OR 2.06 (1.27–3.33)	-
							Adult ADHD Self-Report Scale (ASRS-A)	Attention Deficit Hyperactivity Disorder (ADHD)	full	OR 2.43 (1.44–4.11)	-
							Psychotic-like experiences (PLEs)	Psychoticism	none	-	-
Wang et al., 2018 [39]	cross-sectional	7200	general population 14–39	M/F	South Korea	IGD diagnostic criteria in DSM-5	Patient Health Questionnaire9 (PHQ9)	Depression	full	n/a	-
							Generalized Anxiety Disorder Scale (GAD-7)	Anxiety	n/a	-	-
Wartberg et al., 2017 [40]	cross-sectional	1095	adolescents 13.0 ± 0.82	M/F	Germany	Internet Gaming Disorder Scale (IGDS)	Reynolds Adolescent Adjustment Screening Inventory	Depression and anxiety	full	OR 1.09 (1.02–1.17)	-
								Hyperactivity	full	OR 1.27 (1.16–1.39)	-
Wei et al., 2012 [41]	cross-sectional	722	general population 21.8 ± 4.9	M/F	Taiwan	Chen's Internet Addiction Scale (CIAS)	Depression and Somatic Symptoms Scale (DSSS)	Depression	full	$R^2 = 0.298$	

Table 1. *Cont.*

Source	Study Type	N	Population Age [a]	Sex	Country	IGD Measures	Psychopathology Measures	Psychopathology Outcome	Association	Effect Size	95% CI of d
Panagiotidi, 2017 [42]	cross-sectional	205	adults 27.4 ± 10	M/F	United Kingdom	Problem Video-Game Playing Test (PVGT)	Social Phobia Inventory (SPIN)	Social phobia	full	n/a	-
							ADHD Self-Report Scale (ASRS)	ADHD	full	$R^2 = 0.22$	-
Gentile et al., 2011 [43]	Longitudinal	3034	children, adolescents 11.2 ± 2.06	M/F	Singapore	Pathological Technology Use (PTU)	Asian Adolescent Depression Scale (AADS)	Depression	full	$R^2 = 0.49$	-
							Child Anxiety-Related Emotional Disorders (SCARED)	Anxiety	full	$R^2 = 0.29$	-
							Adult ADHD Self-Report Scale (ASRS-A)	ADHD	none	-	-
							Social Phobia Inventory (SPIN)	Social phobia	full	$R^2 = 0.20$	-
Van Rooij et al., 2011 [44]	Longitudinal	T1 (1572) T2 (1476)	children 13–16	M/F	Deutschland	Compulsive Internet Use Scale (CIUS)	Depressive Mood List	T1: Depression T2: Depression	none full #	n/a	-
Hyun et al., 2015 [45]	case-control	308	general population 21.0 ± 5.9	M/F	South Korea	Young Internet Addiction Scale (YIAS)	Revised Social Anxiety Scale for Children	T1: Social anxiety T2: Social anxiety	none none	-	-
							Beck Depressive Inventory (BDI)	Depression	full	d = 1.09	0.88–1.305
							Beck Anxiety Scale (BAI)	Anxiety	full	d = 0.64	0.437–0.845
							Dupaul's ADHD scale (K-ARS)	ADHD	full	d = 1.05	0.838–1.262
Yen et al., 2016 [46]	case-control	174	adults 23.29 ± 2.34 23.38 ± 2.40	M/F	Taiwan	Semi-structured interview with the DSM-5 IGD criteria	ADHD DSM-IV-TR criteria diagnosis for adult and childhood	ADHD	full	OR 13.51 (4.49–40.64)	-
Brunborg et al., 2014 [47]	cohort	1928	adolescents 13–17	M/F	Norway	Game Addiction Scale for Adolescents (GASA)	Hopkins Symptom Checklist	Depression	T1: full other time: none	$R^2 = 0.25$	-

[a] Age is presented in years as a range or mean with standard deviation (SD). M/F = both males and females analyzed together. * Low severity symptoms. n/a Non-enough data provided to calculate the effect size or not applicable. # When non-addicted heavy gamers and addicted heavy gamers compared. > A difference was found between IGD subjects and non IGD subjects but the psychopathology scores on both groups were not clinical.

3.1. Design of the Included Studies

Nineteen of the 24 articles included were cross-sectional studies [24–42], the rest were two longitudinal studies [43,44], two case-control studies [45,46], and a cohort study [47]. The research was performed, in descending order, in South Korea (4), Australia (3), Germany (3), Norway (2), Taiwan (2), Canada (1), USA (1), Singapore (1), Spain (1), United Kingdom (1), France (1), Finland (1), Deutschland (1) Austria (1) and Sweden (1). Most of the studies were performed in European countries (12).

3.2. Characteristics of the Used Samples

The 24 studies had a total of 53,889 participants. All studies examined both genders. The number of participants in each study ranged from 102 to 12,938 (M = 2155.56; standard deviation (SD): 3176.05). Nine of the studies in this review [24,28,29,33,37,38,40,43,47] targeted adolescent groups, six studies [26,27,30,34,42,46] targeted adults, one [44] targeted children and eight studies [25,31,32,35,36,39,41,45] were carried out in the general population. A total of three studies were conducted in clinical populations, using people in outpatient treatment for IGD [45] or other mental health problems, namely Gambling Disorder [26] and other unspecified psychiatric problems [38].

3.3. Methods of Assessing Internet Gaming Disorder (IGD)

Since 2013, the DSM-5 includes a proposal of diagnostic criteria for IGD. However, only five out of 15 of the reviewed articles published after this year used these criteria [27,29,34,39,46]; three use psychometric questionnaires based on them [30,38,40] to assess the problem.

These diagnostic criteria pertain to repetitive use of Internet-based games, often with other players, that leads to significant issues with functioning. Five of the following criteria must be met within one year: "(i) Preoccupation or obsession with Internet games. (ii) Withdrawal symptoms when not playing Internet games. (iii) A build-up of tolerance (i.e., more time needs to be spent playing the games). (iv) The person has tried to stop or curb playing Internet games but has failed to do so. (v) The person has had a loss of interest in other life activities, such as hobbies. (vi) A person has had continued overuse of Internet games even with awareness of how much they impact a person's life. (vii) The person has lied to others about his or her Internet game usage. (viii) The person uses Internet games to relieve anxiety or guilt (i.e., it is a way to escape). (ix) The person has lost or put at risk opportunities or relationships because of Internet games".

The questionnaires based on these criteria were the Internet Gaming Disorder Test-10 (IGDT-10) [48]; the Gaming Addiction Identification (GAIT) [49] and the Internet Gaming Disorder Scale (IGDS) [50].

The IGDT-10 includes the nine diagnostic criteria of the DSM-5. Each criterion was operationalized using a single item, except for the last criterion referring to "jeopardy or losing a significant relationship, job, or educational or career opportunity because of participation in Internet games." This criterion was operationalized with two items, given its complexity and description of more than one construct.

The GAIT is a screening instrument used to identify addictive factors related to gaming addiction in adolescents. Primarily developed based on items from the AUDIT Alcohol Consumption Questions (AUDIT-C) [51], and the criteria for gambling disorder suggested by the DSM-5, GAIT covers seven of the nine criteria in the proposed IGD criteria. These items are: preoccupation, withdrawal, tolerance, unsuccessful attempts to control the behavior, loss of interests, harm, and loss of a significant relationship or educational opportunity due to gaming. Questions regarding lying/deception to hide the gaming, and escape/mood modification, are not included.

Finally, the IGDS measures each of the nine DSM-5 definitions with three items, either through separating core aspects of a criterion into different items or by applying changes in phrasing or synonyms. Furthermore, the proposed terms "Internet gaming" or "Internet games" were replaced with "gaming" or "games."

The remaining studies employed either measures based on the DSM-IV Gambling Disorder criteria (Pathological Technology Use (PTU), Gaming Addiction Scale (GAS)) or based on DSM-IV Addiction criteria (Gaming Addiction Scale for Adolescents (GASA), Video-game Dependency Test (VDT), Assessment of Internet and Computer Game Addiction (AICGA), Video-Game Use Questionnaire (VGUQ)), or questionnaires used to measure IA problems (Computer/Gaming-station Addiction Scale (CGAS), Generalized Problematic Internet Use Scale (GPIUS), Young Internet Addiction Scale (YIAS), Compulsive Internet Use Scale (CIUS), Problematic Internet use scale (ISS-20), Young Diagnostic Questionnaire (YDQ), Chen's Internet Addiction Scale (CIAS), and Problem Video-Game Playing Test (PVGT)).

3.4. Methods Assessing Psychopathology

Different psychometric assessments were used in the reviewed articles to measure psychopathology.

Depression was measured using various assessment tools, i.e., the Hopkins Symptom Checklist [52], the Asian Adolescent Depression Scale [53], the Beck Depressive Inventory [54], the Beck Depressive Inventory-II [55], the Center for Epidemiologic Studies-Depression Scale-10 [56], the Depressive Mood List [57], the Questionnaire for Depression Diagnostics [58], the Depression Self-Rating Scale [59], the Patient Health Questionnaire-9 [60] and the Depression and Somatic Symptoms Scale [61].

To assess anxiety, in each study, different measures were used, these are the State-Trait Anxiety Inventory [62], the Screen for Child Anxiety-Related Emotional Disorders [63], the Beck Anxiety Scale [64], the Spence Children's Anxiety Scale [65], and the Generalized Anxiety Disorder Scale-7 [66]. In addition, some authors used questionnaires evaluating both depression and anxiety, the Revised Children's Anxiety and Depression Scale [67], the School Health Promotion [68], the Hospital Anxiety and Depression Scale [69], the Youth Self-Report [70] and the Reynolds Adolescent Adjustment Screening Inventory [71].

To measure ADHD symptoms or hyperactivity, three authors [38,42,43] used the ADHD Self-Report Scale [72], two authors [24,37] used the Strengths and Difficulties Questionnaire [73], one author [45] used the Dupaul's ADHD scale [74], and one author [46] used the ADHD DSM-IV-TR criteria diagnosis for adult and childhood [75].

To assess social phobia and social anxiety, two studies [41,43] used the Social Phobia Inventory [76], one study [25] used the Social Phobia Scale [77], and one study [44] used the Revised Social Anxiety Scale for Children [78].

Several studies used questionnaires to assess multiple conditions: in three articles [26,34,35] the Symptom Checklist 90-Revision [79] was employed to assess several conditions (somatization, obsessive-compulsive disorder, interpersonal sensitivity, depression, anxiety, hostility, phobic anxiety, paranoid ideation, and psychoticism), and one study [27] used the Brief Symptoms Inventory [80] to measure the same psychopathologies. Another study [28] evaluated depression, anxiety and obsessive-compulsive disorder through the Revised Children's Anxiety and Depression Scale [67]. Finally, one article [24] assessed emotional problems and hyperactivity using the Strengths and Difficulties Questionnaire [73].

Finally, in one study [38] the association between IGD and psychoticism was explored through the Psychotic-like Experiences Test [81].

3.5. Effect Size of the Associations of Psychopathology with IGD

Regarding the associations between the analyzed mental disorders and IGD, the effect sizes reported in the reviewed papers comprised different levels of association: 35 large [24–27,30,31,41–43,45–47,82], 13 moderate [26,29,31,37,45], eight small [25,33,38,40], and seven non-association [36,38,43,44,83]. In order to summarize these results, Table 2 shows the observed associations identified between IGD and psychopathology only for the main four outcomes. The largest correlations were identified between IGD and anxiety and depression and ADHD, whereas the weakest were observed between IGD and obsessive-compulsive disorder.

Table 2. Number of observed associations identified between IGD and psychopathology stratified by effect size for the four main outcomes.

Effect Size	Depression	Anxiety	ADHD/Hyper-Activity	Social Phobia/Anxiety
Small [a]	2	2	2	0
Moderate [b]	3	5	1	0
Large [c]	8	2	4	2
None	2	1	1	1
Total	15	10	8	3

[a] $d = 0.2$, $R^2 = 0.01$, OR = 1.45. [b] $d = 0.5$, $R^2 = 0.06$, OR = 2.50. [c] $d = 0.8$, $R^2 = 0.14$, OR = 4.25.

3.6. Psychopathology, IGD and Sample Characteristics (Age, Gender)

Twenty-one studies were conducted in healthy populations; only three analyzed clinical populations (IGD or other mental health problems).

Regarding age, the analyzed studies included in the present review focused on three age groups as target populations: general population, adolescents and adults.

Eight articles examined groups of general population formed by children, adolescents and adults together, exploring the association between IGD and 1 depression and anxiety [31,32,39,45], depression [36,41], anxiety [25], social phobia [25,41], ADHD [45] and several psychiatric symptoms using the SCL-90-R [35]. One of these studies focused on a clinical sample of IGD patients [45]. All studies found a large effect size in the correlation between IGD in the general population and depression, except for one that found a non-correlation between both disorders. Large correlation effects with IGD in the general population were also found with ADHD and social phobia. Two studies analyzing anxiety found large effect sizes and two found moderate effect sizes. Large effect sizes were also found with the remaining SCL-90-R scales.

Six studies were focused on adults, analyzing the association between IGD and depression and anxiety [34], depression [30], ADHD [42,46] and several psychiatric symptoms [26,27]; here the SCL-90-R and the Brief Symptom Inventory (BSI) questionnaires were used. One of these studies focused on a clinical sample of pathological gamblers [26]. The authors identified correlations between IGD and depression and anxiety with large and moderate effect sizes, large effect sizes with ADHD, paranoid ideation and obsessive-compulsive symptoms, and finally, large and moderate effect sizes with the remaining SCL-90-R scales.

Adolescent participant groups were used in the remaining 10 studies. One of these studies [38] focused on adolescents with unspecified psychiatric problems. An association between depression and IGD in adolescents was found in seven articles and non-association in one; the effect sizes varied between large (2), moderate (2) and small (2) and no association (1). Anxiety correlated with IGD in adolescents in four of the five studies exploring this relationship; the sizes of the effects varied between large (1), moderate (1) and small (2). The association with ADHD was found in four out of five studies, with effect sizes: large (1), moderate (1) and small (2). Social phobia or social anxiety showed a large association and no association in two studies. Finally, non-association was found with obsessive-compulsive disorder (OCD) and psychoticism in the adolescent population.

With respect to gender, all studies reported higher video-game use among males. Seventeen studies [25–28,30,32–35,37–40,42,43,45,46] found higher rates of IGD among males. Two [24,29] reported no gender differences. The association between psychopathology and IGD was found for both sexes in all the articles (full association), except one [35] that only analyzed the relationship between males.

3.7. IGD and Depression

Nineteen of the 21 studies examined some form of depression as a comorbid symptom. Thirteen studies found a full association [26,27,29–31,37,38,40,41,43,45,47,82], and two [28,36] found no association. Specifically, King et al. [28] reported association with depression in PIU groups, demonstrating significantly more severe depression and anxiety symptoms than either the non-problematic user's group or the pathological video gamers group. In contrast, the pathological video gamers group scores did not differ significantly from the non-problematic users group.

Four studies were not cross-sectional, there were two longitudinal studies [43,44], one cohort study [47], and one case-control [45]. The results of these studies showed large effect size associations with depression. In the case of the longitudinal studies, Gentile et al. [43] reported elevated depressive symptoms after the pathological video-gaming problems started and these symptoms persisted and increased only if the pathological abuse persisted, while Van Rooij et al. [44], in their longitudinal study exploring two different times (years 2008 and 2009) found correlations with depressive mood only in Time 2 when comparing addicted heavy gamers with non-addicted heavy gamers. In the cohort study, the authors reported a correlation between video game addiction and depression with a large effect size only in Time 1, but they did not find any significant correlation between these two variables two years later. Among the rest of correlations detected, the effect sizes for the association with depression comprised eight large [27,30,31,41,43,45,47,82], three moderate [26,29,37], and two small [38,40] observed effects.

3.8. IGD and Anxiety

Regarding the correlation between IGD and anxiety, 11 studies found a full association, one study found a partial association, and one study found no association. The studies finding full association were: a longitudinal study [43] identifying a large effect size; a case-control study [45] identifying a moderate effect size; a cross-sectional study [25], where the authors reported a large effect size in the correlation with the anxiety trait, but a small effect size with anxiety state; and eight cross-sectional studies [26,27,29,31,32,34,38,40] identifying large effect sizes (1), moderate effect sizes (3), and small effect sizes (2). Just as in the case of depression, in the longitudinal study carried out by Gentile et al. [43], the anxiety symptoms appeared after pathological video-gaming problems. A partial association only in males was found in a study [35] and here there was a moderate effect size. Finally, no association with anxiety was found in one cross-sectional study [28].

3.9. IGD and Attention Deficit Hyperactivity Disorder (ADHD)

The relationship between IGD and ADHD and hyperactivity symptoms were analyzed in eight studies. Seven of them reported full association, with four finding large [24,42,45,46], two finding small [38,40], and one reporting moderate, effect sizes [37]. The studies comprised two case-control, five cross-sectional and one longitudinal design; the latter found no association between the two variables [43].

3.10. IGD and Social Phobia and Social Anxiety

Four studies included social phobia or social anxiety as a comorbid symptom in their studies. These studies comprised two longitudinal [43,44] and three cross-sectional designs [25,41,44]. One longitudinal and two cross-sectional studies found full association with IGD, reporting large effect sizes. Furthermore, the longitudinal study, similar to the results found regarding anxiety and depression, found that social phobia symptoms worsen after a youth becomes a pathological gamer, and improve if an individual stops this activity. In the remaining longitudinal study, no association was found between social anxiety and IGD.

3.11. IGD and Obsessive-Compulsive Symptoms

Four studies examined obsessive-compulsive symptoms as a comorbid problem. Three studies [26,27,35] found a full association with large effect sizes, and one [28] found no association.

3.12. Publication Bias

In order to detect possible publication bias, a funnel plot was conducted for depression and anxiety, as there was only a sufficient number of studies reporting results for these two pathologies (according to Grading of Recommendations, Assessment, Development and Evaluation Working Group (GRADE guides), a minimum of five to 10 studies with the same statistic reported are needed). A total of seven studies analyzing the relationship between depression and IGD, and a total of five analyzing anxiety and IGD, reported d values or data to calculate them. Figure 2 depicts the distribution of the reported or calculated correlations for depression and anxiety. The x-axis and y-axis represent the reported d values and the inverse of the sample size, respectively.

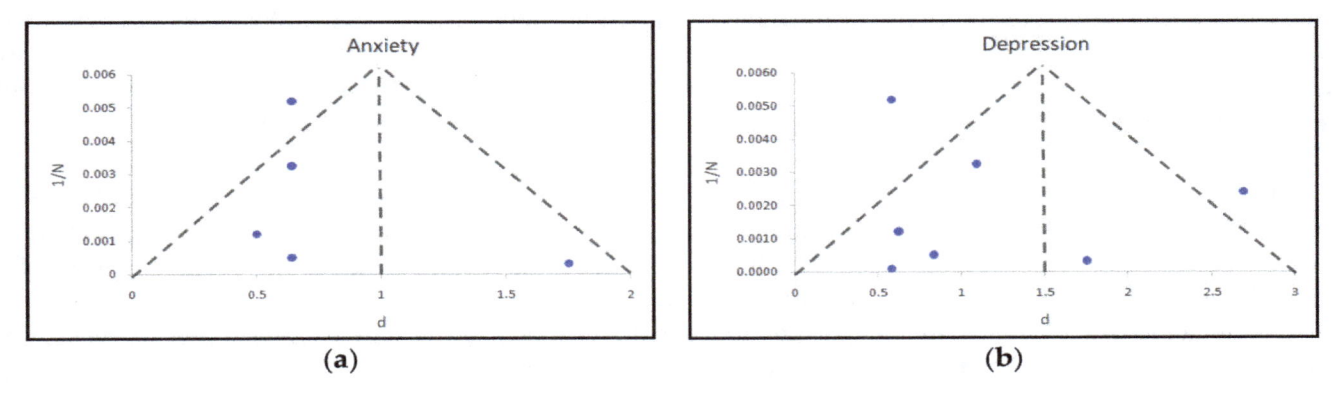

(a) (b)

Figure 2. Funnel plots with pseudo-95% confidence limits: (a) anxiety, (b) depression.

The location of the studies shows a bias towards the left side of the funnel plot, i.e., low values of d, indicating a possible publication bias. Even so, we would like to remark that the number of studies is very small to conclude with definitive results in both psychopathologies [84,85], and thus this information must be interpreted cautiously.

4. Discussion

The main purpose of this review was to explore the state of current literature about the relationship between IGD and comorbid psychopathologies, as this knowledge is crucial to the positioning of the disorder as a behavioral addiction. A secondary aim was to analyze the effect size of these correlations and the potential effect of publication bias. In the reviewed papers on IGD and comorbid psychological pathologies, 92% of the studies describe significant correlations with anxiety, 89% with depression, 87% with ADHD or hyperactivity symptoms, and 75% with social phobia/anxiety and obsessive-compulsive symptoms. However, the potential publication bias detected in the preliminary analysis demands caution in interpretation of the results. Notwithstanding this, it should be noted that despite the inclusion of IGD in Section III of the Diagnostic and Statistical Manual DSM-5 [7] and in the beta version of the ICD-11 (International Classification of Diseases) [8], only a marginally small number of publications were centered on IGD in the literature, and several authors continue analyzing IA or PIU as a whole, without distinguishing the different possible problematic activities that users experience with this medium.

With regard to the main purpose, IGD showed strong correlations with most of the analyzed psychopathologies, in comparison with PIU, where the strongest association was found with depression [14]. The effect sizes examined indicated that the strongest associations were found with anxiety, depression, and ADHD or hyperactivity symptoms and social phobia/anxiety.

The fact as to whether the addictive behaviors (with or without substance use) may be a consequence or a trigger of psychopathology [15] cannot be unraveled yet. The lack of longitudinal studies analyzing the temporal linearity of these events in AI or PIU precludes clarifying whether a specific psychiatric problem helps to develop an AI or, alternatively, a person with a diagnosis of AI —due to negative consequences stemming from it—later developed a comorbid psychiatric disorder. A third possibility is that both problems share underlying biological, sociodemographic or psychological mechanisms that make people vulnerable to both pathologies (which manifest at the same time). In the case of this review, two longitudinal studies and one cohort study required data on whether IGD was the cause or consequence of psychopathological problems; as a result, contradictory results were obtained. On the one hand, the results of the longitudinal study performed by Gentile et al. [43] showed that the adolescents who became and stayed pathological gamers during the study period, in the last time measured, ended up with increased levels of depression, anxiety and social phobia, while those who were pathological at the start but stopped being pathological, ended up with reduced levels of depression, anxiety and social phobia. These results seem to demonstrate that gaming predicts other mental health disorders longitudinally, rather than simply being correlated with them. On the other hand, van Rooij et al. [44] found a relation between addicted heavy gamers and depression in the second year, but no correlation with social anxiety at any time. Finally, Brunborg et al. [47] only found a correlation between depression and IGD at Time 1, but not at other times.

These ambiguous results show the complex relationship between the intrinsic characteristics of online video games, the consequences of their abuse, and associated psychopathologies. The literature shows that adolescents with high scores in IGD also have negative consequences at the psychosocial level: fewer recreational activities, fewer social activities and contacts, and diminished academic performance [86,87]. These abnormalities in "real-world" social support can affect people with different personality profiles in different ways. Generally, each online video game has an associated players' community. This may lead players to find people online with similar interests and, thus, expand or replace their "real-life" social network. As these online relationships spend more and more time, "real-world" social relations will tend to deteriorate or disappear and this lack of "real-life" social support can lead some players to develop symptomatology. But in other cases, establishing this type of online relationships can help alleviate the psychological distress of some players, helping the person to establish social relationships through the Internet and build their lives around it. Some authors provide evidence that personality characteristics (e.g., extraversion, introversion) affect the choice of online or offline options for relationships [88].

Finally, age could be another key factor influencing comorbid psychopathology. In the present review, the strongest associations were found in the adult population. Results focusing on other behavioral addictions (i.e., Gambling Disorder), shows that younger adults, as opposed to older patients, only experience the symptoms of the addiction as psychological discomfort [89], without another comorbid psychopathology. One possible explanation is that older gamblers have experienced the negative consequences of the disorder for a longer period, and this has led them to develop comorbid psychopathology. It is also possible that the psychological symptoms associated with IGD require a longer time period to appear in certain subjects. Another hypothesis is that, first, children and adolescents tend to underestimate the long-term negative consequences of risky or prejudicial behaviors; and second, compared with adults, when making decisions adolescents tend to give more weight to short-term rewards compared with attendant risks [90]. Future research should analyze the differences in the perception of the negative consequences caused by IGD among adults and adolescents.

In relation to gender differences, similar to IA results all the reviewed studies reported higher video-game use among males, and most of the articles found a higher prevalence of IGD in males. Other authors have found that female respondents report less frequent play and less orientation to game genres featuring competition and three-dimensional rotation [91,92]. These characteristics in women players may be a protective factor against IGD. Regarding the amount of time spent playing, although contradictory results have been found regarding the relationship between this factor and IGD [31,42], some authors suggest that its control could be a protective factor in its appearance [93]. With respect to the type of video game chosen, it is likely that both the competitive factor and the immersive factor (in this case favored by a three-dimensional environment) of the online games, characteristics that women do not usually choose, may influence the development of IGD [94–96].

In order to clarify these points, future studies should focus on an analysis of the relationships between the personality of the affected people, the video-game preferences (e.g., massively multiplayer online role-playing game or MMORPG, multiplayer online battle arena or MOBA, first-person shooter gamers), the perception of the negative consequences generated by the problematic use, and the associated psychopathology.

The geographical distribution of the research in IGD seems to be more homogeneous than in IA; 50% of the included studies were developed in Europe and 50% were conducted in the rest of the world (29% in Asia, 30% in Australia, and 8% in North America). The prevalence of the problem and its correlation with psychopathology has been reported in all countries; therefore, it seems that it is a global problem and independent of cultural variation.

In contrast to IA, where there is a lack of common diagnostic criteria [14], in the case of IGD there are several questionnaires available based on the proposed diagnostic criteria for the disorder in the DSM-5. Despite this inclusion, the debate about the adequacy of these criteria and the emphasis upon online gaming rather than "general" gaming addiction is still active [97,98]. Therefore, although there is no gold standard questionnaire for IGD, the authors have a diagnostic base in which to frame their research. In the present review, of the 15 included articles published after the appearance of the DSM-5, only eight authors used these criteria or questionnaires based on them. The rest of the published research is based on measures for IA problems or questionnaires adapted from Gambling Disorder and general addiction criteria. This variability in evaluation methods, and basing the division of the comparison groups (IGD problems vs. no IGD problems) exclusively in the results of auto-administered data, could in part explain the variability found between IGD and comorbid psychopathology.

A consensus on the evaluation method of the problem is critical; in addition, studies focused on clinical populations with a diagnosis confirmed by professionals are needed. The data based on self-reports may not be accurate and may be limited in how they diagnose people [99]; therefore, in future research it would be helpful to complement the results of self-report questionnaires with clinical interviews (at least for the positive cases).

5. Limitations

The results of this review should be interpreted with several limitations in mind. First (as noted), some of the studies were published before the inclusion of IGD as a diagnostic category in the DSM-5. Thus, inconsistencies in clinical definitions and evaluations should be expected. Second, restrictions applied to the language of the articles, and heterogeneity in the nomenclature surrounding IGD across the different studies, suggests a potential risk that a relevant article was missed. However, articles written in other languages (with abstracts in English) were included in the review process; furthermore, a search in the citations of the selected literature was carried out. Third, reviewing only the first 30 pages of results in Google Scholar may have produced some bias; however, this method has been shown to be commonly used [100] and seems not to influence the results of the reviews. In addition, searches in other search engines and citations of included articles may have reduced that risk.

6. Conclusions

The present review included 24 studies analyzing the association between IGD and psychopathology. Compared with IA (which showed strong correlations only with depression), IGD showed strong correlations with anxiety, depression, ADHD or hyperactivity symptoms, social phobia/anxiety, and obsessive-compulsive symptoms. The lack of longitudinal studies and the contradictory results obtained makes it difficult to detect the directionality of these associations and shows the existing complexity of the relationship between IGD and psychopathology. In addition, due to a possible publication bias, the results should be interpreted with caution.

For future research, it would be helpful to investigate the relationships between personality styles, type of video-game problem, negative consequences, and associated psychopathology. It is also necessary to reach a consensus on the diagnostic criteria of IGD and on psychometric instruments used to research the subject. Studies centered in the clinical population, with diagnostic interviews that confirm the presence of the disorder, are critically needed.

Acknowledgments: This work was funded by an AIS (Atención e InvestigaciónenSocioaddiciones) intramural research program. This research has been partially supported by the Marsden grant number E2987-3648 (Royal Society of New Zealand). This partial funder had no role in the study design, data collection, and analysis, decision to publish, or preparation of the manuscript.

Author Contributions: Vega González-Bueso and Juan José Santamaría conceived and planned the review. Vega González-Bueso and Juan José Santamaría carried out the search and revision of the literature. Juan José Santamaría and Daniel Fernández analyzed the data. Vega González-Bueso and Juan José Santamaría drafted the study. All authors (Vega González-Bueso, Juan José Santamaría, Daniel Fernández, Laura Merino, Elena Montero and Joan Ribas) revised the article critically for important intellectual content. All authors (Vega González-Bueso, Juan José Santamaría, Daniel Fernández, Laura Merino, Elena Montero and Joan Ribas) commented on and approved the final manuscript and are accountable for all aspects of the work.

References

1. King, D.L.; Haagsma, M.C.; Delfabbro, P.H.; Gradisar, M.; Griffiths, M.D. Toward a consensus definition of pathological video-gaming: A systematic review of psychometric assessment tools. *Clin. Psychol. Rev.* **2013**, *33*, 331–342. [CrossRef] [PubMed]

2. Sim, T.; Gentile, D.A.; Bricolo, F.; Serpelloni, G.; Gulamoydeen, F. A Conceptual Review of Research on the Pathological Use of Computers, Video Games, and the Internet. *Int. J. Ment. Health Addict.* **2012**, *10*, 748–769. [CrossRef]

3. King, D.L.; Delfabbro, P.H. Issues for DSM-5: Video-gaming disorder? *Aust. N. Z. J. Psychiatry* **2013**, *47*, 20–22. [CrossRef] [PubMed]

4. Starcevic, V.; Aboujaoude, E. Internet addiction: Reappraisal of an increasingly inadequate concept. *CNS Spectr.* **2017**, *22*, 7–13. [CrossRef] [PubMed]

5. Thompson, T. Demographic and motivation variables associated with Internet usage activities. *Internet Res.* **2001**, *11*, 125–137. [CrossRef]

6. Weiser, E.B. Gender Differences in Internet Use Patterns and Internet Application Preferences: A Two-Sample Comparison. *CyberPsychol. Behav.* **2000**, *3*, 167–178. [CrossRef]

7. American Psychiatric Association. *Diagnostic and Statistical Manual of Mental Disorders (DSM-5)*, 5th ed.; American Psychiatric Association: Washington, DC, USA, 2013.

8. ICD-11 Beta Draft—Mortality and Morbidity Statistics. Available online: https://icd.who.int/dev11/l-m/en (accessed on 17 November 2017).

9. Saban, A.; Flisher, A.J. The Association between Psychopathology and Substance Use in Young People: A Review of the Literature. *J. Psychoact. Drugs* **2010**, *42*, 37–47. [CrossRef] [PubMed]

10. Petit, A.; Karila, L.; Chalmin, F.; Lejoyeux, M. Methamphetamine Addiction: A Review of the Literature. *J. Addict. Res. Ther.* **2012**, *1*, 2–7. [CrossRef]

11. Anthony, J.C. Epidemiology of drug dependence and illicit drug use. *Curr. Opin. Psychiatry* **1991**, *4*, 435–439. [CrossRef]

12. Kosten, T.R.; Ziedonis, D.M. Substance abuse and schizophrenia: Editors' introduction. *Schizophr. Bull.* **1997**, *23*, 181–186. [CrossRef] [PubMed]

13. Lehman, A.F.; Myers, C.P.; Corty, E. Assessment and classification of patients with psychiatric and substance abuse syndromes. *Hosp. Community Psychiatry* **1989**, *40*, 1019–1025. [CrossRef] [PubMed]

14. Carli, V.; Durkee, T.; Wasserman, D.; Hadlaczky, G.; Despalins, R.; Kramarz, E.; Wasserman, C.; Sarchiapone, M.; Hoven, C.W.; Brunner, R.; et al. The association between pathological internet use and comorbid psychopathology: A systematic review. *Psychopathology* **2013**, *46*, 1–13. [CrossRef] [PubMed]

15. Dong, G.; Lu, Q.; Zhou, H.; Zhao, X. Precursor or Sequela: Pathological Disorders in People with Internet Addiction Disorder. *PLoS ONE* **2011**, *6*, e14703. [CrossRef] [PubMed]
16. Floros, G.; Siomos, K.; Stogiannidou, A.; Giouzepas, I.; Garyfallos, G. Comorbidity of psychiatric disorders with Internet addiction in a clinical sample: The effect of personality, defense style and psychopathology. *Addict. Behav.* **2014**, *39*, 1839–1845. [CrossRef] [PubMed]
17. Young, K.S. Cognitive behavior therapy with Internet addicts: Treatment outcomes and implications. *Cyberpsychol. Behav.* **2007**, *10*, 671–679. [CrossRef] [PubMed]
18. Chang, F.-C.; Chiu, C.-H.; Lee, C.-M.; Chen, P.-H.; Miao, N.-F. Predictors of the initiation and persistence of Internet addiction among adolescents in Taiwan. *Addict. Behav.* **2014**, *39*, 1434–1440. [CrossRef] [PubMed]
19. Durkee, T.; Kaess, M.; Carli, V.; Parzer, P.; Wasserman, C.; Floderus, B.; Apter, A.; Balazs, J.; Barzilay, S.; Bobes, J.; et al. Prevalence of pathological internet use among adolescents in Europe: Demographic and social factors. *Addiction* **2012**, *107*, 2210–2222. [CrossRef] [PubMed]
20. Moher, D.; Shamseer, L.; Clarke, M.; Ghersi, D.; Liberati, A.; Petticrew, M.; Shekelle, P.; Stewart, L.A. PRISMA-P Group Preferred reporting items for systematic review and meta-analysis protocols (PRISMA-P) 2015 statement. *Syst. Rev.* **2015**, *4*, 1. [CrossRef] [PubMed]
21. Available online: https://www.crd.york.ac.uk/PROSPERO/ (accessed on 17 November 2017).
22. Cohen, J. *Statistical Power Analysis for the Behavioral Sciences*, 2nd ed.; L. Erlbaum Associates: Hillsdale, NJ, USA, 1988; ISBN 9780805802832.
23. Chinn, S. A simple method for converting an odds ratio to effect size for use in meta-analysis. *Stat. Med.* **2000**, *19*, 3127–3131. [CrossRef]
24. Baer, S.; Bogusz, E.; Green, D.A. Stuck on screens: Patterns of computer and gaming station use in youth seen in a psychiatric clinic. *J. Can. Acad. Child Adolesc. Psychiatry* **2011**, *20*, 86–94. [PubMed]
25. Cole, S.H.; Hooley, J.M. Clinical and Personality Correlates of MMO Gaming. *Soc. Sci. Comput. Rev.* **2013**, *31*, 424–436. [CrossRef]
26. Jiménez-Murcia, S.; Fernández-Aranda, F.; Granero, R.; Chóliz, M.; La Verde, M.; Aguglia, E.; Signorelli, M.S.; Sá, G.M.; Aymamí, N.; Gómez-Peña, M.; et al. Video game addiction in gambling disorder: Clinical, psychopathological, and personality correlates. *Biomed. Res. Int.* **2014**, *7*, 105–110. [CrossRef] [PubMed]
27. Kim, N.R.; Hwang, S.S.-H.; Choi, J.-S.; Kim, D.-J.; Demetrovics, Z.; Király, O.; Nagygyörgy, K.; Griffiths, M.D.; Hyun, S.Y.; Youn, H.C.; et al. Characteristics and Psychiatric Symptoms of Internet Gaming Disorder among Adults Using Self-Reported DSM-5 Criteria. *Psychiatry Investig.* **2016**, *13*, 58. [CrossRef] [PubMed]
28. King, D.L.; Delfabbro, P.H.; Zwaans, T.; Kaptsis, D. Clinical features and axis I comorbidity of Australian adolescent pathological Internet and video game users. *Aust. N. Z. J. Psychiatry* **2013**, *47*, 1058–1067. [CrossRef] [PubMed]
29. King, D.L.; Delfabbro, P.H. The Cognitive Psychopathology of Internet Gaming Disorder in Adolescence. *J. Abnorm. Child Psychol.* **2016**, *44*, 1635–1645. [CrossRef] [PubMed]
30. Laconi, S.; Pirès, S.; Chabrol, H. Internet gaming disorder, motives, game genres and psychopathology. *Comput. Hum. Behav.* **2017**, *75*, 652–659. [CrossRef]
31. Männikkö, N.; Billieux, J.; Kääriäinen, M. Problematic digital gaming behavior and its relation to the psychological, social and physical health of Finnish adolescents and young adults. *J. Behav. Addict.* **2015**, *4*, 281–288. [CrossRef] [PubMed]
32. Mentzoni, R.A.; Brunborg, G.S.; Molde, H.; Myrseth, H.; Skouverøe, K.J.M.; Hetland, J.; Pallesen, S. Problematic Video Game Use: Estimated Prevalence and Associations with Mental and Physical Health. *Cyberpsychol. Behav. Soc. Netw.* **2011**, *14*, 591–596. [CrossRef] [PubMed]
33. Müller, K.W.; Janikian, M.; Dreier, M.; Wölfling, K.; Beutel, M.E.; Tzavara, C.; Richardson, C.; Tsitsika, A. Regular gaming behavior and internet gaming disorder in European adolescents: Results from a cross-national representative survey of prevalence, predictors, and psychopathological correlates. *Eur. Child Adolesc. Psychiatry* **2015**, *24*, 565–574. [CrossRef] [PubMed]
34. Na, E.; Lee, H.; Choi, I.; Kim, D.-J. Comorbidity of Internet gaming disorder and alcohol use disorder: A focus on clinical characteristics and gaming patterns. *Am. J. Addict.* **2017**, *26*, 326–334. [CrossRef] [PubMed]
35. Starcevic, V.; Berle, D.; Porter, G.; Fenech, P. Problem Video Game Use and Dimensions of Psychopathology. *Int. J. Ment. Health Addict.* **2011**, *9*, 248–256. [CrossRef]

36. Stetina, B.U.; Kothgassner, O.D.; Lehenbauer, M.; Kryspin-Exner, I. Beyond the fascination of online-games: Probing addictive behavior and depression in the world of online-gaming. *Comput. Hum. Behav.* **2011**, *27*, 473–479. [CrossRef]

37. Strittmatter, E.; Kaess, M.; Parzer, P.; Fischer, G.; Carli, V.; Hoven, C.W.; Wasserman, C.; Sarchiapone, M.; Durkee, T.; Apter, A.; et al. Pathological Internet use among adolescents: Comparing gamers and non-gamers. *Psychiatry Res.* **2015**, *228*, 128–135. [CrossRef] [PubMed]

38. Vadlin, S.; Åslund, C.; Hellström, C.; Nilsson, K.W. Associations between problematic gaming and psychiatric symptoms among adolescents in two samples. *Addict. Behav.* **2016**, *61*, 8–15. [CrossRef] [PubMed]

39. Wang, H.R.; Cho, H.; Kim, D.-J. Prevalence and correlates of comorbid depression in a nonclinical online sample with DSM-5 internet gaming disorder. *J. Affect. Disord.* **2018**, *226*, 1–5. [CrossRef] [PubMed]

40. Wartberg, L.; Kriston, L.; Kramer, M.; Schwedler, A.; Lincoln, T.M.; Kammerl, R. Internet gaming disorder in early adolescence: Associations with parental and adolescent mental health. *Eur. Psychiatry* **2017**, *43*, 14–18. [CrossRef] [PubMed]

41. Wei, H.-T.; Chen, M.-H.; Huang, P.-C.; Bai, Y.-M. The association between online gaming, social phobia, and depression: An internet survey. *BMC Psychiatry* **2012**, *12*, 92. [CrossRef] [PubMed]

42. Panagiotidi, M. Problematic Video Game Play and ADHD Traits in an Adult Population. *Cyberpsychol. Behav. Soc. Netw.* **2017**, *20*, 292–295. [CrossRef] [PubMed]

43. Gentile, D.A.; Choo, H.; Liau, A.; Sim, T.; Li, D.; Fung, D.; Khoo, A. Pathological video game use among youths: A two-year longitudinal study. *Pediatrics* **2011**, *127*, e319–e329. [CrossRef] [PubMed]

44. Van Rooij, A.J.; Schoenmakers, T.M.; Vermulst, A.A.; Van Den Eijnden, R.J.J.M.; Van De Mheen, D. Online video game addiction: Identification of addicted adolescent gamers. *Addiction* **2011**, *106*, 205–212. [CrossRef] [PubMed]

45. Hyun, G.J.; Han, D.H.; Lee, Y.S.; Kang, K.D.; Yoo, S.K.; Chung, U.-S.; Renshaw, P.F. Risk factors associated with online game addiction: A hierarchical model. *Comput. Hum. Behav.* **2015**, *48*, 706–713. [CrossRef]

46. Yen, J.-Y.; Liu, T.-L.; Wang, P.-W.; Chen, C.-S.; Yen, C.-F.; Ko, C.-H. Association between Internet gaming disorder and adult attention deficit and hyperactivity disorder and their correlates: Impulsivity and hostility. *Addict. Behav.* **2017**, *64*, 308–313. [CrossRef] [PubMed]

47. Brunborg, G.S.; Mentzoni, R.A.; Frøyland, L.R. Is video gaming, or video game addiction, associated with depression, academic achievement, heavy episodic drinking, or conduct problems? *J. Behav. Addict.* **2014**, *3*, 27–32. [CrossRef] [PubMed]

48. Király, O.; Sleczka, P.; Pontes, H.M.; Urbán, R.; Griffiths, M.D.; Demetrovics, Z. Validation of the Ten-Item Internet Gaming Disorder Test (IGDT-10) and evaluation of the nine DSM-5 Internet Gaming Disorder criteria. *Addict. Behav.* **2017**, *64*, 253–260. [CrossRef] [PubMed]

49. Vadlin, S.; Åslund, C.; Nilsson, K.W. Development and content validity of a screening instrument for gamingaddiction in adolescents: The Gaming Addiction Identification Test (GAIT). *Scand. J. Psychol.* **2015**, *56*, 458–466. [CrossRef] [PubMed]

50. Lemmens, J.S.; Valkenburg, P.M.; Gentile, D.A. The Internet Gaming Disorder Scale. *Psychol. Assess.* **2015**, *27*, 567–582. [CrossRef] [PubMed]

51. Bush, K.; Kivlahan, D.R.; McDonell, M.B.; Fihn, S.D.; Bradley, K.A. The AUDIT alcohol consumption questions (AUDIT-C): An effective brief screening test for problem drinking. Ambulatory Care Quality Improvement Project (ACQUIP). Alcohol Use Disorders Identification Test. *Arch. Intern. Med.* **1998**, *158*, 1789–1795. [CrossRef] [PubMed]

52. Derogatis, L.R.; Lipman, R.S.; Rickels, K.; Uhlenhuth, E.H.; Covi, L. The Hopkins Symptom Checklist (HSCL): A self-report symptom inventory. *Behav. Sci.* **1974**, *19*, 1–15. [CrossRef] [PubMed]

53. Woo, B.S.C.; Chang, W.C.; Fung, D.S.S.; Koh, J.B.K.; Leong, J.S.F.; Kee, C.H.Y.; Seah, C.K.F. Development and validation of a depression scale for Asian adolescents. *J. Adolesc.* **2004**, *27*, 677–689. [CrossRef] [PubMed]

54. Beck, A.T.; Ward, C.H.; Mendelson, M.; Mock, J.; Erbaugh, J. An inventory for measuring depression. *Arch. Gen. Psychiatry* **1961**, *4*, 561–571. [CrossRef] [PubMed]

55. Beck, A.T.; Steer, R.A.; Ball, R.; Ranieri, W.F. Comparison of Beck Depression Inventories-IA and-II in Psychiatric Outpatients. *J. Pers. Assess.* **1996**, *67*, 588–597. [CrossRef] [PubMed]

56. Andresen, E.M.; Malmgren, J.A.; Carter, W.B.; Patrick, D.L. Screening for depression in well older adults: Evaluation of a short form of the CES-D (Center for Epidemiologic Studies Depression Scale). *Am. J. Prev. Med.* **1994**, *10*, 77–84. [CrossRef]

57. Kandel, D.B.; Davies, M. Epidemiology of depressive mood in adolescents: An empirical study. *Arch. Gen. Psychiatry* **1982**, *39*, 1205–1212. [CrossRef] [PubMed]

58. Kühner, C. *Fragebogen zur Depressionsdiagnostik nach DSM-IV (FDD-DSMIV)*; Hogrefe: Göttingen, Germany, 1997.

59. Svanborg, P.; Ekselius, L. Self-assessment of DSM-IV criteria for major depression in psychiatric out- and inpatients. *Nord. J. Psychiatry* **2003**, *57*, 291–296. [CrossRef] [PubMed]

60. Spitzer, R.L.; Kroenke, K.; Williams, J.B. Validation and utility of a self-report version of PRIME-MD: The PHQ primary care study. Primary Care Evaluation of Mental Disorders. Patient Health Questionnaire. *JAMA* **1999**, *282*, 1737–1744. [CrossRef] [PubMed]

61. Hung, C.-I.; Wang, S.-J.; Liu, C.-Y. Validation of the Depression and Somatic Symptoms Scale by comparison with the Short Form 36 scale among psychiatric outpatients with major depressive disorder. *Depress. Anxiety* **2009**, *26*, 583–591. [CrossRef] [PubMed]

62. Spielberger, C.; Gorsuch, R.L.; Lushene, R.E. *Manual for the State/Trait Anxiety Inventory*; Consulting Psychologists Press: Palo Alto, CA, USA, 1970.

63. Birmaher, B.; Khetarpal, S.; Brent, D.; Cully, M.; Balach, L.; Kaufman, J.; Neer, S.M. The Screen for Child Anxiety Related Emotional Disorders (SCARED): Scale construction and psychometric characteristics. *J. Am. Acad. Child Adolesc. Psychiatry* **1997**, *36*, 545–553. [CrossRef] [PubMed]

64. Beck, A.T.; Epstein, N.; Brown, G.; Steer, R.A. An inventory for measuring clinical anxiety: Psychometric properties. *J. Consult. Clin. Psychol.* **1988**, *56*, 893–897. [CrossRef] [PubMed]

65. Spence, S.H. A measure of anxiety symptoms among children. *Behav. Res. Ther.* **1998**, *36*, 545–566. [CrossRef]

66. Spitzer, R.L.; Kroenke, K.; Williams, J.B.W.; Löwe, B. A Brief Measure for Assessing Generalized Anxiety Disorder. *Arch. Intern. Med.* **2006**, *166*, 1092. [CrossRef] [PubMed]

67. Chorpita, B.F.; Yim, L.; Moffitt, C.; Umemoto, L.A.; Francis, S.E. Assessment of symptoms of DSM-IV anxiety and depression in children: A revised child anxiety and depression scale. *Behav. Res. Ther.* **2000**, *38*, 835–855. [CrossRef]

68. Kunttu, K.; Pesonen, T. *Student Health Survey 2012: A National Survey among Finnish University Students*; Finnish Student Health Service; Ylioppilaiden Terveydenhoitosäätiön Tutkimuksia 47: Helsinki, Finland, 2013.

69. Zigmond, A.S.; Snaith, R.P. The hospital anxiety and depression scale. *Acta Psychiatr. Scand.* **1983**, *67*, 361–370. [CrossRef] [PubMed]

70. Achenbach, T. *Manual for the Youth Self-Report and 1991 Profile*; Department of Psychiatry, University of Vermont: Burlington, VT, USA, 1999.

71. Reynolds, W. *Reynolds Adolescent Adjustment Screening InventoryTM (RAASITM): Professional Manual*; Psychological Assessment Resources: Lutz, FL, USA, 2001.

72. Kessler, R.C.; Adler, L.; Ames, M.; Demler, O.; Faraone, S.; Hiripi, E.; Howes, M.J.; Jin, R.; Secnik, K.; Spencer, T.; et al. The World Health Organization Adult ADHD Self-Report Scale (ASRS): A short screening scale for use in the general population. *Psychol. Med.* **2005**, *35*, 245–256. [CrossRef] [PubMed]

73. Goodman, R. The Strengths and Difficulties Questionnaire: A research note. *J. Child Psychol. Psychiatry* **1997**, *38*, 581–586. [CrossRef] [PubMed]

74. DuPaul, G.J. Parent and Teacher Ratings of ADHD Symptoms: Psychometric Properties in a Community-Based Sample. *J. Clin. Child Psychol.* **1991**, *20*, 245–253. [CrossRef]

75. American Psychiatric Association. *Diagnostic and Statistical Manual of Mental Disorders*, 4th ed.; American Psychiatric Association Text Revision: Arlington, TA, USA, 2000.

76. Connor, K.M.; Davidson, J.R.; Churchill, L.E.; Sherwood, A.; Foa, E.; Weisler, R.H. Psychometric properties of the Social Phobia Inventory (SPIN). New self-rating scale. *Br. J. Psychiatry* **2000**, *176*, 379–386. [CrossRef] [PubMed]

77. Mattick, R.P.; Clarke, J.C. Development and validation of measures of social phobia scrutiny fear and social interaction anxiety. *Behav. Res. Ther.* **1998**, *36*, 455–470. [CrossRef]

78. La Greca, A.M.; Stone, W.L. Social Anxiety Scale for Children-Revised: Factor Structure and Concurrent Validity. *J. Clin. Child Psychol.* **1993**, *22*, 17–27. [CrossRef]

79. Derogatis, L.R. *SCL-90-R. Administration, Scoring and Procedures Manual*; Clinical Psychometric Research Inc.: Baltimore, MD, USA, 1990.

80. Derogatis, L.R.; Melisaratos, N. The Brief Symptom Inventory: An introductory report. *Psychol. Med.* **1983**, *13*, 595–605. [CrossRef] [PubMed]

81. Laurens, K.; Hodgins, S.; MaughanN, B.; Murray, R.; Rutter, M.; Taylor, E. Community screening for psychotic-like experiences and other putative antecedents of schizophrenia in children aged 9–12 years. *Schizophr. Res.* **2007**, *90*, 130–146. [CrossRef] [PubMed]

82. STARCEVIC, V. Problematic Internet use: A distinct disorder, a manifestation of an underlying psychopathology, or a troublesome behaviour? *World Psychiatry* **2010**, *9*, 92–93. [CrossRef] [PubMed]

83. King, D.L.; Delfabbro, P.H.; Griffiths, M.D. Trajectories of Problem Video Gaming Among Adult Regular Gamers: An 18-Month Longitudinal Study. *Cyberpsychol. Behav. Soc. Netw.* **2013**, *16*, 72–76. [CrossRef] [PubMed]

84. Monroe, J. *Meta-Analysis for Observational Studies: Statistical Methods for Heterogeneity, Publication Bias and Combining Studies: Statistics*; University of California: Los Angeles, CA, USA, 2007.

85. Sutton, A.J. *Methods for Meta-Analysis in Medical Research*; J. Wiley: Chichester, UK, 2000; ISBN 9780471490661.

86. Beutel, M.E.; Hoch, C.; Wölfling, K.; Müller, K.W. Clinical characteristics of computer game and internet addiction in persons seeking treatment in an outpatient clinic for computer game addiction. *Z. Psychosom. Med. Psychother.* **2011**, *57*, 77–90. [CrossRef] [PubMed]

87. Batthyány, D.; Müller, K.W.; Benker, F.; Wölfling, K. Computer game playing: Clinical characteristics of dependence and abuse among adolescents. *Wien. Klin. Wochenschr.* **2009**, *121*, 502–509. [CrossRef] [PubMed]

88. Goby, V.P. Personality and Online/Offline Choices: MBTI Profiles and Favored Communication Modes in a Singapore Study. *Cyberpsychol. Behav.* **2006**, *9*, 5–13. [CrossRef] [PubMed]

89. González-Ibáñez, A.; Mora, M.; Gutiérrez-Maldonado, J.; Ariza, A.; Lourido-Ferreira, M.R. Pathological gambling and age: Differences in personality, psychopathology, and response to treatment variables. *Addict. Behav.* **2005**, *30*, 383–388. [CrossRef] [PubMed]

90. Halpern-Felsher, B.L.; Cauffman, E. Costs and benefits of a decision: Decision-making competence in adolescents and adults. *J. Appl. Dev. Psychol.* **2001**, *22*, 257–273. [CrossRef]

91. Lucas, K.; Sherry, J.L. Sex Differences in Video Game Play. *Commun. Res.* **2004**, *31*, 499–523. [CrossRef]

92. Greenberg, B.S.; Sherry, J.; Lachlan, K.; Lucas, K.; Holmstrom, A. Orientations to Video Games Among Gender and Age Groups. *Simul. Gaming* **2010**, *41*, 238–259. [CrossRef]

93. Young, K. Understanding Online Gaming Addiction and Treatment Issues for Adolescents. *Am. J. Fam. Ther.* **2009**, *37*, 355–372. [CrossRef]

94. Floros, G.; Siomos, K. Patterns of Choices on Video Game Genres and Internet Addiction. *Cyberpsychol. Behav. Soc. Netw.* **2012**, *15*, 417–424. [CrossRef] [PubMed]

95. Elliott, L.; Golub, A.; Ream, G.; Dunlap, E. Video Game Genre as a Predictor of Problem Use. *Cyberpsychol. Behav. Soc. Netw.* **2012**, *15*, 155–161. [CrossRef] [PubMed]

96. King, D.; Delfabbro, P.; Griffiths, M. Video Game Structural Characteristics: A New Psychological Taxonomy. *Int. J. Ment. Health Addict.* **2010**, *8*, 90–106. [CrossRef]

97. Petry, N.M.; Rehbein, F.; Gentile, D.A.; Lemmens, J.S.; Rumpf, H.-J.; Mößle, T.; Bischof, G.; Tao, R.; Fung, D.S.S.; Borges, G.; et al. An international consensus for assessing internet gaming disorder using the new DSM-5 approach. *Addiction* **2014**, *109*, 1399–1406. [CrossRef] [PubMed]

98. Kuss, D.J.; Griffiths, M.D.; Pontes, H.M. Chaos and confusion in DSM-5 diagnosis of Internet Gaming Disorder: Issues, concerns, and recommendations for clarity in the field. *J. Behav. Addict.* **2017**, *6*, 103–109. [CrossRef] [PubMed]

99. Bhandari, A.; Wagner, T. Self-Reported Utilization of Health Care Services: Improving Measurement and Accuracy. *Med. Care Res. Rev.* **2006**, *63*, 217–235. [CrossRef] [PubMed]

100. Kaptsis, D.; King, D.; Delfabbro, P.; Gradisar, M. Withdrawal symptoms in internet gaming disorder: A systematic review. *Clin. Psychol. Rev.* **2016**, *43*, 58–66. [CrossRef] [PubMed]

11

The Relationship between Impulsivity and Internet Gaming Disorder in Young Adults: Mediating Effects of Interpersonal Relationships and Depression

Hyera Ryu [1], Ji-Yoon Lee [1], Aruem Choi [1], Sunyoung Park [1], Dai-Jin Kim [2] and Jung-Seok Choi [1,3,*]

[1] Department of Psychiatry, SMG-SMU Boramae Medical Center, Seoul 07061, Korea; hyera.ryu12@gmail.com (H.R.); idiyuni91@gmail.com (J.-Y.L.); choiar90@gmail.com (A.C.); spark.37eme@gmail.com (S.P.)

[2] Department of Psychiatry, Seoul St. Mary's Hospital, College of Medicine, The Catholic University of Korea, Seoul 06591, Korea; kdj922@catholic.ac.kr

[3] Department of Psychiatry and Behavioral Science, Seoul National University College of Medicine, Seoul 03080, Korea

* Correspondence: choijs73@gmail.com

Abstract: *Background:* This study aimed to explore relationships between impulsivity, interpersonal relationships, depression, and Internet Gaming Disorder (IGD) symptoms. *Methods:* A total of 118 young adults participated in this study: 67 IGD patients who met five or more of the DSM-5 diagnostic criteria for IGD and 56 healthy controls. We administered questionnaires to assess IGD symptoms (Young's Internet Addiction Test; Y-IAT), impulsivity (Barratt Impulsiveness Scale; BIS-11), interpersonal relationship (Relationship Change Scale; RCS), and depression (Beck Depression Inventory; BDI). We used PROCESS macro in SPSS to perform mediation analysis. *Results:* IGD symptom was positively related to depression and impulsivity, and negatively related to the quality of interpersonal relationships. Mediation analysis revealed full mediation effects of interpersonal relationships and depression on the association between impulsivity and IGD symptoms in the IGD group. Specifically, even after adjusting for gender as a covariate, high impulsivity was associated with greater difficulty with interpersonal relationships; which further affected depression and increased the risk of IGD. *Conclusions:* These results demonstrate the importance of early intervention in IGD patients, particularly in young adults with high impulsivity. When intervening in adults' IGD, we should consider not only individual factors (e.g., depression) but also socioenvironmental factors (e.g., interpersonal relationships).

Keywords: internet gaming disorder; impulsivity; depression; interpersonal relationships; serial mediation

1. Introduction

Internet Gaming Disorder (IGD) is a kind of behavioral addiction that has been defined as a loss of control, and persistent and recurrent use of internet games leading to significant impairment in psychosocial functioning [1]. In particular, Diagnostic and Statistical Manual of Mental Disorders-Fifth Edition (DSM-5) has added an IGD as one of the conditions for further study in Section 3 [1], due to increased social interest worldwide. In previous studies, the prevalence of IGD, diagnosed according to DSM-5 criteria, was 1.16% in Germany [2], 2.5% in Slovenia [3], and 2.9% in Hungary [4]. However, higher estimates of prevalence (5.9% [5] and 10.8% [6]), have been reported in Korea. Because the risk of IGD is high in Korea, there is an urgent need to explore the characteristics of IGD in Korea, with further research in particular with respect to personal and environmental factors.

Choi [7] and Choi et al. [8], who proposed an integrated pathway model of IGD based on the model of gambling problems developed by Blaszczynski and Nower [9], suggested that IGD is a complex disorder caused by interactions among different bio-psycho-social factors. One of the biological factors is trait impulsiveness. The impulsivity is a tendency to behave voluntarily with little or no prior consideration of consequences [10], and could be measured by the Barratt Impulsiveness Scale (BIS-11), which is one of the oldest and most widely used a measurement of impulsive personality traits. In the BIS-11, impulsivity could be classified cognitive, motor, and nonplanning impulsiveness. Cognitive impulsiveness is the propensity to respond or make decisions during problem solving without thinking; motor impulsiveness is the tendency of impulsive behaviors, such as manifesting difficulty with impulse control or acting without thinking. Finally, nonplanning impulsiveness is a lack of foresight and a tendency not to plan or consider consequences before starting something [11]. In many previous studies, impulsivity has been regarded as a marker for vulnerability to IGD [12–16]. Dalbudak et al. found that IGD was correlated with the severity of impulsivity among Turkish university students, and Lee et al. showed that trait impulsivity is a vulnerable factor of IGD in young adults. In particular, impulsivity assessed by neuropsychological tests, such as the Stop Signal Test and Go/No-Go Task, was related to IGD symptoms [13,17,18]. In addition, several studies showed that impulsivity is related to depression [19,20] and that it indirectly predicts loneliness and poor interpersonal relationships [21]. Thus, impulsivity is not only a core feature of IGD symptoms but also an important factor affecting individuals' emotional and social functioning.

The quality of interpersonal relationships such as deficient social support and loneliness is among the social factors reported to be risk factors for IGD [22–24]. Previous studies have shown that loneliness increases the difficulty of maintaining healthy social interactions and may increase a preference for online social interaction, which can lead to IGD [22,25–28]. Furthermore, social contacts with family and friends help to reduce IGD symptoms [24,29]. In previous studies, loneliness, lack of social support, and lack of a sense of belonging have been shown to predict depression [30,31]. Thus, IGD could be assumed to be related to poor interpersonal relationships, which is a risk factor for depression and IGD symptoms.

Depression is one of the psychological factors associated with IGD. Prior research has shown that depression is a psychiatric disorder that is often comorbid with IGD [29,32,33]. In one study, 7% of adult IGD patients had a comorbid dysthymic disorder [34], and Ko et al. [35] identified a relationship between IGD and major depressive disorder or dysthymic disorder in college students. However, some studies have reported inconsistent results regarding the relationship between depression and IGD symptoms [29,36–40]. Ha et al. [41] suggested that participants who reported depression tended to seek cyberspace to avoid negative emotions and difficulties in daily life, and they had a high likelihood of being addicted to internet games because of the emotional support they found in cyberspace. Furthermore, a 2-year longitudinal study found that participants who overused internet games tended to be more depressed than those who did not [42]. Given these inconsistent results, it is necessary to clarify the relationship between depression and IGD. In addition, no previous studies have examined the relationship between bio-psycho-social factors and IGD symptoms by distinguishing between IGD and HC groups. Thus, it is important to examine the pathways connecting impulsivity, interpersonal relationships, depression, and IGD symptoms.

This study aimed to clarify relationships between impulsivity, interpersonal relationships, depression, and IGD symptoms and to identify the mediating effects of interpersonal relationships and depression on the relationship between impulsivity and IGD symptoms by distinguishing between IGD and HC group. We hypothesized that participants in the IGD group who also showed higher impulsivity would have more difficulty in interpersonal relationships, which would increase depression and increase the risk of IGD symptoms.

2. Materials and Methods

2.1. Participants and Procedure

A total of 123 young adults participated in this study, including 67 patients diagnosed with IGD and 56 healthy controls. The patients with IGD were seeking treatment at the outpatient clinics of SMG-SNU Boramae Medical Center in Seoul due to excessive internet gaming. They were diagnosed with IGD by a clinically experienced psychiatrist according to the DSM-5 criteria (more than five items). Also, the Structured Clinical interview was administered by a psychiatrist to identify past and current psychiatric disorders and only individuals with a history of intellectual disability or psychotic disorder were excluded. Of 67 patients with IGD, 10 had major depressive disorders, and two and one displayed social anxiety disorder and bipolar I disorder, respectively. Healthy controls (HC), who were recruited through advertisements, had no history of any psychiatric disorder.

To screen for the participants' intelligence quotient (IQ), the Korean-Wechsler Adult Intelligence Scale-IV (K-WAIS-IV) was administered, and five subjects with an IQ < 80 were excluded. Thus, 118 participants were included in the final analyses, including 62 in the IGD (male = 55; age = 25.54 $\pm$ 5.29 years) and 56 in the HC group (male = 38; age = 24.23 $\pm$ 3.92 years). All subjects completed informed consent forms before participating in the study. This study was conducted in accordance with the Declaration of Helsinki, and the protocol was approved by the Institutional Review Board of the SMG-SNU Boramae Medical Center (16-2014-139).

2.2. Measures

2.2.1. Demographic Variables

All participants answered a questionnaire to provide basic information such as age, gender, education year, and Internet use time (weekday and weekend).

2.2.2. Young's Internet Addiction Test (Y-IAT)

The Y-IAT was developed by Young (1998) [28], and has been validated in Korea [43]. It is 20-item self-report questionnaire and each item was answered using a 5-point scale ranging from 1 (very rarely) to 5 (very frequently). The total score ranged from 20 to 100, with higher scores reflecting a greater tendency of IGD symptoms. Cronbach's alpha was 0.96 in this study.

2.2.3. Barratt Impulsiveness Scale-11 (BIS-11)

The BIS-11 is an 11-item, revised version of the original Barratt Impulsiveness Scale, which is used to assess the degree of impulsivity [11]. This scale includes three subscales: cognitive, motor, and nonplanning impulsiveness. Cronbach's alpha was 0.76 in this study.

2.2.4. Relationship Change Scale (RCS)

The RCS consists of 25-item and 5-point Likert scale, which was originally developed by Schlein et al. [44], and was later translated into Korean by Mun (1980) and revised according to the Korean culture by Chun [45]. The RCS measures interpersonal relationships, and higher scores indicate better interpersonal relationships. The total score ranges from 25 to 125. Cronbach's alpha was 0.93 in this study.

2.2.5. Beck Depression Inventory-II (BDI-II)

The BDI, developed by Beck et al. [46], is a 21-item self-report questionnaire that measures the severity of particular symptoms experienced over the past week. Total scores range from 0 to 63, and higher scores reflect more severe depression. The BDI-II has previously been validated in Korean [47]. Cronbach's alpha was 0.92 in this study.

2.3. Statistical Analysis

Chi-square and t-tests were performed to compare the demographic and clinical characteristics of the HC and IGD groups. Pearson's correlation analysis was conducted to examine relationships between IGD symptoms (Y-IAT), impulsivity (BIS-11), depression (BDI), and interpersonal relationships (RCS) in the HC and IGD groups, respectively. To examine whether the quality of interpersonal relationships and depression mediated the relationship between impulsivity and IGD symptoms, we performed serial mediation analysis using the SPSS PROCESS macro, version 2.16 (model 6), developed by Hayes [48]. Serial mediation assumes a causal chain linking the mediators, with a specified direction of causal flow [49]. In particular, we analyzed using bootstrapping method, because there were limitations of Sobel's test (e.g., need a large sample). 5000 bootstrapping was used to identify indirect effects in the mediation models and analyzed with 95% confidence interval. SPSS software version 21.0 (SPSS, Inc., Chicago, IL, USA) was used for all data analyses.

3. Results

3.1. Demographic and Clinical Characteristics

In the total group, the mean age was 24.92 ± 4.71 years, and 78.8% ($n = 93$) of the sample were male. A comparison of the demographic and clinical characteristics of the IGD and HC groups showed that the percentage of males [$x^2(1) = 7.662$, $p < 0.05$], the internet gaming use time on weekdays [$t(69.23) = 9.088$, $p < 0.001$], internet gaming use time on weekends [$t(71.52) = 10.979$, $p < 0.001$], Y-IAT scores [$t(99.305) = 9.855$, $p < 0.001$], BIS-11 scores [$t(116) = 4.673$, $p < 0.001$], and BDI scores [$t(89.97) = 6.261$, $p < 0.001$] were significantly higher in the IGD than in the HC group, and the RCS score [$t(108.75) = -5.033$, $p < 0.001$] was significantly lower in the IGD group. Results are shown in Table 1.

Table 1. Demographics and Clinical characteristics ($n = 118$).

Variables	IGD ($n = 62$) M $\pm$ SD	HC ($n = 56$) M $\pm$ SD	$\varnothing^2 / t$	p Value
Gender (male, %)	55 (88.7%)	38 (67.9%)	7.662 *	0.007
Age (years)	25.54 ± 5.29	24.23 ± 3.92	1.545	0.125
Education (years)	13.88 ± 1.70	13.92 ± 1.51	−0.139	0.890
Time for weekday (h/day)	3.89 ± 3.02	0.28 ± 0.73	9.088 **	<0.001
Time for weekend (h/day)	5.72 ± 3.53	0.44 ± 1.09	10.979 **	<0.001
Y-IAT	53.71 ± 15.93	30.34 ± 9.15	9.855 **	<0.001
RCS	83.43 ± 14.48	94.87 ± 9.99	−5.033 **	<0.001
BIS-11	64.87 ± 9.65	57.33 ± 7.59	4.673 **	<0.001
BIS-11_Cognitive	19.03 ± 2.98	17.60 ± 2.39	2.840 *	0.005
BIS-11_Motor	18.09 ± 4.12	14.17 ± 2.84	6.053 **	<0.001
BIS-11_Nonplanning	27.74 ± 4.75	25.55 ± 3.82	2.735 *	0.007
BDI	12.04 ± 8.58	4.28 ± 4.30	6.261 **	<0.001

* $p < 0.05$, ** $p < 0.001$. Time for weekday/weekend = Average internet gaming use time per day on weekday and weekend; IGD = Internet Gaming Disorders; HC = Healthy Control; Y-IAT = Young's Internet Addiction Test; RCS = Relationship Change scale; BIS-11 = Barratt Impulsiveness Scale; BDI = Beck Depression Inventory.

3.2. Association between IGD Symptoms and Clinical Variables in the IGD and HC Groups

In both IGD and HC group, IGD symptoms as measured by Y-IAT were significantly correlated with depression (IGD: $r = 0.472$, $p < 0.001$; HC: $r = 0.363$, $p < 0.001$), and interpersonal problems (IGD: $r = -0.285$, $p < 0.05$; HC: $r = -0.268$, $p < 0.05$). However, there was a significant relationship between IGD symptoms and impulsivity only in the IGD group ($r = 0.306$, $p < 0.05$), specifically, IGD symptoms were related to cognitive impulsiveness ($r = 0.375$, $p < 0.001$) and nonplanning impulsiveness ($r = 0.275$, $p < 0.05$), but not to motor impulsiveness ($r = 0.129$, $p = 0.318$). In the HC group, impulsivity was not related to the IGD symptoms (Table 2).

Table 2. Correlation Analysis among the variables in IGD and HC group.

IGD (n = 62)	Y-IAT	BIS-11	BIS-11_Cognitive	BIS-11_Motor	BIS-11_Nonplanning	BDI	RCS
Y-IAT	1						
BIS-11	0.306 *	1					
BIS_cognitive	0.375 **	0.783 **	1				
BIS_Motor	0.129	0.765 **	0.388 **	1			
BIS_Nonplanning	0.275 *	0.875 **	0.626 **	0.441 **	1		
BDI	0.472 **	0.334 **	0.407 **	0.136	0.308 *	1	
RCS	−0.285 *	−0.407 **	−0.487 **	−0.103	−0.432 **	−0.641 **	1

HC (n = 56)	Y-IAT	BIS-11	BIS-11_Cognitive	BIS-11_Motor	BIS-11_Nonplanning	BDI	RCS
Y-IAT	1						
BIS-11	−0.023	1					
BIS-11_cognitive	0.070	0.744 **	1				
BIS-11_Motor	0.062	0.845 **	0.489 **	1			
BIS-11_Nonplanning	−0.136	0.893 **	0.489 **	0.630 **	1		
BDI	0.393 **	0.340 *	0.414 **	0.369 **	0.143	1	
RCS	−0.323 *	−0.317 *	−0.453 **	−0.289 *	−0.133	−0.586 **	1

* $p < 0.05$, ** $p < 0.001$. IGD = Internet Gaming Disorders; HC = Healthy Control; Y-IAT = Young's Internet Addiction Test; RCS = Relationship Change scale; BIS-11 = Barratt Impulsiveness Scale; BDI = Beck Depression Inventory.

3.3. Relationships between Impulsivity, Interpersonal Relationships, Depression, and IGD Symptoms

The model depicting serial mediation of the relationship between impulsivity and IGD symptoms by interpersonal relationships and depression in the IGD group is shown in Figure 1. We added sex as a covariate in the model. The serial mediation model was significant [$F(2,58)$ = 5.9481, $p < 0.05$] and explained about 17% of the variance in IGD symptoms in the IGD group. Specifically, both the total effect of impulsivity on IGD (c = 0.47, SE = 0.19, t = 2.39, $p < 0.05$) and the direct effect of impulsivity on interpersonal relationships (a_1 = −0.60, SE = 0.17, t = −3.39, $p < 0.05$) as mediating variables were significant. However, there was no significant direct effect of impulsivity on depression (path a_2 in Figure 1). The direct effect of interpersonal relationships, the first mediating variable, on depression (d_{21} = −0.35, SE = 0.06, t = −5.53, $p < 0.001$), the second mediating variable, was also significant. Furthermore, the direct effect of depression on IGD symptoms (b_2 = 0.76, SE = 0.28, t = 2.65, $p < 0.05$) was also statistically significant, whereas that of interpersonal relationships (path b_1 in Figure 1) was not. Finally, no significant direct effect of impulsivity on IGD was found (c' = 0.29, SE = 0.20, t = 1.42, p = 0.16) when impulsivity and both mediating variables were simultaneously entered into the equation. These results showed that interpersonal relationships and depression fully mediated the relationship between impulsivity and IGD symptoms in IGD group. Furthermore, the findings suggest that, in the IGD group only, high impulsivity leads to poor interpersonal relationships, and increasing depression, which in turn increases IGD symptoms. Additionally, the results of the bootstrapping to verify the indirect effects were significant only for the impact of impulsivity on IGD symptoms through interpersonal relationships and depression (B = 0.10, BCa 95% CI [0.0282, 0.2573]). In contrast, in the HC group, relationships between impulsivity, interpersonal relationships, depression, and IGD symptoms were not significant. A summary of the serial mediation results in the IGD group is shown in Table 3.

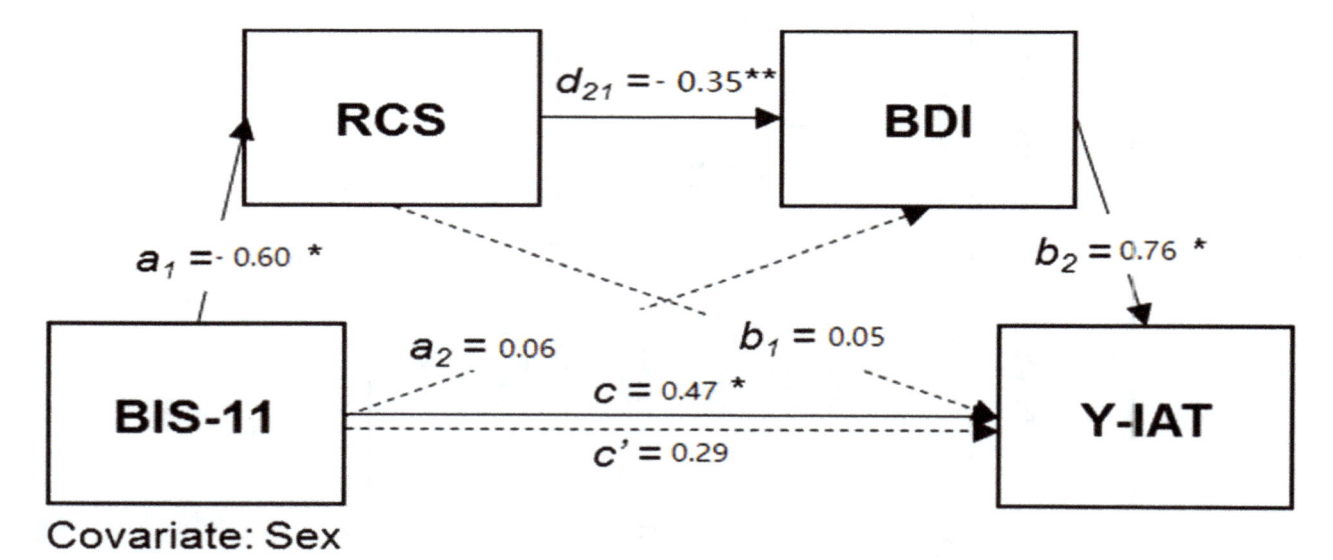

Figure 1. Serial mediation effects on problematic internet use in IGD group (n = 61). BIS-11 = Barratt Impulsiveness Scale; RCS = Relationship Change scale; BDI = Beck Depression Inventory; Y-IAT = Young's Internet Addiction Test; Solid lines showed significant paths with standardized path coefficients and dashed line represents a nonsignificant path. c' means direct effect of impulsivity (X) on internet addiction (Y) and c means indirect effect of impulsivity (X) on internet addiction (Y) through interpersonal relationship (M1) and depression (M2) in serial. Results showed that high impulsivity affected more difficulty in interpersonal relationships, which further affected depression and increased the risk of internet gaming disorder symptoms in IGD group. * $p < 0.05$, ** $p < 0.001$.

Table 3. Summary of serial mediation analysis of interpersonal relationship and depression between impulsivity and IGD symptoms in IGD group. ($n = 61$, bootstrap = 5000).

Effect	Paths	B	SE	t	BCa 95% CI	
					Lower	Upper
Direct effects	Impulsivity → Relationship	−0.60	0.17	−3.39 *		
	Impulsivity → Depression	0.06	0.09	0.72		
	Relationship → Depression	−0.35	0.06	−5.53 **		
	Relationship → Internet Addiction	0.05	0.16	0.30		
	Depression → Internet Addiction	0.76	0.28	2.65 *		
	Impulsivity → Internet Addiction	0.29	0.20	1.42		
Indirect effect	Impulsivity → Relationship → Internet Addiction	−0.01	0.07		−0.1759	0.1243
	Impulsivity → Relationship → Depression → Internet Addiction	0.10	0.05		0.0282	0.2573
	Impulsivity → Depression → Internet Addiction	0.03	0.04		−0.0268	0.1514

* $p < 0.05$, ** $p < 0.001$. BCa = Biased-Corrected and Accelerated 5000 bootstrapping; Covariate = sex.

4. Discussion

In this study, we investigated the well-known association between impulsivity and IGD symptoms by examining a mechanism linking interpersonal relationships and depression by distinguishing between the IGD and HC groups. As no previous studies have examined the pathways between impulsivity, interpersonal relationship, depression, and IGD symptoms by distinguishing between IGD and HC groups, the main purpose of this study was to examine the mechanism of association among these variables. The findings revealed serial mediation effects of depression and difficulty with interpersonal relationships on the relationship between impulsivity and IGD symptoms in the IGD group, but not in HC group. Furthermore, there were only full mediation effects. These results suggest a pathway in the IGD group whereby high impulsivity was related to difficulty with interpersonal relationships, which increased depression and, thereby, the risk of IGD symptoms. Thus, impulsivity was identified as one of the reasons for problems with interpersonal relationships among IGD patients, and the effect on IGD symptoms is mediated by difficulties with interpersonal relationships and depression, rather than having direct effects on IGD symptoms. This result suggests that IGD symptoms can be alleviated by reducing interpersonal problems and depression. This conclusion should be considered in developing treatment programs for IGD patients who report high impulsivity. In particular, Cognitive-Behavioral Therapy (CBT), Interpersonal Psychotherapy of Depression, Acceptance and commitment (ACT), and group therapy might be included as an element of treatment programs to alleviate interpersonal problems and depression.

In addition, one of the main results of our study was those that differentiated between the IGD and HC groups. Participants with IGD were significantly more likely to be male. They reported significantly higher rates of IGD symptoms including internet gaming use time on weekdays and weekends, poor interpersonal relationships, high impulsivity, and depressive symptoms compared with the healthy control group. Bakken et al. [50] and Tsai et al. [51] found that male gender was a predictor of IGD symptoms, with a higher proportion of males in the IGD than in the normal group.

Choi (2012) [7] argued that IGD could be caused by bio-psycho-social factors. In keeping with that study, IGD symptoms were related to impulsivity as a biological factor, interpersonal relationships as a social factor, and depression as a psychological factor in the present study. Specifically, consistent with previous studies, our results showed significant relationships among IGD symptoms measured by the Y-IAT, depression, and difficulty in interpersonal relationships in both the IGD and HC group. Dalbudak et al. [14] found that depression, as measured by the Symptom Checklist-revised (SCL-90-R) was related to the risk for IGD. Similarly, IGD has been found to be associated with many psychiatric disorders and symptoms, including depression, anxiety, ADHD, hostility, interpersonal sensitivity, and paranoid ideation [32,33,41,52,53]. In addition, interpersonal relationships were also associated with IGD symptoms in our study, suggesting that poor interpersonal relationships are associated with IGD. Several previous studies have also found that interpersonal problems were known to cause IGD symptoms [24,31], and Caplan [54] found that people who had psychological problems preferred online interaction and used the internet to cope with loneliness.

However, the relationship between impulsivity, including all subscales, and IGD symptoms was significant in the IGD group, but not in the HC group. In many previous studies, impulsivity was a significant risk factor for IGD [13,14,16,55]. In particular, high impulsivity has been shown to increase the severity of IGD symptoms; this relationship was also found in a study of Korean adults by Lee et al. [15]. However, our results showed that there was no significant correlation between impulsivity and IGD symptoms in HC group. In the previous studies, impulsivity differed significantly by gender, being more common among males [56,57]. The ratio of males to females in the HC group was significantly lower than that in the IGD group in this study. Therefore, the non-significant correlation between impulsivity and IGD symptoms in the HC group may reflect differences between groups in the gender ratio.

There are several limitations to this study. First, it is difficult to generalize the results to other populations because this study was conducted with a small sample of young adults. Thus, it is necessary to include larger and more diverse samples in future studies. Second, this was a cross-sectional study, and all variables were measured at one point in time. MacKinnon et al. [58] suggested that longitudinal research would provide richer information about mediation and would be useful to identify causal relationships when analyzing mediation effects. Therefore, future studies should be longitudinal study so that clear pathways and causal relationships could be more readily identified.

5. Conclusions

The findings of this study clarify the main factors to be considered when intervening in IGD, particularly in the case of IGD patients with high impulsivity. Additionally, the present findings highlight the importance of the role of bio-psycho-social factors in relation to IGD symptoms. Thus, we should focus on reducing interpersonal problems and depression when performing interventions to improve IGD symptoms in individuals with high impulsivity.

Acknowledgments: This study was funded by the National Research Foundation of Korea (NRF-2014M3C7A1062894), Republic of Korea.

Author Contributions: All authors participated in the study and read the final manuscript; Hyera Ryu analyzed and interpreted the data and drafted the manuscript; Ji-Yoon Lee, Aruem Choi, and Sunyoung Park participated in collecting the data; Dai Jin Kim and Jung-Seok Choi conceived and designed the experiments, and the result interpretation and discussion; Jung-Seok Choi reviewed and edited the manuscript.

References

1. American Psychiatric Association. *Diagnostic and Statistical Manual of Mental Disorders (DSM-5®)*, 5th ed.; American Psychiatric Association: Washington, DC, USA, 2013, ISBN 978-0-89042-555-8.
2. Rehbein, F.; Kliem, S.; Baier, D.; Mossle, T.; Petry, N.M. Prevalence of internet gaming disorder in German adolescents: Diagnostic contribution of the nine DSM-5 criteria in a state-wide representative sample. *Addiction* **2015**, *110*, 842–851. [CrossRef] [PubMed]
3. Pontes, H.M.; Macur, M.; Griffiths, M.D. Internet gaming disorder among Slovenian primary schoolchildren: Findings from a nationally representative sample of adolescents. *J. Behav. Addict.* **2016**, *5*, 304–310. [CrossRef] [PubMed]
4. Király, O.; Sleczka, P.; Pontes, H.M.; Urbán, R.; Griffiths, M.D.; Demetrovics, Z. Validation of the ten-item Internet Gaming Disorder gest (IGDT-10) and evaluation of the nine DSM-5 Internet Gaming Disorder criteria. *Addict. Behav.* **2017**, *64*, 253–260. [CrossRef] [PubMed]
5. Yu, H.; Cho, J. Prevalence of internet gaming disorder among Korean adolescents and associations with non-psychotic psychological symptoms, and physical aggression. *Am. J. Health Behav.* **2016**, *40*, 705–716. [CrossRef] [PubMed]
6. Wang, H.R.; Cho, H.; Kim, D.J. Prevalence and correlates of comorbid depression in a nonclinical online sample with DSM-5 Internet Gaming Disorder. *J. Affect. Disord.* **2018**, *226*, 1–5. [CrossRef] [PubMed]

7. Choi, S.W. Internet addiction: Why we become addicted to the internet? *Asia Pac. J. Clin. Oncol.* **2012**, *4*, 12.
8. Choi, S.W.; Lee, H.K.; Kim, H.S.; Lee, K.S. In the modified integrated pathways model of internet addiction. *J. Behav. Addict.* **2013**, *2*, 10.
9. Blaszczynski, A.; Nower, L. A pathways model of problem and pathological gambling. *Addiction* **2002**, *97*, 487–499. [CrossRef] [PubMed]
10. VandenBos, G.R. *APA Dictionary of Psychology*; APA: Washington, DC, USA, 2007.
11. Patton, J.H.; Stanford, M.S.; Barratt, E.S. Factor structure of the Barratt Impulsiveness Scale. *J. Clin. Psychol.* **1995**, *51*, 768–774. [CrossRef]
12. Cao, F.; Su, L.; Liu, T.; Gao, X. The relationship between impulsivity and internet addiction in a sample of Chinese adolescents. *Eur. Psychiatry* **2007**, *22*, 466–471. [CrossRef] [PubMed]
13. Choi, J.S.; Park, S.M.; Roh, M.S.; Lee, J.Y.; Park, C.B.; Hwang, J.Y.; Gwak, A.R.; Jung, H.Y. Dysfunctional inhibitory control and impulsivity in internet addiction. *Psychiatry Res.* **2014**, *215*, 424–428. [CrossRef] [PubMed]
14. Dalbudak, E.; Evren, C.; Topcu, M.; Aldemir, S.; Coskun, K.S.; Bozkurt, M.; Evren, B.; Canbal, M. Relationship of internet addiction with impulsivity and severity of psychopathology among Turkish university students. *Psychiatry Res.* **2013**, *210*, 1086–1091. [CrossRef] [PubMed]
15. Lee, H.W.; Choi, J.S.; Shin, Y.C.; Lee, J.Y.; Jung, H.Y.; Kwon, J.S. Impulsivity in internet addiction: A comparison with pathological gambling. *Cyberpsychol. Behav. Soc. Netw.* **2012**, *15*, 373–377. [CrossRef] [PubMed]
16. Lin, M.P.; Ko, H.C.; Wu, J.Y. Prevalence and psychosocial risk factors associated with internet addiction in a nationally representative sample of college students in Taiwan. *Cyberpsychol. Behav. Soc. Netw.* **2011**, *14*, 741–746. [CrossRef] [PubMed]
17. Ding, W.N.; Sun, J.H.; Sun, Y.W.; Chen, X.; Zhou, Y.; Zhuang, Z.G.; Li, L.; Zhang, Y.; Xu, J.R.; Du, Y.S. Trait impulsivity and impaired prefrontal impulse inhibition function in adolescents with internet gaming addiction revealed by a go/no-go fMRI study. *Behav. Brain Funct.* **2014**, *10*, 20. [CrossRef] [PubMed]
18. Dong, G.; Zhou, H.; Zhao, X. Impulse inhibition in people with internet addiction disorder: Electrophysiological evidence from a go/nogo study. *Neurosci. Lett.* **2010**, *485*, 138–142. [CrossRef] [PubMed]
19. Granö, N.; Keltikangas-Jarvinen, L.; Kouvonen, A.; Virtanen, M.; Elovainio, M.; Vahtera, J.; Kivimäki, M. Impulsivity as a predictor of newly diagnosed depression. *Scand. J. Psychol.* **2007**, *48*, 173–179. [CrossRef] [PubMed]
20. Swann, A.C.; Steinberg, J.L.; Lijffijt, M.; Moeller, F.G. Impulsivity: Differential relationship to depression and mania in bipolar disorder. *J. Affect. Disord.* **2008**, *106*, 241–248. [CrossRef] [PubMed]
21. Savci, M.; Aysan, F. Relationship between impulsivity, social media usage and loneliness. *Educ. Process Int. J.* **2016**, *5*, 106–115. [CrossRef]
22. Kim, J.; LaRose, R.; Peng, W. Loneliness as the cause and the effect of problematic internet use: The relationship between internet use and psychological well-being. *Cyberpsychol. Behav.* **2009**, *12*, 451–455. [CrossRef] [PubMed]
23. Nalwa, K.; Anand, A.P. Internet addiction in students: A cause of concern. *Cyberpsychol. Behav.* **2003**, *6*, 653–656. [CrossRef] [PubMed]
24. Yao, M.Z.; Zhong, Z.-J. Loneliness, social contacts and internet addiction: A cross-lagged panel study. *Comput. Hum. Behav.* **2014**, *30*, 164–170. [CrossRef]
25. Ceyhan, A.A.; Ceyhan, E. Loneliness, depression, and computer self-efficacy as predictors of problematic internet use. *Cyberpsychol. Behav.* **2008**, *11*, 699–701. [CrossRef] [PubMed]
26. Meerkerk, G.J.; Van Den Eijnden, R.J.; Vermulst, A.A.; Garretsen, H.F. The compulsive internet use scale (CIUS): Some psychometric properties. *Cyberpsychol. Behav.* **2009**, *12*, 1–6. [CrossRef] [PubMed]
27. Thatcher, A.; Goolam, S. Defining the South African internet 'addict': Prevalence and biographical profiling of problematic internet users in South Africa. *S. Afr. J. Psychol.* **2005**, *35*, 766–792. [CrossRef]
28. Young, K.S. Internet addiction: The emergence of a new clinical disorder. *Cyberpsychol. Behav.* **1998**, *1*, 237–244. [CrossRef]
29. Young, K.S.; Rogers, R.C. The relationship between depression and internet addiction. *Cyberpsychol. Behav.* **1998**, *1*, 25–28. [CrossRef]
30. Adams, K.B.; Sanders, S.; Auth, E.A. Loneliness and depression in independent living retirement communities: Risk and resilience factors. *Aging Ment. Health* **2004**, *8*, 475–485. [CrossRef] [PubMed]

31. Hagerty, B.M.; Williams, R.A. The effects of sense of belonging, social support, conflict, and loneliness on depression. *Nurs. Res.* **1999**, *48*, 215–219. [CrossRef] [PubMed]

32. Ko, C.H.; Yen, J.Y.; Yen, C.F.; Chen, C.S.; Chen, C.C. The association between internet addiction and psychiatric disorder: A review of the literature. *Eur. Psychiatry* **2012**, *27*, 1–8. [CrossRef] [PubMed]

33. Yen, J.Y.; Ko, C.H.; Yen, C.F.; Wu, H.Y.; Yang, M.J. The comorbid psychiatric symptoms of internet addiction: Attention deficit and hyperactivity disorder (ADHD), depression, social phobia, and hostility. *J. Adolesc. Health* **2007**, *41*, 93–98. [CrossRef] [PubMed]

34. Bernardi, S.; Pallanti, S. Internet addiction: A descriptive clinical study focusing on comorbidities and dissociative symptoms. *Compr. Psychiatry* **2009**, *50*, 510–516. [CrossRef] [PubMed]

35. Ko, C.H.; Yen, J.Y.; Chen, C.S.; Chen, C.C.; Yen, C.F. Psychiatric comorbidity of internet addiction in college students: An interview study. *CNS Spectr.* **2008**, *13*, 147–153. [CrossRef] [PubMed]

36. Bahrainian, S.A.; Alizadeh, K.H.; Raeisoon, M.R.; Gorji, O.H.; Khazaee, A. Relationship of internet addiction with self-esteem and depression in university students. *J. Prev. Med. Hyg.* **2014**, *55*, 86–89. [PubMed]

37. Dieris-Hirche, J.; Bottel, L.; Bielefeld, M.; Steinbüchel, T.; Kehyayan, A.; Dieris, B.; Te Wildt, B. Media use and internet addiction in adult depression: A case-control study. *Comput. Hum. Behav.* **2017**, *68*, 96–103. [CrossRef]

38. Jang, K.S.; Hwang, S.Y.; Choi, J.Y. Internet addiction and psychiatric symptoms among Korean adolescents. *J. Sch. Health* **2008**, *78*, 165–171. [CrossRef] [PubMed]

39. Seifi, A.; Ayati, M.; Fadaei, M. The study of the relationship between internet addiction and depression, anxiety and stress among students of Islamic Azad University of Birjand. *Int. J. Econ. Manag. Soc. Sci.* **2014**, *3*, 28–32.

40. Shapira, N.A.; Goldsmith, T.D.; Keck, P.E.; Khosla, U.M.; McElroy, S.L. Psychiatric features of individuals with problematic internet use. *J. Affect. Disord.* **2000**, *57*, 267–272. [CrossRef]

41. Ha, J.H.; Yoo, H.J.; Cho, I.H.; Chin, B.; Shin, D.; Kim, J.H. Psychiatric comorbidity assessed in Korean children and adolescents who screen positive for internet addiction. *J. Clin. Psychiatry* **2006**, *67*, 821–826. [CrossRef] [PubMed]

42. Ko, C.H.; Yen, J.Y.; Chen, C.S.; Yeh, Y.C.; Yen, C.F. Predictive values of psychiatric symptoms for internet addiction in adolescents: A 2-year prospective study. *Arch. Pediatr. Adolesc. Med.* **2009**, *163*, 937–943. [CrossRef] [PubMed]

43. Kim, E.; Lee, S.; Oh, S. The validation of korean adolescent internet addiction scale (K-AIAS). *Korean J. Clin. Psychol.* **2003**, *22*, 125–139.

44. Schlein, S.; Guerney, B.; Stover, L. The Interpersonal Relationship Scale. Ph.D. Thesis, Pennsylvania State University, State College, PA, USA, 1971. Unpublished work.

45. Chun, S. The social skills training for social adjustment of the schizophrenic patients. *Ment. Health Soc. Work* **1995**, *2*, 33–50.

46. Beck, A.T.; Steer, R.A.; Brown, G.K. *Manual for the Beck Depression Inventory-II*; Psychological Corporation: San Antonio, TX, USA, 1996.

47. Sung, H.; Kim, J.; Park, Y.; Bai, D.; Lee, S.; Ahn, H. A study on the reliability and the validity of Korean version of the beck depression inventory-II (BDI-II). *J. Korean Soc. Biol. Ther. Psychiatry* **2008**, *14*, 201–212.

48. Hayes, A. *Process for SPSS (Version 2.16) [Macros]*; The Guilford Press: New York, NY, USA, 2016.

49. Hayes, A. PROCESS: A Versatile Computational Tool for Observed Variable Mediation, Moderation, and Conditional Process Modeling. 2012. Available online: http://www.afhayes.com/public/process2012.pdf (accessed on 16 May 2016).

50. Bakken, I.J.; Wenzel, H.G.; Götestam, K.G.; Johansson, A.; ØREN, A. Internet addiction among Norwegian adults: A stratified probability sample study. *Scand. J. Psychol.* **2009**, *50*, 121–127. [CrossRef] [PubMed]

51. Tsai, H.F.; Cheng, S.H.; Yeh, T.L.; Shih, C.-C.; Chen, K.C.; Yang, Y.C.; Yang, Y.K. The risk factors of internet addiction—A survey of university freshmen. *Psychiatry Res.* **2009**, *167*, 294–299. [CrossRef] [PubMed]

52. Carli, V.; Durkee, T.; Wasserman, D.; Hadlaczky, G.; Despalins, R.; Kramarz, E.; Wasserman, C.; Sarchiapone, M.; Hoven, C.W.; Brunner, R. The association between pathological internet use and comorbid psychopathology: A systematic review. *Psychopathology* **2013**, *46*, 1–13. [CrossRef] [PubMed]

53. Koc, M. Internet addiction and psychopathology. *Turk. Online J. Educ. Technol.* **2011**, *10*, 143–148.

54. Caplan, S.E. Preference for online social interaction: A theory of problematic internet use and psychosocial well-being. *Commun. Res.* **2003**, *30*, 625–648. [CrossRef]

55. Bargeron, A.H.; Hormes, J.M. Psychosocial correlates of internet gaming disorder: Psychopathology, life satisfaction, and impulsivity. *Comput. Hum. Behav.* **2017**, *68*, 388–394. [CrossRef]

56. Chapple, C.L.; Johnson, K.A. Gender differences in impulsivity. *Youth Violence Juv. Justice* **2007**, *5*, 221–234. [CrossRef]

57. Cross, C.P.; Copping, L.T.; Campbell, A. Sex differences in impulsivity: A meta-analysis. *Psychol. Bull.* **2011**, *137*, 97–130. [CrossRef] [PubMed]

58. MacKinnon, D.P.; Fairchild, A.J.; Fritz, M.S. Mediation analysis. *Annu. Rev. Psychol.* **2007**, *58*, 593–614. [CrossRef] [PubMed]

12

Spanish Validation of the Internet Gaming Disorder Scale–Short Form (IGDS9-SF): Prevalence and Relationship with Online Gambling and Quality of Life

Marta Beranuy [1], **Juan M. Machimbarrena** [2], **M. Asunción Vega-Osés** [3], **Xavier Carbonell** [4], **Mark D. Griffiths** [5], **Halley M. Pontes** [6,7] **and Joaquín González-Cabrera** [1,*]

[1] Faculty of Education, Universidad Internacional de la Rioja (UNIR), Avenida de la Paz, 137, 26006 Logroño, Spain; marta.beranuy@unir.net

[2] Faculty of Psychology, University of the Basque Country (UPV/EHU), Avenida de Tolosa, 70, 20018 Donostia, Spain; juanmanuel.machimbarrena@ehu.eus

[3] Faculty of Health Sciences, Universidad Pública de Navarra (UPNA), Calle Cataluña, s/n, 31006 Pamplona, Navarra, Spain; mvegaose@educacion.navarra.es

[4] Faculty of Psychology, Education and Sport Blanquerna, Universitat Ramon Llull. Calle Císter, 34, 08022 Barcelona, Spain; xaviercs@blanquerna.url.edu

[5] International Gaming Research Unit, Psychology Department, Nottingham Trent University, Nottingham NG11 8NS, UK; mark.griffiths@ntu.ac.uk

[6] University of Tasmania, School of Psychological Sciences, Newnham Campus, Building O, Launceston TAS 7250, Australia; contactme@halleypontes.com

[7] The International Cyberpsychology and Addictions Research Laboratory (iCARL), University of Tasmania, Launceston TAS 7250, Australia

* Correspondence: joaquin.gonzalez@unir.net

Abstract: Online gaming is a very common form of leisure among adolescents and young people, although its excessive and/or compulsive use is associated with psychological impairments in a minority of gamers. The latest (fifth) edition of the Diagnostic and Statistical Manual of Mental Disorders (DSM-5, Section III) tentatively introduced Internet Gaming Disorder (IGD). Since then, a number of evaluation tools using the DSM-5 criteria have been developed, including the Internet Gaming Disorder Scale–Short Form (IGDS9-SF). The main objective of this study was to translate and adapt the IGDS9-SF into Spanish, as well as to obtain indicators relating to its validity and reliability. The Spanish version of four scales were administered: IGDS9-SF, Mobile Phone-Related Experiences Questionnaire (CERM), Online Gambling Disorder Questionnaire (OGD-Q), and KIDSCREEN-27. The sample comprised 535 Vocational Training students (mean age 18.35 years; SD±2.13; 78.5% males) who reported playing video games in the past 12 months. Confirmatory factor analysis yielded a one-dimensional model with a good fit while the reliability indicators were satisfactory. Findings indicated that 1.9% of gamers were classified with IGD (meeting five or more criteria for more than 12 months). Additionally, another 1.9% were considered gamers 'at-risk' because they endorsed four criteria. Positive and significant relationships were found between the IGDS9-SF, the CERM, and the OGD-Q. Participants classified with IGD had poorer health-related quality of life. In conclusion, the Spanish IGDS9-SF is a valid and reliable instrument to assess IGD according to the DSM-5.

Keywords: Internet Gaming Disorder; gaming disorder; gaming addiction; behavioral addiction; Internet Gaming Disorder Scale-Short Form

1. Introduction

The way in which individuals interact with technology is constantly evolving. New behaviors have emerged, communication and leisure activities have changed, and new psychological problems arose. In the late 1990s, concerns about the addictive use of the internet [1,2] were discussed and, since then, the concept has been extensively studied and debated [3–6]. Although it has been addressed from multiple perspectives and researchers have used different terms, 'internet addiction' has been one of the most commonly used terms, along with 'problematic internet use' [7–9]. Early research focused on internet-related and mobile-related behavior in general terms. However, over the years, studies have focused on more specific uses. This approach has been defined as the move from general problematic internet use (GPIU) to specific problematic internet use (SPIU) (e.g., [5]). Consequently, research has especially focused on internet gaming [10–12], online gambling [13–15], online sex/cybersex [16,17], and social media use [18–20].

Among the aforementioned problems, 'Gaming Disorder' (GD) has recently been introduced in the nosological manuals (American Psychiatric Association [APA], and World Health Organization [WHO],) by being included as a disorder under the heading of addictive behaviors. The DSM-5 [21] places the 'Internet Gaming Disorder' (IGD) in Section III (disorders requiring further investigation) and the International Classification of Diseases 11th (ICD-11) [22] considers GD among non-substance addictions.

IGD is considered an addictive behavior that does not involve the ingestion of a psychoactive substance, and is mainly characterized by recurrent and persistent participation in online video games, leading to clinically significant distress [21]. The nine IGD criteria contain the characteristics indicated in the components model of addiction [23], including salience, mood modification, tolerance, withdrawal, the conflicts it generates (whether interpersonal and/or intrapersonal), and the risk of relapse. The theoretical overlap between the components model of addiction and the nine IGD criteria has been previously ascertained empirically in earlier studies [24]. Despite this definition, the use of different theoretical frameworks has created difficulties in the conceptualization of a problem with worrisome prevalence data and which also produces harmful effects on those who suffer from it, making it a possible public health problem [25].

The video game industry generates millions of Euros in revenue every year (1.530 million Euros in 2018, 12.6% more than the previous year) as video gaming is considered one of the main forms of leisure for many audiences across all stages of life. According to the Spanish Video Game Association [26], the total number of gamers in 2018 amounted to 16.8 million (41% female). Their age ranged from 6 to 64 years old, although the youngest (6–14 years) stand out, and they played for an average of 6.2 h per week. Studies on participation in video games indicate the highest prevalence among younger populations [27], which appears to be an at-risk population due to specific features associated with adolescence (i.e., being at a developmental stage where there is little thought given to the long-term consequences of their actions [28]) and membership of the Z Generation (i.e., born during the early years of the 21st century comprising individuals who have never known a world without the internet and mobile phones [29]).

Adolescent studies indicate a prevalence of IGD ranging from 1.7% to 10% [4,30–33]. According to the meta-analytical study by Fam [27], the prevalence of IGD among male adolescents is 6.8%, and 1.3% among females. In international samples, and without an established age range, the percentage ranges from 0.7% to 15.6% [34] or slightly higher in Chinese studies (from 3.5% to 17% [35]).

In Spain (where the present study was carried out), a study with a school sample of 708 students reported 72.8% online gamers [36] of whom 8.3% met five or more of the nine criteria for IGD (86.44% were male). Another study conducted with Spanish-speaking online gamers reported a prevalence of 2.6% disordered gamers [37]. This same study found that 6.5% were "engaged gamers at high risk", and 11.9% were "engaged gamers at low risk", with the remainder classified as "regular" or "casual" gamers. In a clinical sample of 86 disordered adolescent gamers, it was found that 96.6% were male [38].

In terms of comorbidity, IGD has been associated with a wide spectrum of psychological problems including depression, anxiety, social phobias, poorer school performance, and sleep disorders [36,39–42]. In addition, studies have begun to appear comprising clinical samples demanding psychological treatment, which meet the criteria for the disorder [38,43]. In the study by Martín-Fernández et al. [38], all participants had diagnostic comorbidity, in accordance with other studies [44,45]. The most prevalent comorbidities with IGD were found to be depression, social anxiety, ADHD, and aggressive behaviors [46,47]. Additionally, it is also important to examine the relationship of IGD with other non-substance addictions (particularly gambling) because several studies have established common risk factors such as personality traits [48], levels of impulsivity and compulsivity [49], and similarities in the neurobiological functioning of patients with IGD and patients with pathological gambling [50]. It is relevant to relate IGD with online gambling disorder or other problematic behaviors such as problematic smartphone use, because these three behaviors occur via Information and Communications Technologies (ICTs) and which typically meet addiction criteria similar to IGD (i.e., salience, mood modification, tolerance, withdrawal, conflict, and relapse) when people present with a clinical problem. Currently, there are psychometric tests that evaluate online gambling disorder specifically in adolescent populations [14]. In addition, the most used device to play or connect to the internet is via smartphone. Although a decade ago, gaming consoles and computers were the only technological hardware available to play online, in recent years, the use of the smartphone has significantly increased [51]. Currently smartphones are used by 21% of almost 17 million players in Spain (only surpassed by gaming consoles; 26%). This percentage increases considerably (up to 40%) in the 15–24-year age range. It should also be noted that in the Spanish context, the average time spent weekly with mobile gaming is 5.1 h, compared to 3.9 h on gaming consoles and the 4.9 h on computers [26]).

Many studies have focused on the negative effects of IGD on psychological health and other health-related problems, but fewer studies have linked it to more global general well-being constructs (such as health-related quality of life [HRQoL]). HRQoL is defined as a state of complete physical, mental, and social well-being that is perceived by individuals and by those around them (for more information see the review by Wallander and Koot [52]). The evaluation of HRQoL is complex because it is a polyhedral construct that presents multiple conceptual approaches although one of the best approaches for examining the infant-juvenile stage is with the KIDSCREEN [53], a psychometric test adapted in almost 30 languages. The HRQoL provides general indicators on the impact of a problem in areas relevant to an adolescent's life, such as physical and psychological well-being or the relationship with parents and peers. Several studies indicate that inadequate use of the internet is related to low scores on HRQoL, in addition to a lower self-perceived social support and more friends only known through the internet [54,55]. Similarly, other studies indicate that both HRQoL and social aspects are affected among people presenting problems related to the use of video games in adolescence [31,36].

The APA's [21] operationalization of IGD has arguably reduced the diversity in the assessment instruments as well as the number of items contained in each of these instruments, providing more uniform measures with high internal consistency and adequate criterion validity. A systematic review [56] indicated the nine-item Internet Gaming Disorder Scale-Sort Form (IGDS9-SF) [57] as the most reviewed and translated instrument to assess IGD based on the nine IGD criteria developed by the APA. In fact, since its publication, the IGDS9-SF has been translated into at least nine languages: Chinese [58], German [59], Czech [60], Slovenian [61], Italian [62], Persian [63], Turkish [64,65], Polish [66], European and South American Portuguese [67,68]. Therefore, it is a cross-culturally suitable psychometric tool to assess IGD that allows framing the problem uniformly and inter-culturally with adequate psychometric properties.

This IGDS9-SF is based on the nine criteria suggested by the DSM-5 for IGD that includes: (i) preoccupation with gaming; (ii) withdrawal symptoms; (iii) tolerance; (iv) unsuccessful attempts to reduce or quit gaming; (v) loss of interest in previous activities or entertainments as a result of (and with the exception of) gaming; (vi) continuing to game despite knowing the associated psychosocial problems; (vii) deceiving family members, therapists, or others about the amount of time spent on gaming; (viii) playing video games to evade or relieve negative moods; and (ix) jeopardizing or losing a meaningful relationship, job, or educational or employment opportunity due to gaming.

As aforementioned, the use of different theoretical frameworks to assess IGD generated problems in conceptualization and, given the broad international acceptance of the IGDS9-SF and its robust psychometric properties, the objective of the present study was to extend the cross-cultural psychometric assessment evidence-base related to the assessment of IGD by translating and adapting the IGDS9-SF into Spanish to ascertain its psychometric suitability to this specific cultural context in terms of the validity and reliability of its scores. The validation in this cultural context for the Spanish language is a priority, given that Spanish is the third most spoken language in the world (534 million speakers [69,70]) and there are 21 countries where Spanish is the official language [70]. Consequently, a Spanish version of the most used IGD assessment tool is needed to encourage and improve research investigating IGD in Spanish-speaking countries and to facilitate cross-culturally unified research of this emerging public health issue.

The secondary objectives of this study were to: (a) to obtain indicators of validity and reliability of the Spanish version of IGDS9-SF, including the confirmatory study of its factor structure; (b) to test whether the newly developed psychometric test works equally in both men and women, as well as in adolescences and young adults; (c) establish the prevalence of IGD in a sample of adolescents and young Vocational Training (VT) students aged between 15 and 25 years; and (d) examine the relationship between the IGD and HRQoL. To achieve the aforementioned objective, it was hypothesized that: (i) the IGDS9-SF would show adequate psychometric properties in the sample recruited, similarly to previous IGDS9-SF psychometric validation studies conducted in different countries [58,59,61,67]; (ii) the measurement model would be invariant across both genders [57]; (iii) the prevalence of IGD would be between 2% and 4%, which is referred to in other national and international studies [27,37]; and (iv) those who met the IGD criteria within the sample recruited would present lower scores on the different HRQoL dimensions [31].

2. Materials and Methods

2.1. Design and Participants

The instrument validation study was conducted from February to May 2019. The sample was recruited from 17 VT centers in the Autonomous Community of Navarre by means of non-parametric incidental sampling. The distribution of students by cycles and school stages was as follows: basic VT (152 first-grade students, 14.2%; 70 second-grade students, 6.5%); middle degree VT (433 first-grade students, 40.4%; 56 second-grade students, 5.2%); and higher degree VT (325 first-grade students, 30.3%; 35 second-grade students, 3.4%). The initial number of participants was 1064 (593 males and 471 females), of whom 535 reported playing video games in the last 12 months. Of this final sample, 420 were males (78.5%) and 115 were females (21.5%). The mean and standard deviation of age was 18.35 years (±2.13), with a range of 15–25 years.

2.2. Instruments

The participants provided information about demographic variables including gender, grade, school, and age. They also indicated the name of the video game they spent the most hours on in the past 12 months and whether or not they considered themselves addicted to online video games. In addition, they completed the following assessment tools.

Spanish translation of the IGDS9-SF [57,61] (see the Spanish version in Appendix A). The IGDS9-SF assesses the severity of IGD and its detrimental effects, examining online and/or offline gaming activities that occur over a 12-month period with nine questions based on the DSM-5 IGD criteria that are rated on a five-point Likert scale: 1 (never), 2 (rarely), 3 (sometimes), 4 (often), and 5 (very often). Participants' total scores are obtained by adding the score of each answer (ranging from 9 to 45). Higher scores typically indicate a higher level of IGD symptom-severity and greater incidence of problems related to gaming behaviors. For the Spanish adaptation, three experts evaluated (through a table of test specifications) each of the translations and psychological adaptations of the nine items. High inter-rater reliability was recorded throughout the process (> 0.9) on all the items [71]. The set of items is shown in Table 1, however the whole questionnaire including instructions and response scale can be found in Appendix A. In addition, initial piloting was carried out on a sample of 30 participants, providing adequate indicators of reliability and content and internal validity, and not reporting any comprehension or reading problems. The pilot participants were not included in the final sample.

Table 1. Means, standard deviations, item-total correlation, positive response percentage, and factorial loads of the Internet Gaming Disorder Scale–Short Form (IGDS9-SF) items ($n = 9$).

IGDS9-SF Items	M	SD	IT	%+	CFE
1. ¿Te sientes preocupado por tu comportamiento con el juego? (Algunos ejemplos: ¿Piensas en exceso cuando no estás jugando o anticipas en exceso a la próxima sesión de juego?, ¿Crees que el juego se ha convertido en la actividad dominante en tu vida diaria?)	1.74	0.95	0.53	48.0	0.58
2. ¿Sientes irritabilidad, ansiedad o incluso tristeza cuando intentas reducir o detener tu actividad de juego?	1.45	0.79	0.64	32.5	0.71
3. ¿Sientes la necesidad de pasar cada vez más tiempo jugando para lograr satisfacción o placer?	1.57	0.97	0.67	34.3	0.74
4. ¿Fallas sistemáticamente al intentar controlar o terminar tu actividad de juego?	1.64	0.89	0.63	43.2	0.69
5. ¿Has perdido intereses en aficiones anteriores y otras actividades de entretenimiento como resultado de tu compromiso con el juego?	1.56	0.93	0.61	34.3	0.66
6. ¿Has continuado jugando a pesar de saber que te estaba causando problemas con otras personas? (pareja, amistad o familia)	1.45	0.88	0.65	27.2	0.71
7. ¿Has engañado a alguno de tus familiares, terapeutas o amigos sobre el tiempo que pasas jugando?	1.57	0.99	0.47	33.6	0.51
8. ¿Juegas para escapar temporalmente o aliviar un estado de ánimo negativo (por ejemplo, desesperanza, tristeza, culpa o ansiedad)?	1.94	1.20	0.47	49.0	0.50
9. ¿Has comprometido o perdido una relación importante, un trabajo o una oportunidad educativa debido a tu actividad de juego?	1.23	0.64	0.58	14.8	0.63

Note: For original items see Pontes and Griffiths [57]; M = Arithmetic mean; SD = Standard deviation; IT = corrected item-total correlation; %+ Percentage that has responded positively (at least once); CFE = Standardized factorial loads.

Cuestionario de Experiencias Relacionadas con el teléfono móvil (CERM [Mobile Phone-Related Experiences Questionnaire] [72]). This instrument has 10 items that evaluate two factors: (i) conflicts related to mobile phone abuse and (ii) problems due to the emotional and communicational use of the mobile phone. The items of this instrument are rated on a four-point Likert scale, ranging from 1 (hardly ever) to 4 (almost always). The CERM has been previously shown to have adequate indicators of reliability and validity in Spanish adolescents. In the present sample, the Cronbach's alpha reliability coefficient for the CERM was 0.78 and the Omega coefficient was 0.79.

Online Gambling Disorder Questionnaire (OGD-Q) [14]. This instrument was designed to evaluate online gambling disorder using a total of 11 items that are rated on a five-point Likert scale ranging from 1 (never) to 5 (every day). The total OGD-Q score varies between 11 and 55, with higher scores indicating higher levels of online disordered gambling. The questionnaire has been validated for a Spanish sample of adolescents and presents adequate indicators of reliability and validity. In the present sample, the Cronbach's alpha reliability coefficient for the OGD-Q was 0.91 and Omega coefficient was 0.92.

Spanish version of the KIDSCREEN-27 [53]. This instrument assesses HRQoL in children and adolescents between ages 8 and 18 years. This version assesses five dimensions by using 27 items: physical well-being, psychological well-being, autonomy and relationship with parents, peers and social support, and school environment. The development of the KIDCREEN was based on the probabilistic partial credit model (PCM) which pertains to the family of Rasch models. PCM explains the actual behavior of the responders in the testing situation by the estimated person parameter and the location of the item-answers-category-thresholds. The PCM assumes all items of a scale to be the indicators of a single unidimensional latent trait [53]. For the KIDSCREEN-27, the mean scores varied around 50 (SD = 10) due to T-value standardization. There are standardized data for the Spanish infant-juvenile population. The reliability of the each dimension was as follows: physical well-being (α= 0.86; ω = 0.86); psychological well-being (α= 0.84; ω = 0.84), autonomy and relationship with parents (α= 0.84; ω = 0.84), peers and social support (α= 0.88; ω = 0.88), and school environment (α= 0.80; ω = 0.80). Due to the nature of the KIDSCREEN (designed for children and adolescents), responses from participants over 18 years were not considered in the analyses of this instrument in the present study.

2.3. Procedure

The battery of questionnaires was applied in an online format utilizing Survey Monkey©. Participants completed the questionnaires in the different computer technology classrooms coordinated by the guidance departments of each center, and under the supervision of the classroom tutor. At the outset of the study participants were advised to answer all questions truthfully and to not stop at any particular question for a long time. The overall average time needed to complete the survey ranged between 15 and 25 min, depending on students' age and reading ability.

2.4. Ethical Considerations

The study was conducted with the informed consent of the participants and the directors of the schools. Through the official communication channels with the families, the schools sent a consent form that informed either the legal tutors or the students themselves (if they were at least 18 years old) about the purpose of the study and its characteristics, its promoters, and their right not to participate without penalties. Those parents/tutors who did not wish to allow participation returned the signed consent. This occurred in less than 1% of the sample. The study was approved by the Research Ethics Committee of the research from Universidad Internacional de la Rioja (UNIR) (PI:008/2019). There were no exclusion criteria, except for the refusal to participate by the legal guardians or by the students themselves.

2.5. Data Analysis

Statistical analyses were carried out using the Statistical Package for the Social Sciences (SPSS) [73] program, the R software, the psych package [74], the Lavaan package [75], and the equaltestMI [76]. Firstly, regarding internal validity, an analysis of the psychometric properties of each item was performed, indicating the arithmetic mean, standard deviation, item-total correlation, percentage of positive responses to each item, and the factorial loadings of each item (see Table 1). The multiple criterion for the selection of items without technical deficiencies was that none of them could fail to meet two of the following three statistical indices: (i) a mean between 1.5 and 2.5; (ii) a standard deviation equal to or greater than 1; and (iii) an item-total correlation equal to or greater than 0.35.

To ensure better comparability between the present study and the original IGDS9-SF study, the structure of the IGDS9-SF was initially examined with Exploratory Factor Analysis (EFA) of the items, following the verification of the assumptions (Kaiser-Meyer-Olkin index and Bartlett sphericity test). The factor extraction method used was Principal Axis Factoring with Oblimin rotation. Confirmatory Factor Analysis (CFA) was then performed using Weighted Least Squares Median adjusted method (WLSM). Following the recommendations of Hu and Bentler [77], goodness of fit was assessed using the chi-squared statistic, the comparative fit index (CFI), Tucker-Lewis Index (TLI), the root mean square error of approximation (RMSEA), and the standardized root mean square residual (SRMR). In general, CFI and TLI values of 0.95 or higher reflect a good fit while RMSEA values between 0.06 and 0.08 indicate acceptable fit. Finally, SRMR values lower than 0.08 indicate adequate fit [78]. The hypothesized model was unidimensional, in which all nine items would load on the same latent factor. To determine the internal consistency of the instruments employed, the Cronbach's alpha, McDonald's Omega, greatest Lower Bound (GBL), Gutmann's λ6, Average Variance Explained (AVE) and Composite Reliability (CR) coefficients were estimated. To calculate Measurement Invariance (MI) the sample was split by gender (males and females) and age (under 18 years old and 18 years old or older). MI across age and gender was evaluated through the following steps: (a) testing for the invariance of number of factors (configural invariance); (b) testing for the equality of factor loadings (weak or metric invariance); and (c) testing for the equality of indicator intercepts (strong or scalar invariance). Given that chi-square is sensitive to sample size and non-normality conditions, it was assumed that the model is invariant if the ΔCFI is not above 0.01 [79].

Finally, the following analyses were performed in relation to the secondary objectives of the study: (i) analysis of frequencies and central tendency and dispersion measurements of the study variables; (ii) t-test for independent samples (or failing that, Welch's test); (iii) calculation of the effect size with Cohen's d or Hedges' g, as appropriate; (iv) Pearson correlations; (v) analysis of variance with post-hoc Games-Howell comparisons; and (vi) Mann-Whitney U-test for independent samples. A value of less than $p=.05$ was considered significant.

To obtain the prevalence rate of IGD in the past 12 months, the indications of the APA [21] and Pontes et al. [67] were followed (i.e., endorsing five or more items in classifying individuals with IGD). To establish item endorsement, the items of the IGDS9-SF were dichotomized so that response categories as 4 (often) and 5 (very often) were used to classify the item as a problem (i.e., endorsement of the specific criterion). The remainder of the responses were classified as 'no problem' (i.e., no endorsement of the specific criterion). In addition, participants who endorsed four items were considered 'at-risk' of IGD while participants' preferred video game genre was classified in the following categories: action/shooter (FPS (First-Person Shooter), TPS (Three-Person Shooter), etc.), strategy (4x, RTS (Real-Time Strategy), etc.), role-playing (ARPG (Action Role-Playing Games), JRPG (Japanese Role-Playing Game), RPG (Role-Playing Game), etc.), fighting, MOBA (Multiplayer Online Battle Arena), MMORPG (Massive Multiplayer Online Role-Playing Game), simulators, letters, sports, musical, and casual.

3. Results

The scores of Items 1, 4, 6, 7, and 9 showed significant differences as a function of gender, with higher scores in males than in females ($p < 0.05$). The rest of the items did not present significant gender differences. The effect sizes were small in most cases ($d < 0.3$), except for Item 1 ($d = 0.31$). Additionally, in relation to the differences according to class year, significant differences were only found on Item 6 ($p < 0.05$) between the students of first basic VT and first middle degree, with a small effect size ($d < 0.3$). No significant differences were observed in the remaining items for the class year variable.

3.1. Evidence of Validity of the IGDS9-SF Scores

Table 1 shows the different psychometric indicators for each of the IGDS9-SF items, namely the mean, standard deviation, item-total correlation, percentage of positive response on each item, and factor loadings for each item. At the psychometric level, the scores obtained revealed problems in the mean and standard deviation of all the items, although the item-total correlations in all the items were satisfactory. Items with at least one positive value ranged from 14.8% for Item 9 to 49% for Item 1.

With regards to the EFA results, the data of the Kaiser-Meyer-Olkin index and the Bartlett sphericity test produced values of 0.909 and $\chi^2 = 1629.36$, $p < 0.001$. The correlation matrix between the items was appropriate for the EFA. The results further indicated a single latent factor explaining 47.49% of the total sample variance. Regarding the CFA, the hypothesized unidimensional model yielded adequate fit indices: χ^2 (27, n = 532) = 9.908., $p < 0.001$, RMSEA = 0.019 (95% CI [0.000, 0.026], CFI = 0.995, NNFI = 0.993, and SRMR = 0.035. The standardized factor loadings (see Table 1) were statistically significant and notable in all items, ranging from 0.50 to 0.74. The Cronbach's alpha was 0.85 and Omega coefficients for the IGDS9-SF were both 0.85 (IC: [0.83, 0.87]). The Greatest Lower Bound was 0.88 and Gutmann's λ was 0.85. Finally, the average variance extracted was 0.5 and the Composite Reliability was 0.88.

3.2. Measurement Invariance

To evaluate the generalizability of the model across males and females, participants under 18 years old and 18 years old or older, two multi-group CFAs were performed. For each analysis, an unconstrained model with factor loadings free to vary between subgroups was compared with a more constrained model, in which the factor loadings were held constant across subgroups. Before conducting multi-group analyses, separate CFAs were performed for gender and age subgroups. Regarding gender, the model for females offered a lower fit in general than that of males or the overall model. However, the indicators still presented adequate threshold and the MI analyses were performed. The MI of the single-factor solution was supported at the configural and metric levels. However, the increase in the CFI and RMSEA prevented testing the model any further for gender. Regarding age, both subgroups showed a good fit for the data, in the case of age the MI supported the structure of the single-factor solution across all three levels (configural, metric, and scalar). The results obtained for the different models are displayed in Table 2.

Table 2. Invariance analyses across gender and age.

Model	χ^2	df	Com. Md	ΔSB χ^2	Δdf	p	CFI	ΔCFI	RMSEA	ΔRMSEA	SRMR
1.Overall model	9.91	27	–	–	–	–	0.995	–	0.019	–	0.035
Gender											
2. Men Model	9.08	27	–	–	–	–	0.994	–	0.02	–	0.037
3. Women Model	12.95	27	–	–	–	–	0.984	–	0.035	–	0.072
4. Configural Model	22.03	54	–	–	–	–	0.992	–	0.024	–	0.044
5. Metric Model	39.05	62	4–5	9.57	8	0.296	0.989	−0.003	0.026	0.002	0.058
6. Scalar Model	57.11	70	5–6	26.81	8	>0.001	0.976	−0.013	0.036	0.010	0.062
Age											
7. ≤17 Model	5.38	27	–	–	–	–	0.998	–	0.012	–	0.035
8.≥18 Model	11.93	27	–	–	–	–	0.988	–	0.029	–	0.049
9. Configural Model	17.33	54	–	–	–	–	0.992	–	0.023	–	0.043
10. Metric Model	28.85	62	9–10	11.99	8	0.151	0.988	−0.004	0.026	0.003	0.056
11. Scalar Model	37.40	70	10–11	14.60	8	0.464	0.983	−0.005	0.029	0.003	0.058

Note: n for Men's model = 419; n for women's model = 113; n for ≤ 17's Model = 296; n for ≥ 18's model = 236; χ^2 = Chi-Squared; df = Degrees of freedom; Comp. Md = Compared models; Δ SBχ^2 = differences in Satorra-Bentler Scaled Chi-Squared; Δdf = difference in number of degrees of freedom; p = significance value for the Scaled Chi-Squared Difference Test; CFI: Comparative Fit Index; ΔCFI = differences in Comparative Fit Index; RMSEA = Root Mean Square Error of Approximation; SRMR = Standardized Root Mean Square Residual;.

3.3. Convergent Validity

In relation to convergent validity, the Pearson's bivariate correlation carried out between the total IGDS9-SF scores and the OGD-Q scores had a value of r = 0.440, $p < 0.001$ ($n = 101$); with the CERM, it was $r = 0.553$, $p = 0.001$. Additionally, IGDS9-SF correlated with the five dimensions of the KIDSCREEN-27 as follows: physical well-being ($r = -0.164$, $p = 0.001$), psychological well-being ($r = -0.315$, $p = 0.001$), autonomy and relationship with parents ($r = -0.167$, $p = 0.001$), peers and social support ($r = -0.257$, $p = 0.001$), and school environment ($r = -0.176$, $p = 0.001$).

It was also found that gamers who preferably played the MOBA-, RPG-, or MMORPG-type game genres reported higher scores on the IGDS9-SF (15.21 ± 6.14) than those who played other genres (FPS, action/platforms, musical, sports simulators, fighting, or casual) (13.81 ± 4.55) ($t = 2.679$, $p < 0.008$, $d = 0.26$). Additionally, in response to the question '*I am addicted to video games*', 65 answered 'yes', and 473 replied 'no'. Those who self-reported that they were addicted had a significantly higher mean score on the IGDS9-SF (19.19 ± 8.30) compared to those who did not (13.43 ± 4.73) ($t = 8.233$, $p < 0.001$, d = 0.85).

3.4. Prevalence and Psychological Involvement of Internet Gaming Disorder

Following the diagnostic approach suggested by Pontes et al., [61], the participants who were classified with IGD (i.e., endorsing at least five of the criteria within the last 12 months) accounted for 1.9% of the sample of gamers ($n = 10$; see Table 3) and almost 1% of the total study sample. Of these 10 participants, nine were male and one was female. In addition, 1.9% endorsed four diagnostic criteria ($n = 10$) and were classed as 'at-risk' of developing IGD. It should also be noted that 76.2% ($n = 410$) did not endorse any diagnostic criteria.

Table 3. Number of participants who meet between 1 and 9 of the Internet Gaming Disorder criteria (adapted from Pontes, et al. [61]).

Number of Criteria Endorsed	Number of Participants	Total % of the Sample (n = 1064)	Total % of Online Gamers (n = 535)
1	71	6.67	13.2
2	27	2.54	5
3	10	0.94	1.9
4	10	0.94	1.9
5	1	0.09	0.2
6	1	0.09	0.2
7	2	0.19	0.4
8	2	0.19	0.4
9	4	0.38	0.8

Table 4 shows the psychological involvement of players with IGD (those with five or more symptoms) compared to those with four or fewer symptoms in relation to HRQoL. The loss of physical ($p = 0.011$) and psychological well-being ($p = 0.018$) is especially notable. There was also a loss of autonomy and relationship with parents ($p = 0.047$) and worse school environment ($p = 0.038$). There were no differences for the dimension of peers and social support ($p = 0.080$). The effect sizes for all contrasts were greater than $g > 0.42$.

Table 4. Comparison between gamers with Internet Gaming Disorder (IGD) (endorsing five or more criteria) versus those endorsing four criteria or fewer with respect to the five dimensions of the KIDSCREEN-27.

Instrument	n (< 5 symptoms)	M ± SD (< 5 symptoms)	n (≥ 5 symptoms)	M ± SD (≥ 5 symptoms)	Mann-Whitney U (p)	Effect Size (Hedges' g)
KD Phy-Wb	341	45.40 ± 11.39	7	33.92 ± 10.51	2.529 (.011)	1.00
KD Psy-Wb	341	46.70 ± 9.47	7	38.00 ± 8.88	2.370 (.018)	0.92
KD A and Pr	341	48.51 ± 10.91	7	39.75 ± 21.70	1.749 (.080)	0.78
KD SS and P	341	50.97 ± 11.31	7	37.81 ± 20.06	1.988 (.047)	1.14
KD SE	341	46.19 ± 9.10	7	42.31 ± 13.26	2.076 (.038)	0.42

Note: n (< 5 symptoms): participants with fewer than four problem criteria/items; n (≥ 5 symptoms) participants with four or more problem criteria/items; KD Phy-Wb = Physical well-being; KD Psy-Wb = Psychological well-being; KD A and Pr = Autonomy and relations with parents; KD SS and P = Social Support and Peers; KD SE = School Environment; M = arithmetic mean; SD = standard deviation.

4. Discussion

The IGDS9-SF is a sound psychometric test that assesses IGD, and it is one of the most frequently used instruments as it had the greatest number of adaptations to different languages and cultural contexts [56]. In the present study, the development of the Spanish IGDS9-SF was carried out through a rigorous conceptual and methodological procedure that followed conventional international standards [71]. Appropriate indicators of validity and reliability were obtained in a sample of adolescents and young people. Factor analysis confirmed a single-factor solution with adequate goodness of fit, the item-total correlations were also high, and the factor loadings of all the items were satisfactory. Furthermore, the unidimensional factor model was found to be gender and age invariant across the metric level, which is considered a prerequisite for meaningful cross-group comparisons [80]. The present study adopted a similar procedure to studies conducted for different constructs, such as nomophobia [81–83], online gambling disorder [14], and previous validations of the IGDS9-SF in other languages such as Portuguese [67], Slovenian [61], and Italian [62], among others.

The prevalence rate of IGD in the present sample was 1.9%, which is similar to the 2.6% found in another Spanish sample by Fuster et al. [37] but noticeably lower than that of 8.3% reported by Buiza-Aguado et al. [36]. These discrepancies may be due to the use of different psychometric tools in assessing IGD. In other studies that have utilized the IGDS9-SF, the prevalence rates of disordered gaming were reported to be between 3% to 5% [59,61]. The results of the present study fall within the prevalence rate range reported by other international studies [31]. Finally, it also corroborates the fact that males are more frequently classified with IGD than females [31,37,38].

In relation to other validity indicators, the present study sought to evaluate the relationship between the IGDS9-SF and instruments assessing conceptually similar psychological problems such as the CERM [72] and the OGD-Q [14]. The results obtained indicated high correlations between these constructs, suggesting a convergent relationship with other relevant problems related to maladaptive use of technology and the internet such as problematic smartphone use and online gambling disorder. In addition, indicators relating to the relationship between IGDS9-SF and HRQoL allowed the examination of five key dimensions in adolescence (i.e., physical well-being; psychological well-being; autonomy and relationship with parents; peers and social support; and the school environment). Inverse and significant relationships were found between all five aforementioned dimensions, which means that higher level problems with online gaming associate with poorer self-reported quality of life. It is especially interesting to compare participants categorized as gamers with IGD or who are at risk with those who are not, because there was a significant decrease in quality of life scores in the former. Overall, the effects sizes of these correlations were high (i.e., most were greater than 0.80). These results are consistent with those of other studies using the 20-item Internet Gaming Disorder Test (IGD-20 Test [24]) and the KIDSCREEN-27 [31]. This finding also has a theoretical-conceptual relationship with the components model of addiction by Griffiths [23], which highlights the importance relating to the negative effects of the symptoms of addiction. In addition, it also supports the notion of other more general conceptualizations of problematic use of the internet [8], in which problems are related to poorer social and personal functioning, as well as to compulsive use and negative consequences.

Limitations and Future Lines of Research

The study conducted presents with several potential limitations worth discussing. Firstly, the IGDS9-SF is a self-report psychometric tool, so the potential for confounding effects stemming from response biases and social desirability by the adolescents and young people who completed it cannot be completely ruled out. This could be improved in the future by developing complementary measures combining behavioral tracking data (e.g., actual time spent playing and in-game preferences) to enhance self-report data. Secondly, the sample recruited was not randomly selected. However, the sample size of the present study was significantly large, especially in the context of a psychometric study. Nevertheless, caution is suggested when extrapolating the prevalence rates reported in the present study and considering them as a first approximation to the problem. Thirdly, although the diagnostic approach of the APA [21] and the recommendation of the original authors of the IGDS9-SF were followed when classifying disordered gamers, the authors have sought to establish a less conservative diagnostic approach which requires further discussion and analyses. Fourthly, whereas adequate indicators of validity and reliability were obtained, other important measures such as test-retest were not considered due to the imperatives of fieldwork. Fifthly, the KIDSCREEN-27 is a tool designed to evaluate HRQoL in the infantile-juvenile population, and the sample here included some participants over age 18 years. Thus, participants over 18 years were not considered in the analyses related to this construct, which reduced the sample size. It would be of interest for future research to use developmentally specific quality of life assessment tools for those over 18 years. It would also be fruitful to explore in future research other processes that favor the diagnostic accuracy of this scale, such as Receiver Operating Characteristic (ROC) curves (as demonstrated by Severo et al. [68] and Monacis et al. [62]), and other diagnostic elements, such as interviewing or complementary measures, should be used in the future in order to establish a robust clinically-driven gold standard diagnosis. Finally, according to the data obtained, the possible relationship between IGD and online gambling disorder with the advent of gambling-type elements in video games (e.g., loot boxes) should be noted for future lines of research to be explored. Legally, loot boxes are not considered online gambling, but at a psychosocial level, they meet the characteristics to be defined as a type of gambling [84].

5. Conclusions

The present study corroborates the psychometric properties of the scores obtained on the IGDS9-SF. In addition, preliminary data on the prevalence of the disordered gaming were obtained, which are useful for knowledge of an emerging global health challenge. The findings reported here will be particularly useful to pediatric and psychological care units, as well as for those in charge of school orientation at schools. All the above is also of special interest to parents, because education and parental supervision can play a very important role in the prevention of these problems associated with the internet, and in particular, internet gaming.

Author Contributions: Conceptualization, M.B, X.C, and J.G.-C.; Data curation, M.B. and J.M.M.; Formal analysis, J.M.M. and J.G.-C.; Funding acquisition, J.G.-C.; Investigation, M.B., J.M.M., M.A.V.-O., X.C., M.D.G., H.M.P, and J.G.-C.; Methodology, J.M.M. and J.G.-C.; Project administration, J.G.-C.; Resources, M.A.V.-O.; Supervision, X.C., M.D.G., H.M.P., and J.G.-C.; Writing—original draft, M.B., J.M.M., and J.G.-C.; Writing—review and editing, M.B., J.M.M., M.A.V.-O., X.C., M.D.G., H.M.P., and J.G.-C. All authors have read and agreed to the published version of the manuscript.

Appendix A. The Spanish version of IGDS9-SF

Los siguientes ítems hacen referencia a tu actividad con los videojuegos durante el último año (es decir, los últimos 12 meses). Por actividad en los videojuegos entendemos cualquier acción relacionada con los mismos (jugar desde un ordenador/portátil o desde una videoconsola) o desde cualquier otro tipo de dispositivo (por ejemplo, teléfono móvil, tablet, etc.) tanto conectado a Internet como sin estarlo y a cualquier tipo de juego					
Preguntas	**Nunca**	**Raramente**	**Ocasionalmente**	**A menudo**	**Muy a menudo**
1.¿Te sientes preocupado por tu comportamiento con el juego? (Algunos ejemplos: ¿Piensas en exceso cuando no estás jugando o anticipas en exceso a la próxima sesión de juego?, ¿Crees que el juego se ha convertido en la actividad dominante en tu vida diaria?)					
2. ¿Sientes irritabilidad, ansiedad o incluso tristeza cuando intentas reducir o detener tu actividad de juego?					
3. ¿Sientes la necesidad de pasar cada vez más tiempo jugando para lograr satisfacción o placer?					
4. ¿Fallas sistemáticamente al intentar controlar o terminar tu actividad de juego?					
5. ¿ Has perdido intereses en aficiones anteriores y otras actividades de entretenimiento como resultado de tu compromiso con el juego?					
6. ¿ Has continuado jugando a pesar de saber que te estaba causando problemas con otras personas? (pareja, amistad o familia)?					
7. ¿ Has engañado a alguno de tus familiares, terapeutas o amigos sobre el tiempo que pasas jugando?					
8. ¿ Juegas para escapar temporalmente o aliviar un estado de ánimo negativo (por ejemplo, desesperanza, tristeza, culpa o ansiedad)?					
9. ¿ Has comprometido o perdido una relación importante, un trabajo o una oportunidad educativa debido a tu actividad de juego?					

References

1. Griffiths, M.D. Technological addictions. *Clin. Psychol. Forum* **1995**, *76*, 14–19.

2. Young, K.S. Internet addiction: The emergence of a new clinical disorder. *Cyberpsychol. Behav.* **1998**, *1*, 237–244. [CrossRef]

3. Carbonell, X.; Guardiola, E.; Beranuy, M.; Bellés, A. A bibliometric analysis of the scientific literature on Internet, video games, and cell phone addiction. *J. Med. Libr. Assoc. JMLA* **2009**, *97*, 102–107. [CrossRef] [PubMed]

4. Kuss, D.; Griffiths, M.; Karila, L.; Billieux, J. Internet addiction: A systematic review of epidemiological research for the last decade. *Curr. Pharm. Des.* **2014**, *20*, 4026–4052. [CrossRef] [PubMed]

5. Lopez-Fernandez, O. Generalised versus specific internet use-related addiction problems: A mixed methods study on internet, gaming, and social networking behaviours. *Int. J. Environ. Res. Public. Health* **2018**, *15*, 2913. [CrossRef] [PubMed]

6. Paulus, F.W.; Ohmann, S.; von Gontard, A.; Popow, C. Internet gaming disorder in children and adolescents: A systematic review. *Dev. Med. Child Neurol.* **2018**, *60*, 645–659. [CrossRef] [PubMed]

7. Davis, R.A. A cognitive-behavioral model of pathological Internet use. *Comput. Hum. Behav.* **2001**, *17*, 187–195. [CrossRef]

8. Caplan, S.E. Theory and measurement of generalized problematic Internet use: A two-step approach. *Comput. Hum. Behav.* **2010**, *26*, 1089–1097. [CrossRef]

9. Caplan, S.E. Problematic Internet use and psychosocial well-being: Development of a theory-based cognitive–behavioral measurement instrument. *Comput. Hum. Behav.* **2002**, *18*, 553–575. [CrossRef]

10. Kuss, D.J.; Griffiths, M.D. Internet gaming addiction: A systematic review of empirical research. *Int. J. Ment. Health Addict.* **2012**, *10*, 278–296. [CrossRef]

11. Pearcy, B.T.D.; McEvoy, P.M.; Roberts, L.D. Internet gaming disorder explains unique variance in psychological distress and disability after controlling for comorbid depression, OCD, ADHD, and anxiety. *Cyberpsychol. Behav. Soc. Netw.* **2017**, *20*, 126–132. [CrossRef] [PubMed]

12. van Rooij, A.J.; Schoenmakers, T.M.; van de Eijnden, R.J.J.M.; van de Mheen, D. Compulsive internet use: The role of online gaming and other internet applications. *J. Adolesc. Health* **2010**, *47*, 51–57. [CrossRef] [PubMed]

13. Gainsbury, S.M.; Russell, A.; Hing, N.; Wood, R.; Lubman, D.; Blaszczynski, A. How the internet is changing gambling: Findings from an Australian prevalence survey. *J. Gambl. Stud.* **2015**, *31*, 1–15. [CrossRef]

14. González-Cabrera, J.; Machimbarrena, J.M.; Beranuy, M.; Pérez-Rodríguez, P.; Fernández-González, L.; Calvete, E. Design and measurement properties of the Online Gambling Disorder Questionnaire (OGD-Q) in Spanish adolescents. *J. Clin. Med.* **2020**, *9*, 120. [CrossRef] [PubMed]

15. Wood, R.T.; Williams, R.J. A comparative profile of the Internet gambler: Demographic characteristics, game-play patterns, and problem gambling status. *New Media Soc.* **2011**, *13*, 1123–1141. [CrossRef]

16. Griffiths, M.D. Internet sex addiction: A review of empirical research. *Addict. Res. Theory* **2012**, *20*, 111–124. [CrossRef]

17. Meerkerk, G.-J.; Eijnden, R.J.J.M.V.D.; Garretsen, H.F.L. Predicting compulsive internet use: It's all about sex! *Cyberpsychol. Behav.* **2006**, *9*, 95–103. [CrossRef]

18. Hormes, J.M.; Kearns, B.; Timko, C.A. Craving Facebook? Behavioral addiction to online social networking and its association with emotion regulation deficits: Online social networking addiction. *Addiction* **2014**, *109*, 2079–2088. [CrossRef]

19. Ryan, T.; Chester, A.; Reece, J.; Xenos, S. The uses and abuses of Facebook: A review of Facebook addiction. *J. Behav. Addict.* **2014**, *3*, 133–148. [CrossRef]

20. Carbonell, X.; Panova, T. A critical consideration of social networking sites' addiction potential. *Addict. Res. Theory* **2017**, *25*, 48–57. [CrossRef]

21. American Psychiatric Association. *Diagnostic and Statistical Manual of Mental Disorders*, 5th ed.; American Psychiatric Publishing: Washington, DC, USA, 2013.

22. World Health Organization. *The ICD-11 Classification of Mental and Behavioural Disorders*; WHO: Geneva, Switzerland, 2018; Available online: https://icd.who.int/browse11/l-m/en (accessed on 18 January 2020).

23. Griffiths, M. A 'components' model of addiction within a biopsychosocial framework. *J. Subst. Use* **2005**, *10*, 191–197. [CrossRef]

24. Pontes, H.M.; Király, O.; Demetrovics, Z.; Griffiths, M.D. The conceptualisation and measurement of DSM-5 internet gaming disorder: The development of the IGD-20 Test. *PLoS ONE* **2014**, *9*, e110137. [CrossRef]

25. Rumpf, H.-J.; Achab, S.; Billieux, J.; Bowden-Jones, H.; Carragher, N.; Demetrovics, Z.; Higuchi, S.; King, D.L.; Mann, K.; Potenza, M.; et al. Including gaming disorder in the ICD-11: The need to do so from a clinical and public health perspective: Commentary on: A weak scientific basis for gaming disorder: Let us err on the side of caution (van Rooij et al., 2018). *J. Behav. Addict.* **2018**, *7*, 556–561. [CrossRef] [PubMed]

26. Asociación Española de Videojuegos La industria del videojuego en españa. *Anuario 2018*; Asociación Española de Videojuegos: Madrid, España, 2018.

27. Fam, J.Y. Prevalence of internet gaming disorder in adolescents: A meta-analysis across three decades. *Scand. J. Psychol.* **2018**, *59*, 524–531. [CrossRef] [PubMed]

28. Salmela-Aro, K. Stages of Adolescence. In *Encyclopedia of Adolescence*; Elsevier: Oxford, UK, 2011; pp. 360–368. ISBN 978-0-12-373951-3.

29. Mascó, A. *Entre Generaciones [between Generations]*; Temas: Buenos Aires, Argentina, 2013.

30. Petry, N.M.; Rehbein, F.; Gentile, D.A.; Lemmens, J.S.; Rumpf, H.-J.; Mößle, T.; Bischof, G.; Tao, R.; Fung, D.S.S.; Borges, G.; et al. An international consensus for assessing internet gaming disorder using the new DSM-5 approach: Internet gaming disorder. *Addiction* **2014**, *109*, 1399–1406. [CrossRef] [PubMed]

31. Wartberg, L.; Kriston, L.; Thomasius, R. The prevalence and psychosocial correlates of internet gaming disorder. *Dtsch. Aerzteblatt Online* **2017**. [CrossRef]

32. Yau, Y.; Potenza, M. Internet gaming disorder. *Psychiatr. Ann.* **2014**, *44*, 379–383. [CrossRef]

33. Yu, H.; Cho, J. Prevalence of internet gaming disorder among Korean adolescents and associations with non-psychotic psychological symptoms, and physical aggression. *Am. J. Health Behav.* **2016**, *40*, 705–716. [CrossRef]

34. Feng, W.; Ramo, D.E.; Chan, S.R.; Bourgeois, J.A. Internet gaming disorder: Trends in prevalence 1998–2016. *Addict. Behav.* **2017**, *75*, 17–24. [CrossRef]

35. Long, J.; Liu, T.; Liu, Y.; Hao, W.; Maurage, P.; Billieux, J. Prevalence and correlates of problematic online gaming: A systematic review of the evidence published in Chinese. *Curr. Addict. Rep.* **2018**, *5*, 359–371. [CrossRef]

36. Buiza-Aguado, C.; Alonso-Canovas, A.; Conde-Mateos, C.; Buiza-Navarrete, J.J.; Gentile, D. Problematic video gaming in a young Spanish population: Association with psychosocial health. *Cyberpsychol. Behav. Soc. Netw.* **2018**, *21*, 388–394. [CrossRef] [PubMed]

37. Fuster, H.; Carbonell, X.; Pontes, H.M.; Griffiths, M.D. Spanish validation of the Internet Gaming Disorder-20 (IGD-20) Test. *Comput. Hum. Behav.* **2016**, *56*, 215–224. [CrossRef]

38. Martín-Fernández, M.; Matalí, J.L.; García-Sánchez, S.; Pardo, M.; Lleras, M.; Castellano-Tejedor, C. Adolescentes con trastorno por juego en internet (IGD): Perfiles y respuesta al tratamiento. *Adicciones* **2016**, *29*, 125. [CrossRef] [PubMed]

39. Gentile, D.A.; Choo, H.; Liau, A.; Sim, T.; Li, D.; Fung, D.; Khoo, A. Pathological video game use among youths: A two-year longitudinal study. *Pediatrics* **2011**, *127*, e319–e329. [CrossRef] [PubMed]

40. Kim, E.J.; Namkoong, K.; Ku, T.; Kim, S.J. The relationship between online game addiction and aggression, self-control and narcissistic personality traits. *Eur. Psychiatry* **2008**, *23*, 212–218. [CrossRef]

41. Lemmens, J.S.; Valkenburg, P.M.; Gentile, D.A. The Internet Gaming Disorder Scale. *Psychol. Assess.* **2015**, *27*, 567–582. [CrossRef] [PubMed]

42. Thomée, S.; Härenstam, A.; Hagberg, M. Mobile phone use and stress, sleep disturbances, and symptoms of depression among young adults-a prospective cohort study. *BMC Public Health* **2011**, *11*, 66. [CrossRef]

43. Torres-Rodríguez, A.; Griffiths, M.D.; Carbonell, X.; Oberst, U. Treatment efficacy of a specialized psychotherapy program for Internet Gaming Disorder. *J. Behav. Addict.* **2018**, *7*, 939–952. [CrossRef]

44. Ha, J.H.; Yoo, H.J.; Cho, I.H.; Chin, B.; Shin, D.; Kim, J.H. Psychiatric comorbidity assessed in Korean children and adolescents who screen positive for internet addiction. *J. Clin. Psychiatry* **2006**, *67*, 821–826. [CrossRef]

45. Ferguson, C.J.; Coulson, M.; Barnett, J. A meta-analysis of pathological gaming prevalence and comorbidity with mental health, academic and social problems. *J. Psychiatr. Res.* **2011**, *45*, 1573–1578. [CrossRef]

46. Fernández-Villa, T.; Alguacil Ojeda, J.; Almaraz Gómez, A.; Cancela Carral, J.M.; Delgado-Rodríguez, M.; García-Martín, M.; Jiménez-Mejías, E.; Llorca, J.; Molina, A.J.; Ortíz Moncada, R.; et al. Uso problemático de internet en estudiantes universitarios: Factores asociados y diferencias de género. *Adicciones* **2015**, *27*, 265. [CrossRef] [PubMed]

47. Ko, C.-H.; Yen, J.-Y.; Yen, C.-F.; Chen, C.-S.; Chen, C.-C. The association between Internet addiction and psychiatric disorder: A review of the literature. *Eur. Psychiatry* **2012**, *27*, 1–8. [CrossRef] [PubMed]

48. Müller, K.W.; Beutel, M.E.; Egloff, B.; Wölfling, K. Investigating risk factors for internet gaming disorder: A comparison of patients with addictive gaming, pathological gamblers and healthy controls regarding the big five personality traits. *Eur. Addict. Res.* **2014**, *20*, 129–136. [CrossRef] [PubMed]

49. Choi, S.-W.; Kim, H.; Kim, G.-Y.; Jeon, Y.; Park, S.; Lee, J.-Y.; Jung, H.; Sohn, B.; Choi, J.-S.; Kim, D.-J. Similarities and differences among Internet gaming disorder, gambling disorder and alcohol use disorder: A focus on impulsivity and compulsivity. *J. Behav. Addict.* **2014**, *3*, 246–253. [CrossRef] [PubMed]

50. Fauth-Bühler, M.; Mann, K. Neurobiological correlates of internet gaming disorder: Similarities to pathological gambling. *Addict. Behav.* **2017**, *64*, 349–356. [CrossRef]

51. Liu, C.-H.; Lin, S.-H.; Pan, Y.-C.; Lin, Y.-H. Smartphone gaming and frequent use pattern associated with smartphone addiction. *Medicine* **2016**, *95*, e4068. [CrossRef]

52. Wallander, J.L.; Koot, H.M. Quality of life in children: A critical examination of concepts, approaches, issues, and future directions. *Clin. Psychol. Rev.* **2016**, *45*, 131–143. [CrossRef]

53. Kidscreen Group Europe. *The KIDSCREEN Questionnaires-Quality of Life Questionnaires for Children and Adolescents, Handbook*; Pabst Science Publishers: Lengerich, Germany, 2006.

54. Takahashi, M.; Adachi, M.; Nishimura, T.; Hirota, T.; Yasuda, S.; Kuribayashi, M.; Nakamura, K. Prevalence of pathological and maladaptive Internet use and the association with depression and health-related quality of life in Japanese elementary and junior high school-aged children. *Soc. Psychiatry Psychiatr. Epidemiol.* **2018**, *53*, 1349–1359. [CrossRef]

55. Barayan, S.; Al Dabal, B.; Abdelwahab, M.; Shafey, M.; Al Omar, R. Health-related quality of life among female university students in Dammam district: Is Internet use related? *J. Fam. Community Med.* **2018**, *25*, 20. [CrossRef]

56. Bernaldo-de-Quirós, M.; Labrador-Méndez, M.; Sánchez-Iglesias, I.; Labrador, F.J. Instrumentos de medida del trastorno de juego en internet en adolescentes y jóvenes según criterios DSM-5: Una revisión sistemática [Measuring instruments for internet gambling disorder in adolescents and young people according to DSM-5 criteria: A systematic review]. *Adicciones* **2019**. [CrossRef]

57. Pontes, H.M.; Griffiths, M.D. Measuring DSM-5 internet gaming disorder: Development and validation of a short psychometric scale. *Comput. Hum. Behav.* **2015**, *45*, 137–143. [CrossRef]

58. Yam, C.-W.; Pakpour, A.H.; Griffiths, M.D.; Yau, W.-Y.; Lo, C.-L.M.; Ng, J.M.T.; Lin, C.-Y.; Leung, H. Psychometric testing of three Chinese online-related addictive behavior instruments among Hong Kong university students. *Psychiatr. Q.* **2019**, *90*, 117–128. [CrossRef] [PubMed]

59. Montag, C.; Schivinski, B.; Sariyska, R.; Kannen, C.; Demetrovics, Z.; Pontes, H.M. Psychopathological symptoms and gaming motives in disordered gaming—A psychometric comparison between the WHO and APA diagnostic frameworks. *J. Clin. Med.* **2019**, *8*, 1691. [CrossRef] [PubMed]

60. Suchá, J.; Dolejš, M.; Pipová, H.; Maierová, E.; Cakirpaloglu, P. *Hraní digitálních her českými adolescenty*, 1st ed.; Univerzita Palackého v Olomouci: Křížkovského: Olomouc, Czech, 2018; ISBN 978-80-244-5424-5.

61. Pontes, H.M.; Macur, M.; Griffiths, M.D. Internet gaming disorder among Slovenian primary schoolchildren: Findings from a nationally representative sample of adolescents. *J. Behav. Addict.* **2016**, *5*, 304–310. [CrossRef]

62. Monacis, L.; Palo, d.V.; Griffiths, M.D.; Sinatra, M. Validation of the Internet Gaming Disorder Scale—Short-Form (IGDS9-SF) in an Italian-speaking sample. *J. Behav. Addict.* **2016**, *5*, 683–690. [CrossRef]

63. Wu, T.-Y.; Lin, C.-Y.; Årestedt, K.; Griffiths, M.D.; Broström, A.; Pakpour, A.H. Psychometric validation of the Persian nine-item Internet Gaming Disorder Scale–Short Form: Does gender and hours spent online gaming affect the interpretations of item descriptions? *J. Behav. Addict.* **2017**, *6*, 256–263. [CrossRef]

64. Aricak, O.T. Psychiatric Symptomatology as a predictor of cyberbullying among university students. *Eurasian J. Educ. Res.* **2009**, *34*, 167–184.

65. Evren, C.; Dalbudak, E.; Topcu, M.; Kutlu, N.; Evren, B.; Pontes, H.M. Psychometric validation of the Turkish nine-item Internet Gaming Disorder Scale–Short Form (IGDS9-SF). *Psychiatry Res.* **2018**, *265*, 349–354. [CrossRef]

66. Schivinski, B.; Brzozowska-Woś, M.; Buchanan, E.M.; Griffiths, M.D.; Pontes, H.M. Psychometric assessment of the internet gaming disorder diagnostic criteria: An item response theory study. *Addict. Behav. Rep.* **2018**, *8*, 176–184. [CrossRef]

67. Pontes, H.M.; Griffiths, M.D. Portuguese validation of the Internet Gaming Disorder Scale–Short-Form. *Cyberpsychol. Behav. Soc. Netw.* **2016**, *19*, 288–293. [CrossRef]

68. Severo, R.B.; Barbosa, A.P.P.N.; Fouchy, D.R.C.; Coelho, F.M.d.C.; Pinheiro, R.T.; de Figueiredo, V.L.M.; de Siqueira Afonso, V.; Pontes, H.M.; Pinheiro, K.A.T. Development and psychometric validation of Internet Gaming Disorder Scale-Short-Form (IGDS9-SF) in a Brazilian sample. *Addict. Behav.* **2020**, *103*, 106191. [CrossRef] [PubMed]

69. Ethnologue What are the top 200 most spoken languages? Available online: https://www.ethnologue.com/guides/ethnologue200 (accessed on 18 January 2020).

70. Instituto Cervantes. El español: Una lengua viva. Informe 2019 [Spanish: A Living Language. 2019 report]. Available online: https://www.cervantes.es/imagenes/File/espanol_lengua_viva_2019.pdf (accessed on 20 February 2020).

71. Muñiz, J.; Fonseca-Pedrero, E. Diez pasos para la construcción de un test. *Psicothema* **2019**, 7–16. [CrossRef]

72. Beranuy, M.; Chamarro, A.; Graner, C.; Carbonell, X. Validación de dos escalas breves para evaluar la adicción a Internet y el abuso de móvil [Validation of two short scales to assess Internet addiction and mobile abuse]. *Psicothema* **2009**, *21*, 480–485.

73. *IBM Corp Statistical Package for the Social Sciences for Windows*; IBM Corp: Armonk, NY, USA, 2015.

74. Revelle, W. *Psych: Procedures for Personality and Psychological Research*, R package version 1.9.12; Northwestern University: Evanston, IL, USA, 2015; Available online: https://CRAN.R-project.org/package=psych (accessed on 27 February 2020).

75. Rosseel, Y. lavaan: An *R* Package for structural equation modeling. *J. Stat. Softw.* **2012**, *48*. [CrossRef]

76. Giang, M.; Mai, Y.; Yuan, K.-H. *equaltestMI: Examine measurement invariance via equivalence testing and projection method*, R package version 0.1.0; 2017. Available online: https://CRAN.R-project.org/package=equaltestMI (accessed on 27 February 2020).

77. Hu, L.; Bentler, P.M. Cutoff criteria for fit indexes in covariance structure analysis: Conventional criteria versus new alternatives. *Struct. Equ. Model. Multidiscip. J.* **1999**, *6*, 1–55. [CrossRef]

78. Byrne, B.M. *Structural equation modeling with EQS: Basic concepts, application, and programming*; Lawrence Elbaum Associates: Mahwah, NJ, USA, 2006.

79. Cheung, G.W.; Rensvold, R.B. Evaluating goodness-of-fit indexes for testing measurement invariance. *Struct. Equ. Model. Multidiscip. J.* **2002**, *9*, 233–255. [CrossRef]

80. Bollen, K.A. *Structural equations with latent variables: Bollen/structural equations with latent variables*; John Wiley & Sons, Inc.: Hoboken, NJ, USA, 1989; ISBN 978-1-118-61917-9. [CrossRef]

81. Yildirim, C.; Correia, A.-P. Exploring the dimensions of nomophobia: Development and validation of a self-reported questionnaire. *Comput. Hum. Behav.* **2015**, *49*, 130–137. [CrossRef]

82. León-Mejía, A.; Calvete, E.; Patino-Alonso, C.; Machimbarrena, J.M.; González-Cabrera, J. Factor structure and sex and age cut-off points for the Spanish version of the Nomophobia Questionnaire. *Adicciones* **2020**. [CrossRef]

83. González-Cabrera, J.; León-Mejía, A.; Pérez-Sancho, C.; Calvete, E. Adaptación al español del cuestionario Nomophobia Questionnaire (NMP-Q) en una muestra de adolescentes [Spanish adaptation of the Nomophobia Questionnaire (NMP-Q) in a sample of adolescents]. *Actas Esp. Psiquiatr.* **2017**, *45*, 137–144.

84. Griffiths, M.D. Is the buying of loot boxes in video games a form of gambling or gaming? *Gaming Law Rev.* **2018**, *22*, 52–54. [CrossRef]

13

Risk Factors for Internet Gaming Disorder: Psychological Factors and Internet Gaming Characteristics

Mi Jung Rho [1,2,†], Hyeseon Lee [3,†], Taek-Ho Lee [3], Hyun Cho [4,5], DongJin Jung [5,6], Dai-Jin Kim [5,6,*,‡] and In Young Choi [1,2,*,‡]

1   Department of Medical Informatics, College of Medicine, The Catholic University of Korea, Seoul 06591, Korea; rhomijung@gmail.com
2   Catholic Institute for Healthcare Management and Graduate School of Healthcare Management and Policy, The Catholic University of Korea, Seoul 06591, Korea
3   Department of Industrial & Management Engineering, Pohang University of Science and Technology, Pohang 37673, Korea; hyelee@postech.ac.kr (H.L.); dlxorgh2@postech.ac.kr (T.-H.L.)
4   Department of Psychology, Korea University, Seoul 02841, Korea; sonap1@hanmail.net
5   Addiction Research Institute, Department of Psychiatry, Seoul St. Mary's Hospital, College of Medicine, The Catholic University of Korea, Seoul 06591, Korea; forever0851@naver.com
6   Department of Psychiatry, Seoul St. Mary's Hospital, College of Medicine, The Catholic University of Korea, Seoul 06591, Korea
*   Correspondence: kdj922@catholic.ac.kr (D.-J.K.); iychoi@catholic.ac.kr (I.Y.C.)
†   Both authors contributed equally to this work.
‡   Both corresponding authors contributed equally to this work.

Abstract: *Background*: Understanding the risk factors associated with Internet gaming disorder (IGD) is important to predict and diagnose the condition. The purpose of this study is to identify risk factors that predict IGD based on psychological factors and Internet gaming characteristics; *Methods*: Online surveys were conducted between 26 November and 26 December 2014. There were 3568 Korean Internet game users among a total of 5003 respondents. We identified 481 IGD gamers and 3087 normal Internet gamers, based on Diagnostic and Statistical Manual for Mental Disorders (DSM-5) criteria. Logistic regression analysis was applied to identify significant risk factors for IGD; *Results*: The following eight risk factors were found to be significantly associated with IGD: functional and dysfunctional impulsivity (odds ratio: 1.138), belief self-control (1.034), anxiety (1.086), pursuit of desired appetitive goals (1.105), money spent on gaming (1.005), weekday game time (1.081), offline community meeting attendance (2.060), and game community membership (1.393; $p < 0.05$ for all eight risk factors); *Conclusions*: These risk factors allow for the prediction and diagnosis of IGD. In the future, these risk factors could also be used to inform clinical services for IGD diagnosis and treatment.

Keywords: internet gaming disorder; Dickman Impulsivity Inventory-Short Version (DII); Brief Self-Control Scale (BSCS); Symptom Checklist-90-Revised (SCL-90-R); Behavioral Inhibition System/Behavioral Activation System (BIS/BAS); Diagnostic and Statistical Manual for Mental Disorders (DSM-5)

1. Introduction

Since Internet games became widespread in the 2000s [1], Internet game usage has experienced rapid growth among both youth and adults. According to a report by the Entertainment Software

Association (ESA) [2], 155 million Americans play video games, of which 42% play video games regularly. In 2015 alone, American game consumers spent more than US$22.41 billion on game content, hardware, and accessories [2]. Worldwide Internet game usage and gaming money has been rapidly increasing. As a result, Internet Gaming Disorder (IGD) has become a major social problem and important research topic. The World Health Organization (WHO) has proposed a new category named "Gaming Disorder" for the 11th Revision of the International Classification of Diseases (ICD-11) [3]. The ability to predict, diagnose, and manage IGD in advance is critical to the prevention of IGD. To do that, the risk factors associated with IGD need to be better understood.

Firstly, the psychological factors associated with IGD need to be understood. IGD can be considered a behavioral addiction [4–8] and has been found to be related to a number of psychological and health problems, including depression, social anxiety, fatigue, loneliness, negative self-esteem, and impulsivity [9–12]. IGD co-occurs with various psychiatric conditions and can lead to a range of negative outcomes. For example, IGD can cause social problems such as lower academic achievement [10,11,13–17]. In addition, IGD shares many similarities with other addictions, such as substance use disorder [18].

Secondly, the Internet gaming characteristics associated with IGD need to be better understood. Research in this area has increased in both quantity and quality. In order to predict, diagnose, and manage IGD, researchers have attempted to identify the causes and negative consequences of excessive gaming as well as risk factors of IGD. Some research, however, has only focused on psychological factors [16,19] or Internet gaming characteristics, such as the level of Internet usage, money spent on gaming, and type of game device [20]. A comprehensive approach based on both psychological factors and Internet gaming characteristics is needed to better understand IGD. Accordingly, the purpose of the present study was to identify risk factors that predict IGD, based on psychological factors and Internet gaming characteristics.

2. Materials and Methods

2.1. Participants

Online surveys were conducted using an existing survey company online panel (Hankook Research, Inc., Seoul, South Korea between 26 November and 26 December 2014. Online informed consent was obtained from all participants, prior to their participation. The online panel consisted of native Koreans aged 20–49 years, from metropolitan areas in South Korea. Among a total of 5003 respondents, 3881 Internet game users were identified. The final sample size comprised 3568 Internet game users, which did not include missing values.

Using the DSM-5 criteria to diagnose IGD is controversial [3,21]. Some researchers have attempted to overcome this confusion [21,22]. Because there are very few criteria for IGD in the DSM-5, it was used to evaluate IGD in the present study. In addition, DSM-5 criteria were validated from discussions among an expert group. Based on DSM-5 criteria, Internet game users with scores above 5 were evaluated as the IGD group [20,23]. Thus, in the final sample, there were 481 IGD gamers (13.48% of the sample) and 3087 normal Internet gamers (86.52%).

2.2. Measures and Procedure

Twenty independent variables were measured as potential risk factors for IGD. Independent variables consisted of participants' demographic characteristics, Internet gaming characteristics, and psychological variables.

In the case of Internet gaming characteristics, there were very few related studies, so related variables could not be chosen from the existing literature. Internet gaming characteristics were therefore derived from the Internet Addiction Survey 2013 conducted by the Korea National Information Society Agency [24]. The specific items were identified from discussions among an expert group. The expert group consisted of psychiatrists, psychologists, and data scientists of medical informatics who had more than 3 years' experience in addiction. Psychological variables were derived from previous research and were again collected from discussions among an expert group. The reliability of all variables was determined by the expert group.

Participants' demographic characteristics consisted of five factors: gender, age, job, score on the Alcohol Use Disorder Identification Test (AUDIT-K) [25], and score on the Fagerström Test for Nicotine Dependence (FTND) [26]. Participant data were divided into three groups based on AUDIT-K and FTND scores, as summarized in Appendix A (Table A1). The AUDIT-K is a ten-item questionnaire developed for male and female drinkers at a high risk of alcohol abuse. It is composed of three scores that are dependent on gender: male (0–9: normal drinker, 10–19: mild-to-moderate drinker, and $\geq$20: heavy drinker) and female (0–5: normal drinker, 6–9: mild-to-moderate drinker, and $\geq$10: heavy drinker). The FTND test is a six-item questionnaire designed to measure nicotine dependence. It is composed of three scores (0–3: low, 4–6: intermediate, and $\geq$7: high).

Seven Internet gaming characteristics were also measured: money spent on gaming, weekday game time, weekend game time, game device, game venue, offline game club attendance, and game club membership status.

Finally, eight psychological variables were measured, including the Dickman Impulsivity Inventory-Short Version (DII), Brief Self-Control Scale (BSCS) [27], Symptom Checklist-90-Revised (SCL-90-R) [28] and Behavioral Inhibition System/Behavioral Activation System (BIS/BAS) [29,30], as summarized in Table 1. The DII measures the personality trait of impulsivity [31]. The response options for each item are true (1) or false (0). The BSCS assesses dispositional self-control [27]. Each BSCS item is rated on a five-point scale, from 1 (strongly disagree) to 5 (strongly agree). The SCL-90-R consists of 90 items and assesses psychological distress [32,33]. Each of the items is rated on a five-point scale of distress, from 0 (no distress) to 4 (extreme distress). In the present study, 23 items from the SCL-90-R were adapted to evaluate depression (13 items) and anxiety (10 items).

The behavioral inhibition system (BIS) and a behavioral activation system (BAS) underlie behavior and affect [30]. The BIS scale estimates reactions to anticipated punishment and the BAS scale assesses positive responses to rewards. The BAS Drive scale estimates the pursuit of desired goals. The BAS Fun Seeking scale examines the tendency to seek and impulsively engage in potentially rewarding activities [30,34]. The BIS/BAS consists of a four-point scale, from 1 (not at all) to 4 (strongly agree). The total scores of the BIS/BAS scales range from zero to 80.

Questions related to cost, gaming time, and age were self-reported questions and free text which yielded a continuous value. The rest were multiple choice questions based on predefined categories.

Table 1. Description of Internet gaming characteristics and psychological factors.

	Variables	# of Items
Demographic characteristics	Gender, age, job	3
	AUDIT-K	10
	FTND	6
Internet gaming characteristics	Money spent on gaming (/month), Weekday game time (/day), Weekend game time (/day), Game device, Game venue, Offline game club attendance, Game club membership status	7
Psychological factors	DII	12
	BSCS	13
	SCL depression	13
	SCL anxiety	10
	BIS	7
	BAS reward responsiveness	5
	BAS drive	4
	BAS fun seeking	4

AUDIT-K: Alcohol Use Disorder Identification Test; FTND: Fagerström Test for Nicotine Dependence; DII: Dickman Impulsivity Inventory-Short Version; BSCS: Brief Self-Control Scale; SCL: Symptom Checklist; BIS: behavioral inhibition system; BAS: behavioral activation system.

2.3. Statistical Analysis

Out of 3881 respondents who identified as Internet game users, cases with missing responses were excluded, and all analyses were performed for 3568 respondents. We conducted t-tests and Chi-square tests to compare the IGD group to the control group in terms of demographic and Internet gaming characteristics. Multiple regression analysis was used to identify risk factors for the IGD group. The data were analyzed using SAS 9.4 (SAS Institute, Inc., Cary, NC, USA).

2.4. Ethics

The study procedures were carried out in accordance with the Declaration of Helsinki and were approved by the Institutional Review Board of Catholic University (IRB number: KC15EISI0103). Participants' data were de-identified.

3. Results

Out of 3568 participants, 481 (13.5%) were included in the IGD group and 3087 (86.5%) were included in the control group. The respondents' age ranged from 20 to 49, and 1559 (43.7%) were between the ages of 30 and 39. There were 2036 (57.1%) males and 1532 (42.9%) females (Table 2). Office workers and professional technicians comprised 67.8% of the sample, and college students comprised 15%. There were similar proportions of individuals in each group with a marital status of either single or married. There were no significant differences in demographic characteristics between the two groups; however, males were more likely to be in the IGD group than females. For income level, there were more people from the control group in the middle class, while low and high income classes showed slightly higher dependence.

Table 2. Participants' characteristics.

Variables		Total n (%)	IGD Group n (%)	Control Group n (%)	Chi-Square (p-Value)
Gender	Mal	2036 (57.1)	290 (60.3)	1746 (56.6)	2.36 (0.124)
	Female	1532 (42.9)	191 (39.7)	1341 (43.4)	
Age	20–29 years	1259 (35.3)	170 (35.3)	1089 (35.3)	0.43 (0.808)
	30–39 years	1559 (43.7)	215 (44.7)	1344 (43.5)	
	40–49 years	750 (21.0)	96 (20.0)	654 (21.2)	
Education	High school graduate or less	1053 (29.5)	134 (27.9)	919 (29.8)	0.76 (0.683)
	College graduate	2130 (59.7)	295 (61.3)	1835 (59.4)	
	Graduate school	385 (10.8)	52 (10.8)	333 (10.8)	
Job	Office worker, et al. [1]	2418 (67.8)	334 (69.4)	2084 (67.5)	0.86 (0.835)
	Student	535 (15.0)	67 (13.9)	468 (15.2)	
	etc.	217 (6.1)	27 (5.6)	190 (6.2)	
	Unemployed/housewife	398 (11.2)	53 (11.0)	345 (11.2)	
Marital status	Couple [2]	1867 (52.3)	241 (50.1)	1626 (52.7)	1.10 (0.294)
	Single [2]	1701 (47.7)	240 (49.9)	1461 (47.3)	
Income level	Low	1567 (43.9)	219 (45.5)	1348 (43.7)	3.52 (0.172)
	Middle	1557 (43.6)	193 (40.1)	1364 (44.2)	
	High	444 (12.4)	69 (14.3)	375 (12.2)	
	Total	3568 (100)	481 (13.5)	3087 (86.5)	

[1] Office worker et al.: office worker, administrative position, service industry, professional technician and production employee; [2] Single: never married, divorced, separated or widowed, Couple: married or living with a partner; IGD: Internet gaming disorder.

Differences in Internet gaming characteristics for all variables except game playing were significant between the IGD group and the control group (Table 3). Among all participants, 57.8% of the IGD group had a game club membership, while 35.4% of the control group had a game club membership. The respondents having a game club membership showed higher IGD than the control group (57.8% vs. 35.4%). Most of the Internet game users played at home, and there was no difference between the IGD group and control group (76.1% vs. 77.2%). In the case of playing in a gaming Internet cafe, the IGD group was much higher than the control group (17.5% vs. 10.2%). For game devices, the IGD group used a personal computer (PC) more than the control group (53.0% vs. 37.9%). For game partners, those playing with friends or online partners showed higher dependence than the control group (29.1% vs. 21.5%). Both the IGD and the control group had perceptions of addictiveness. For offline club game attendance, the IGD group's attendance was much higher than that of the control group (57.3% vs. 26.6%). For the onset of Internet games, 48.3% of respondents began in middle or high school. The IGD group spent more time gaming than the control group (2.85 vs. 1.97 h on weekdays and 4.12 vs. 2.92 h on weekends, respectively) and spent more money on gaming than the control group ($31.4 vs. $11.0, respectively).

Table 3. Internet gaming characteristics.

Variables		Total	IGD Group	Normal Group	Test Statistics
		n (%)	n (%)	n (%)	(p-Value)
Game club membership	No	2198 (61.6)	203 (42.2)	1995 (64.6)	88.45 (<0.001)
	Yes	1370 (38.4)	278 (57.8)	1092 (35.4)	
Game playing	Playing one game intensively	2098 (58.8)	302 (62.8)	1796 (58.2)	3.65 (0.056)
	Playing various games	1470 (41.2)	179 (37.2)	1291 (41.8)	
Game venue	Home	2748 (77.0)	366 (76.1)	2382 (77.2)	32.85 (<0.001)
	Gaming Internet cafe	400 (11.2)	84 (17.5)	316 (10.2)	
	Others [1]	420 (11.8)	31 (6.4)	389 (12.6)	
Game device	PC	1424 (39.9)	255 (53.0)	1169 (37.9)	42.39 (<0.001)
	Console	63 (1.8)	11 (2.3)	52 (1.7)	
	Mobile device [2]	2080 (58.3)	215 (44.7)	1865 (60.4)	
Game partner	Alone	2593 (72.7)	321 (66.7)	2272 (73.6)	14.07 (0.003)
	Family	169 (4.7)	20 (4.2)	149 (4.8)	
	Friends	280 (7.9)	52 (10.8)	228 (7.4)	
	Online partner	526 (14.7)	88 (18.3)	438 (14.2)	
Self-perceptions of addictiveness	Not at all	203 (5.7)	19 (4.0)	184 (6.0)	85.69 (<0.001)
	A little	1077 (30.2)	90 (18.7)	987 (32.0)	
	Much	1979 (55.5)	285 (59.3)	1694 (54.9)	
	Very much	309 (8.7)	87 (18.1)	222 (7.2)	
Offline game club attendance	Not attend	2469 (69.2)	205 (42.6)	2264 (73.3)	185.63 (<0.001)
	Sometimes	1032 (28.9)	256 (53.2)	776 (25.1)	
	Very often	67 (1.9)	20 (4.2)	47 (1.5)	
Onset of Internet game	Under middle school	842 (23.6)	122 (25.4)	720 (23.3)	11.42 (0.009)
	Middle or high school	882 (24.72)	142 (29.5)	740 (24.0)	
	After graduating high school	1056 (29.6)	131 (27.2)	925 (30.0)	
	30s or 40s	788 (22.09)	86 (17.9)	702 (22.7)	
Gaming time/day	Weekdays	2.09	2.85	1.97	7.21 (<0.001)
	Weekends and holidays	3.08	4.12	2.92	7.19 (<0.001)
	Maximum	4.07	5.93	3.78	6.30 (<0.001)
Money spent on gaming/month		$13.76	$31.36	$11.02	8.23 (<0.001)

Time unit: hours, the exchange rate for Korean won to the U.S. dollar is 1100.00 won (September 2016), t-statistics for continuous variable, and chi-square value for categorical variables. [1] Others: School, play station room, the outside including bus, substation; [2] Mobile device: Smartphone and Tablet.

Risk Factors Predicting IGD

The results of the multivariate logistic regression analysis are shown in Table 4. Firstly, demographic characteristics were shown not to be risk factors. All variables included in the logistic regression model do not show muliticollinearity. Secondly, with regard to Internet gaming characteristics, money spent on gaming (OR = 1.005), weekday game time (OR = 1.081), offline game club attendance (OR = 2.060), and game club membership status (OR = 1.393) were significant behavioral factors predicting IGD. Thirdly, DII (OR = 1.138), BSCS (OR = 1.034), anxiety (OR = 1.086), and BAS-Drive (OR = 1.105) were significant psychological predictors of IGD. Those who had one unit score higher for DII were 1.138 times more likely to be dependent. Additionally, with one unit score higher for the BSCS, Anxiety, and BAS-Drive factors, the probability of dependence increased by 1.034, 1.086, and 1.105 times, respectively. One of measures for model performance in a general linear model, Nagelkerke's R^2 is 0.3012 which showed it was a better model than others [35].

Table 4. Risk factors predicting IGD.

	Variables	Estimate (SE)		p-Value	OR 95% CI
	Intercept	−5.452 (0.602)			-
	Gender	0.023 (0.139)		0.869	1.023 (0.779–1.344)
	Age	0.138	0.090	0.125	1.148 (0.962–1.37)
Job	Office worker, et al. [1]	−0.167	0.193	0.387	0.846 (0.579–1.236)
	Student	−0.017	0.248	0.944	0.983 (0.604–1.599)
	etc.	−0.260	0.291	0.373	0.771 (0.436–1.365)
AUDIT	Normal drinker	−0.136	0.163	0.404	0.873 (0.634–1.201)
	Mild-to-moderate drinker	−0.313	0.166	0.059	0.731 (0.528–1.012)
	Heavy drinker	0.171	0.161	0.289	1.186 (0.865–1.626)
FTND	Low	−0.201	0.171	0.240	0.818 (0.585–1.144)
	Intermediate	0.177	0.195	0.362	1.194 (0.815–1.748)
	High	0.358	0.307	0.243	1.431 (0.784–2.611)
	Money spent on gaming ***	0.005	0.002	<0.001 ***	1.005 (1.002–1.008)
	Weekday game time ***	0.078	0.027	0.003 ***	1.081 (1.026–1.139)
	Weekend game time	0.004	0.019	0.843	1.004 (0.968–1.041)
Game device	PC	0.160	0.132	0.224	1.174 (0.907–1.519)
	Console	0.239	0.413	0.563	1.270 (0.565–2.853)
Game venue	Home	0.324	0.217	0.135	1.383 (0.905–2.114)
	Gaming Internet cafe	0.282	0.270	0.296	1.326 (0.781–2.25)
	Offline game club attendance ***	0.723	0.130	<0.001 ***	2.060 (1.597–2.658)
	Game club membership status **	0.332	0.125	0.008 **	1.393 (1.09–1.78)
	DII ***	0.129	0.022	<0.001 ***	1.138 (1.09–1.188)
	BSCS **	0.034	0.012	0.006 **	1.034 (1.01–1.059)
	SCL Depression	−0.008	0.012	0.496	0.992 (0.968–1.016)
	SCL Anxiety ***	0.082	0.015	<0.001 ***	1.086 (1.054–1.118)
	BIS	−0.031	0.025	0.215	0.969 (0.923–1.018)
	BAS reward responsiveness	0.005	0.039	0.908	1.005 (0.93–1.085)
	BAS drive *	0.100	0.041	0.015 *	1.105 (1.02–1.198)
	BAS fun seeking	−0.063	0.042	0.133	0.939 (0.865–1.019)

SE: standard error; * $p < 0.1$, ** $p < 0.05$, *** $p < 0.01$; [1] Office worker, et al.: office worker, administrative position, service industry, professional technician and Production employee.

4. Discussion

We identified risk factors predicting IGD, specifically examining psychological and Internet gaming characteristics as potential risk factors. Based on the results of the present study, we draw the following conclusions.

Firstly, examination of psychological factors yielded meaningful results. Users with IGD perceived themselves as being obsessed with Internet gaming (Table 3) and that they had difficulty quitting the game. Thus, social support may be needed to prevent IGD and support treatment efforts. Psychological risk factors related to IGD included impulsivity, low self-control, anxiety, and pursuit of desired appetitive goals. Past research has shown that IGD has similarities to other addictions, such as gambling and substance use disorder [18,36,37]. In particular, impulsivity and self-control are important psychological factors affecting addiction [38,39]. Impulsivity has been reported as a risk factor in addiction to social networking sites or smartphones [29,40] and lack of self-control is related to addictions such as substance use disorder [27] and Internet use [41–43]. Anxiety may be relevant psychopathological symptom to detect Internet, smartphone, and video game addiction [44–46]. Lastly, BAS Drive was a risk factor associated with IGD. The level of BAS Drive represents the tendency to pursue desired goals actively [34] and has been shown to be one of the personality factors associated with smartphone addiction [29]. This shows that to predict and diagnose IGD, research on the associated psychological risk factors is needed.

Secondly, a number of Internet gaming characteristics were significant in predicting IGD. Users with IGD mainly played games at home. In the case of playing games in a gaming Internet cafe, the proportion of individuals with dependence was higher than normal (17.5% vs. 10.2%). Game users mainly played using a PC compared to a mobile device (53.0% vs. 37.9%) since high specification desktops were needed. However, the control group played games more frequently using mobile devices compared to PCs. With regard to the onset of Internet gaming, 48.3% of respondents began in middle or high school. Users with IGD tended to start playing Internet games at a relatively early age. This finding suggests that early initiation of game playing may be a risk factor for IGD. Accordingly, diverse approaches are needed early on to prevent adolescent and adult IGD. Offline game club attendance and game club membership status were also risk factors for IGD. Users with IGD were more likely to be game club members than those in the control group (57.3% vs. 26.6%) and were more likely to attend offline clubs, with 73.3% of the control group having never attended offline game meetings. On average, users with IGD were thought to have no social relationships and to be more isolated. However, they did attend offline game clubs and have game club memberships. There were some social users with IGD.

Additional risk factors of IGD were money spent on gaming and weekday game time. In the case of game time, Internet game users spent an average of 2.09 h on weekends playing games. Users with IGD spent more time than normal gamers playing Internet games (2.85 vs. 1.97 h on weekdays and 4.12 vs. 2.92 h on weekends). According to the Ministry of Science ICT and Future Planning (MSIP) report, Korean gamers spent an average of 1.1 h on weekends playing games. Users with Internet over-dependence spent 0.3 more hours playing on weekends than normal users (1.4 vs. 1.1 h) [47]. The results from our study show that game time was higher in our sample. The MSIP report focused on individuals ranging in age from early childhood (3 years) to 59 years whereas our results came from a sample of adults between the ages of 20 and 49. This higher game time suggests that IGD is more serious in adults. Users with IGD spent more money on gaming than the control group ($31.4 vs. $11.0). Previous research has reported that spending extreme amounts of time and money is a predictor of IGD [20,48–52]. Lo et al., (2005) found that the amount of time spent playing online games is directly correlated with levels of social anxiety [50]. Rau et al., (2006) proposed that many game players have difficulty in controlling game time [49]. Accordingly, approaches are needed for IGD among adults and controlling time and money is important to preventing and managing IGD.

5. Conclusions

This study had several limitations. Data on Internet gaming characteristics were self-reported, including money spent on gaming, weekday game time, and weekend game time. If technology could be developed, such as the Smartphone Overdependence Management System (SOMS), to collect time or money data automatically [53], future research may provide more accurate and realistic results. We collected data using an online survey. This was based on an existing online panel from a survey company. Online panel respondents were native Koreans aged 20–49 years, from metropolitan areas in South Korea. Using an online survey based on an existing panel was a useful way to collect a large amount of data; however, this may have resulted in some recruitment bias. Future research should involve data collected from the entire Korea area. The present study was designed to be cross-sectional because it is difficult to collect time-series data from Internet gamers. As a result, our findings are limited in their ability to reflect fast-changing Internet gaming trends. Future research could incorporate time-series data from longitudinal studies. Future research could also involve a more accurate diagnosis of IGD based on a clinical interview. The results showed that depression has no significant relationship with IGD. This is contrary to other published studies that have found video or internet game addiction to be related to depression [10,45,54]. We used the SCL-90-L to evaluate depression; however, there are many other scales to measure depression, such as the 21-item Depression Anxiety Stress Scale (DASS-21) [55] and the Hopkins Symptom Checklist (HSCL) [56]. Future studies should evaluate depression using other measures. This study targeted respondents aged between 20 and 49, of which 1559 (43.7%) were between the ages of 30 and 39. Therefore, the reported results could be influenced by demographic characteristics.

Despite these limitations, the present study yielded a valuable contribution to our understanding of risk factors for IGD by using a comprehensive approach based on psychological factors and Internet gaming characteristics. These findings can be used to develop clinical services for the diagnosis and treatment of IGD.

Acknowledgments: This research was supported by the Brain Research Program through the National Research Foundation of Korea (NRF) funded by the Ministry of Science, ICT & Future Planning (NRF-2014M3C7A1062893). In addition, this research by Hyeseon Lee partially was supported by the Basic Science Research Program through the National Research Foundation of Korea (NRF-2017R1A2B4002944).

Author Contributions: All authors participated in the study concept and design. Hyeseon Lee and Taek-Ho Lee performed the statistical analysis. Mi Jung Rho performed interpretation of the data and drafted the manuscript. Hyun Cho and DongJin Jung participated in collecting the data. In Young Choi and Dai-Jin Kim participated in the study supervision.

Appendix A

Table A1. Criteria and score in the AUDIT and the FTND tests.

Category	AUDIT Test		FTND Test	
	Male	Female	Category	Score
	Score			
Normal drinker	≤9	≤5	Low risk	≤3
Mild-to-moderate drinker	10~19	6~9	Intermediate risk	4~6
Heavy drinker	≥20	≥10	High risk	≥7

References

1. Kuss, D.J. Internet gaming addiction: Current perspectives. *Psychol. Res. Behav. Manag.* **2013**, *6*, 125–137. [CrossRef] [PubMed]
2. Entertainment software association (ESA). *2015 Essential Facts about the Computer and Video Game Industry*; ESA: Washington, DC, USA, 2015.
3. Aarseth, E.; Bean, A.M.; Boonen, H.; Colder Carras, M.; Coulson, M.; Das, D.; Deleuze, J.; Dunkels, E.; Edman, J.; Ferguson, C.J. Scholars' open debate paper on the world health organization ICD-11 gaming disorder proposal. *J. Behav. Addict.* **2017**, *6*, 267–270. [CrossRef] [PubMed]
4. Choi, S.-W.; Kim, H.; Kim, G.-Y.; Jeon, Y.; Park, S.; Lee, J.-Y.; Jung, H.; Sohn, B.; Choi, J.-S.; Kim, D.-J. Similarities and differences among internet gaming disorder, gambling disorder and alcohol use disorder: A focus on impulsivity and compulsivity. *J. Behav. Addict.* **2014**, *3*, 246–253. [CrossRef] [PubMed]
5. Na, E.; Lee, H.; Choi, I.; Kim, D.J. Comorbidity of internet gaming disorder and alcohol use disorder: A focus on clinical characteristics and gaming patterns. *Am. J. Addict.* **2017**, *26*, 326–334. [CrossRef] [PubMed]
6. Cho, H.; Kwon, M.; Choi, J.-H.; Lee, S.-K.; Choi, J.S.; Choi, S.-W.; Kim, D.-J. Development of the internet addiction scale based on the internet gaming disorder criteria suggested in DSM-5. *Addict. Behav.* **2014**, *39*, 1361–1366. [CrossRef] [PubMed]

7. Demetrovics, Z.; Urbán, R.; Nagygyörgy, K.; Farkas, J.; Griffiths, M.D.; Pápay, O.; Kökönyei, G.; Felvinczi, K.; Oláh, A. The development of the problematic online gaming questionnaire (POGQ). *PLoS ONE* **2012**, *7*, e36417. [CrossRef] [PubMed]

8. Petry, N.M.; O'brien, C.P. Internet gaming disorder and the DSM-5. *Addiction* **2013**, *108*, 1186–1187. [CrossRef] [PubMed]

9. Männikkö, N.; Billieux, J.; Kääriäinen, M. Problematic digital gaming behavior and its relation to the psychological, social and physical health of finnish adolescents and young adults. *J. Behav. Addict.* **2015**, *4*, 281–288. [CrossRef] [PubMed]

10. Brunborg, G.S.; Mentzoni, R.A.; Frøyland, L.R. Is video gaming, or video game addiction, associated with depression, academic achievement, heavy episodic drinking, or conduct problems? *J. Behav. Addict.* **2014**, *3*, 27–32. [CrossRef] [PubMed]

11. Van Rooij, A.J.; Kuss, D.J.; Griffiths, M.D.; Shorter, G.W.; Schoenmakers, T.M.; Van de Mheen, D. The (co-) occurrence of problematic video gaming, substance use, and psychosocial problems in adolescents. *J. Behav. Addict.* **2014**, *3*, 157–165. [CrossRef] [PubMed]

12. Park, J.H.; Han, D.H.; Kim, B.-N.; Cheong, J.H.; Lee, Y.-S. Correlations among social anxiety, self-esteem, impulsivity, and game genre in patients with problematic online game playing. *Psychiatry Investig.* **2016**, *13*, 297–304. [CrossRef] [PubMed]

13. Kardefelt-Winther, D. A conceptual and methodological critique of internet addiction research: Towards a model of compensatory internet use. *Comput. Hum. Behav.* **2014**, *31*, 351–354. [CrossRef]

14. Lemmens, J.S.; Valkenburg, P.M.; Peter, J. Psychosocial causes and consequences of pathological gaming. *Comput. Hum. Behav.* **2011**, *27*, 144–152. [CrossRef]

15. Liu, M.; Peng, W. Cognitive and psychological predictors of the negative outcomes associated with playing mmogs (massively multiplayer online games). *Comput. Hum. Behav.* **2009**, *25*, 1306–1311. [CrossRef]

16. Caplan, S.E. Relations among loneliness, social anxiety, and problematic internet use. *Cyberpsychol. Behav.* **2006**, *10*, 234–242. [CrossRef] [PubMed]

17. Kuss, D.J.; Griffiths, M.D. Internet gaming addiction: A systematic review of empirical research. *Int. J. Ment. Health Addict.* **2012**, *10*, 278–296. [CrossRef]

18. Kardefelt-Winther, D. A critical account of DSM-5 criteria for internet gaming disorder. *Addict. Res. Theory* **2015**, *23*, 93–98. [CrossRef]

19. Hyun, G.J.; Han, D.H.; Lee, Y.S.; Kang, K.D.; Yoo, S.K.; Chung, U.-S.; Renshaw, P.F. Risk factors associated with online game addiction: A hierarchical model. *Comput. Hum. Behav.* **2015**, *48*, 706–713. [CrossRef]

20. Rho, M.J.; Jeong, J.-E.; Chun, J.-W.; Cho, H.; Jung, D.J.; Choi, I.Y.; Kim, D.-J. Predictors and patterns of problematic internet game use using a decision tree model. *J. Behav. Addict.* **2016**, *5*, 500–509. [CrossRef] [PubMed]

21. Kuss, D.J.; Griffiths, M.D.; Pontes, H.M. Chaos and confusion in DSM-5 diagnosis of internet gaming disorder: Issues, concerns, and recommendations for clarity in the field. *J. Behav. Addict.* **2017**, *6*, 103–109. [CrossRef] [PubMed]

22. Kuss, D.J.; Griffiths, M.D.; Pontes, H.M. DSM-5 diagnosis of internet gaming disorder: Some ways forward in overcoming issues and concerns in the gaming studies field: Response to the commentaries. *J. Behav. Addict.* **2017**, *6*, 133–141. [CrossRef] [PubMed]

23. Petry, N.M.; Rehbein, F.; Gentile, D.A.; Lemmens, J.S.; Rumpf, H.J.; Mößle, T.; Bischof, G.; Tao, R.; Fung, D.S.; Borges, G. An international consensus for assessing internet gaming disorder using the new DSM-5 approach. *Addiction* **2014**, *109*, 1399–1406. [CrossRef] [PubMed]

24. Agency, N.I.A. *Internet Addiction Survey*; NIA: Daegu Metropolitan City, South Korea, 2013.

25. Lee, B.; Lee, C.; Lee, P.; Choi, M.; Namkoong, K. Development of korean version of alcohol use disorders identification test (AUDIT-K): Its reliability and validity. *J. Korean Acad. Addict. Psychiatry* **2000**, *4*, 83–92.

26. Fagerstrom, K.-O.; Schneider, N.G. Measuring nicotine dependence: A review of the fagerstrom tolerance questionnaire. *J. Behav. Med.* **1989**, *12*, 159–182. [CrossRef] [PubMed]

27. Tangney, J.P.; Baumeister, R.F.; Boone, A.L. High self-control predicts good adjustment, less pathology, better grades, and interpersonal success. *J. Personal.* **2004**, *72*, 271–324. [CrossRef]

28. Derogatis, L. *Manual for the Symptom Checklist 90 Revised (SCL-90-R)*; The Johns Hopkins University School of Medicine: Baltimore, MD, USA, 1986.

29. Kim, Y.; Jeong, J.-E.; Cho, H.; Jung, D.-J.; Kwak, M.; Rho, M.J.; Yu, H.; Kim, D.-J.; Choi, I.Y. Personality factors predicting smartphone addiction predisposition: Behavioral inhibition and activation systems, impulsivity, and self-control. *PLoS ONE* **2016**, *11*, e0159788. [CrossRef] [PubMed]

30. Carver, C.S.; White, T.L. Behavioral inhibition, behavioral activation, and affective responses to impending reward and punishment: The BIS/BAS scales. *J. Personal. Soc. Psychol.* **1994**, *67*, 319–333. [CrossRef]

31. Dickman, S.J. Functional and dysfunctional impulsivity: Personality and cognitive correlates. *J. Personal. Soc. Psychol.* **1990**, *58*, 95–102. [CrossRef]

32. Franke, G. *SCL-90-R: Die Symptom-Check-Liste von Derogatis-Deutsche Version*; Beltz Test Gesellschaft Google Scholar: Göttingen, Germany, 1995.

33. Derogatis, L.R.; Cleary, P.A. Factorial invariance across gender for the primary symptom dimensions of the SCL-90. *Br. J. Soc. Clin. Psychol.* **1977**, *16*, 347–356. [CrossRef] [PubMed]

34. Gray, J.A.; McNaughton, N. *The Neuropsychology of Anxiety: An Enquiry into the Function of the Septo-Hippocampal System*; Oxford University Press: Oxford, UK, 2003.

35. Nagelkerke, N.J.D. A note on a general definition of the coefficient of determination. *Biometrika* **1991**, *78*, 691–692. [CrossRef]

36. Kaptsis, D.; King, D.L.; Delfabbro, P.H.; Gradisar, M. Withdrawal symptoms in internet gaming disorder: A systematic review. *Clin. Psychol. Rev.* **2016**, *43*, 58–66. [CrossRef] [PubMed]

37. Yen, J.Y.; Ko, C.H.; Yen, C.F.; Chen, S.H.; Chung, W.L.; Chen, C.C. Psychiatric symptoms in adolescents with internet addiction: Comparison with substance use. *Psychiatry Clin. Neurosci.* **2008**, *62*, 9–16. [CrossRef] [PubMed]

38. Reynolds, B.; Ortengren, A.; Richards, J.B.; de Wit, H. Dimensions of impulsive behavior: Personality and behavioral measures. *Personal. Individ. Differ.* **2006**, *40*, 305–315. [CrossRef]

39. Baumeister, R.F. Ego depletion and self-regulation failure: A resource model of self-control. *Alcohol. Clin. Exp. Res.* **2003**, *27*, 281–284. [CrossRef] [PubMed]

40. Wu, A.M.; Cheung, V.I.; Ku, L.; Hung, E.P. Psychological risk factors of addiction to social networking sites among chinese smartphone users. *J. Behav. Addict.* **2013**, *2*, 160–166. [CrossRef] [PubMed]

41. Mei, S.; Yau, Y.H.; Chai, J.; Guo, J.; Potenza, M.N. Problematic internet use, well-being, self-esteem and self-control: Data from a high-school survey in china. *Addict. Behav.* **2016**, *61*, 74–79. [CrossRef] [PubMed]

42. LaRose, R.; Lin, C.A.; Eastin, M.S. Unregulated internet usage: Addiction, habit, or deficient self-regulation? *Media Psychol.* **2003**, *5*, 225–253. [CrossRef]

43. Park, J.-A.; Park, M.-H.; Shin, J.-H.; Li, B.; Rolfe, D.T.; Yoo, J.-Y.; Dittmore, S.W. Effect of sports participation on internet addiction mediated by self-control: A case of korean adolescents. *Kasetsart J. Soc. Sci.* **2016**, *37*, 164–169. [CrossRef]

44. Tonioni, F.; D'Alessandris, L.; Lai, C.; Martinelli, D.; Corvino, S.; Vasale, M.; Fanella, F.; Aceto, P.; Bria, P. Internet addiction: Hours spent online, behaviors and psychological symptoms. *Gen. Hosp. Psychiatry* **2012**, *34*, 80–87. [CrossRef] [PubMed]

45. Loton, D.; Borkoles, E.; Lubman, D.; Polman, R. Video game addiction, engagement and symptoms of stress, depression and anxiety: The mediating role of coping. *Int. J. Mental Health Addict.* **2016**, *14*, 565–578. [CrossRef]

46. Elhai, J.D.; Dvorak, R.D.; Levine, J.C.; Hall, B.J. Problematic smartphone use: A conceptual overview and systematic review of relations with anxiety and depression psychopathology. *J. Affect. Disord.* **2017**, *207*, 251–259. [CrossRef] [PubMed]

47. The Ministry of Science and ICT. *(The) 2015 Survey on Internet Overdependence*; The Ministry of Science and ICT: Gwacheon-si, Korea, 2016.

48. Allison, S.E.; von Wahlde, L.; Shockley, T.; Gabbard, G.O. The development of the self in the era of the internet and role-playing fantasy games. *Am. J. Psychiatry* **2006**, *163*, 381–385. [CrossRef] [PubMed]

49. Rau, P.-L.P.; Peng, S.-Y.; Yang, C.-C. Time distortion for expert and novice online game players. *Cyberpsychol. Behav.* **2006**, *9*, 396–403. [CrossRef] [PubMed]

50. Lo, S.-K.; Wang, C.-C.; Fang, W. Physical interpersonal relationships and social anxiety among online game players. *Cyberpsychol. Behav.* **2005**, *8*, 15–20. [CrossRef] [PubMed]

51. Wood, R.T.; Griffiths, M.D.; Parke, A. Experiences of time loss among videogame players: An empirical study. *Cyberpsychol. Behav.* **2007**, *10*, 38–44. [CrossRef] [PubMed]

52. Wood, R.T.; Griffiths, M.D. Time loss whilst playing video games: Is there a relationship to addictive behaviours? *Int. J. Ment. Health Addict.* **2007**, *5*, 141–149. [CrossRef]

53. Lee, S.-J.; Rho, M.J.; Yook, I.H.; Park, S.-H.; Jang, K.-S.; Park, B.-J.; Lee, O.; Lee, D.K.; Kim, D.-J.; Choi, I.Y. Design, development and implementation of a smartphone overdependence management system for the self-control of smart devices. *Appl. Sci.* **2016**, *6*, 440. [CrossRef]

54. Kim, D.J.; Kim, K.; Lee, H.-W.; Hong, J.-P.; Cho, M.J.; Fava, M.; Mischoulon, D.; Heo, J.-Y.; Jeon, H.J. Internet game addiction, depression, and escape from negative emotions in adulthood: A nationwide community sample of korea. *J. Nerv. Ment. Dis.* **2017**, *205*, 568–573. [CrossRef] [PubMed]

55. Lovibond, P.F.; Lovibond, S.H. The structure of negative emotional states: Comparison of the depression anxiety stress scales (DASS) with the beck depression and anxiety inventories. *Behav. Res. Ther.* **1995**, *33*, 335–343. [CrossRef]

56. Derogatis, L.R.; Lipman, R.S.; Rickels, K.; Uhlenhuth, E.H.; Covi, L. The hopkins symptom checklist (HSCL): A self-report symptom inventory. *Syst. Res. Behav. Sci.* **1974**, *19*, 1–15. [CrossRef]

14

Measurement Invariance of the Short Version of the Problematic Mobile Phone Use Questionnaire (PMPUQ-SV) across Eight Languages

Olatz Lopez-Fernandez [1,2,*], Daria J. Kuss [1], Halley M. Pontes [1], Mark D. Griffiths [1], Christopher Dawes [1], Lucy V. Justice [1], Niko Männikkö [3], Maria Kääriäinen [4], Hans-Jürgen Rumpf [5], Anja Bischof [5], Ann-Kathrin Gässler [5], Lucia Romo [6], Laurence Kern [7], Yannick Morvan [6], Amélie Rousseau [8], Pierluigi Graziani [9,10], Zsolt Demetrovics [11], Orsolya Király [11], Adriano Schimmenti [12], Alessia Passanisi [12], Bernadeta Lelonek-Kuleta [13], Joanna Chwaszcz [14], Mariano Chóliz [15], Juan José Zacarés [16], Emilia Serra [16], Magali Dufour [17], Lucien Rochat [18], Daniele Zullino [19,20], Sophia Achab [19,20], Nils Inge Landrø [21], Eva Suryani [22], Julia M. Hormes [23], Javier Ponce Terashima [24] and Joël Billieux [2,20,25]

[1] International Gaming Research Unit, Psychology Department, Nottingham Trent University, Nottingham NG1 4FQ, UK; daria.kuss@ntu.ac.uk (D.J.K.); halleypontes@gmail.com (H.M.P.); mark.griffiths@ntu.ac.uk (M.D.G.); lpxcad@nottingham.ac.uk (C.D.); lucy.justice@ntu.ac.uk (L.V.J.)

[2] Laboratory for Experimental Psychopathology, Psychological Sciences Research Institute, Université Catholique de Louvain, 1348 Louvain-la-Neuve, Belgium; joel.billieux@uni.lu

[3] Department of Social Services and Rehabilitation, Oulu University of Applied Sciences, 90220 Oulu, Finland; niko.mannikko@oamk.fi

[4] Research Unit of Nursing Science and Health Management, University of Oulu and Oulu University Hospital, 90014 Oulu, Finland; maria.kaariainen@oulu.fi

[5] Department for Psychiatry and Psychotherapy, University of Lübeck, 23538 Lübeck, Germany; Hans-Juergen.Rumpf@uksh.de (H.-J.R.); Anja.Bischof@uksh.de (A.B.); akgaessler@outlook.de (A.-K.G.)

[6] EA 4430 Clinique Psychanalyse Développement (CLIPSYD), Université Paris Nanterre, France; U894 Centre de Psychiatrie et Neurosciences, (CPN), Inserm, 92000 Paris, France; romodesprez@gmail.com (L.R.); ymorvan@parisnanterre.fr (Y.M.)

[7] EA 2931, Centre de Recherches sur le Sport et le Mouvement (CESRM), Université Paris Nanterre, 92000 Nanterre, France; laurence.kern@gmail.com

[8] Psychology Department, PSITEC EA 4074, Université Lille Nord de France, 59650 Villeneuve d'Ascq, France; amelie.rousseau@univ-lille3.fr

[9] LPS EA 849, Aix-Marseille University, 13007 Marseille, France; pierluigi.graziani@free.fr

[10] Psychologie, Langues, Lettres et Histoire Département, University of Nîmes, 30000 Nîmes, France; pierluigi.graziani@free.fr

[11] Institute of Psychology, ELTE Eötvös Loránd University, 1064 Budapest, Hungary; demetrovics@t-online.hu (Z.D.); orsolya.papay@gmail.com or kiraly.orsolya@ppk.elte.hu (O.K.)

[12] Faculty of Human and Social Sciences, UKE—Kore University of Enna, Cittadella Universitaria, 94100 Enna, Italy; adriano.schimmenti@unikore.it (A.S.); alessia.passanisi@unikore.it (A.P.)

[13] Department of Family Science and Social Work, Katolicki Uniwersytet Lubelski Jana Pawła II, 20-950 Lublin, Poland; bernadetalelonek@kul.lublin.pl

[14] Department of Psychology, Katolicki Uniwersytet Lubelski Jana Pawła II, 20-950 Lublin, Poland; chwaszcz@kul.pl

[15] Department of Basic Psychology, University of Valencia, 46010 Valencia, Spain; Mariano.Choliz@uv.es

[16] Department of Developmental and Educational Psychology, University of Valencia, 46010 Valencia, Spain; Juan.J.Zacares@uv.es (J.J.Z.); Emilia.Serra@uv.es (E.S.)

[17] Service de Toxicomanie, Faculte de medicine Université de Sherbrooke, Longueuil, Qc, J4K 0A8, Canada; magali.dufour@usherbrooke.ca

[18] Department of Psychology and Educational Sciences, University of Geneva, 1205 Geneva, Switzerland; Lucien.Rochat@unige.ch

[19] Department of Psychiatry—Research Unit Addictive Disorders, University of Geneva, 1205 Geneva, Switzerland; Daniele.Zullino@hcuge.ch (D.Z.); Sophia.Achab@hcuge.ch (S.A.)

20   Department of Mental Health and Psychiatry—Addiction Division, University Hospitals of Geneva, 1205 Geneva, Switzerland

21   Clinical Neuroscience Research Group, Department of Psychology, University of Oslo, 0317 Oslo, Norway; n.i.landro@psykologi.uio.no

22   Department Psychiatry and Behavior, School of Medicine and Health Science, Atma Jaya Catholic University of Indonesia, Jakarta 14440, Indonesia; eva.suryani@atmajaya.ac.id or amyeva511@gmail.com

23   Department of Psychology, University at Albany State University of New York, Albany, NY, USA; jhormes@albany.edu

24   University Hospitals Cleveland Medical Center/Case Western Reserve University, Cleveland, OH 44106, USA; javier@incaas.org

25   Addictive and Compulsive Behaviours Lab (ACB-lab), Institute for Health and Behaviour, University of Luxembourg, 4366 Esch-sur-Alzette, Luxembourg

*   Correspondence: olatz.lopez-fernandez@ntu.ac.uk or lopez.olatz@gmail.com

Abstract: The prevalence of mobile phone use across the world has increased greatly over the past two decades. Problematic Mobile Phone Use (PMPU) has been studied in relation to public health and comprises various behaviours, including dangerous, prohibited, and dependent use. These types of problematic mobile phone behaviours are typically assessed with the short version of the Problematic Mobile Phone Use Questionnaire (PMPUQ–SV). However, to date, no study has ever examined the degree to which the PMPU scale assesses the same construct across different languages. The aims of the present study were to (i) determine an optimal factor structure for the PMPUQ–SV among university populations using eight versions of the scale (i.e., French, German, Hungarian, English, Finnish, Italian, Polish, and Spanish); and (ii) simultaneously examine the measurement invariance (MI) of the PMPUQ–SV across all languages. The whole study sample comprised 3038 participants. Descriptive statistics, correlations, and Cronbach's alpha coefficients were extracted from the demographic and PMPUQ-SV items. Individual and multigroup confirmatory factor analyses alongside MI analyses were conducted. Results showed a similar pattern of PMPU across the translated scales. A three-factor model of the PMPUQ-SV fitted the data well and presented with good psychometric properties. Six languages were validated independently, and five were compared via measurement invariance for future cross-cultural comparisons. The present paper contributes to the assessment of problematic mobile phone use because it is the first study to provide a cross-cultural psychometric analysis of the PMPUQ-SV.

Keywords: mobile phone use; smartphone use; Problematic Mobile Phone Use; Problematic Mobile Phone Use Questionnaire; psychometric testing; measurement invariance

---

1. Introduction

Mobile phones have become a ubiquitous technology and their use is widespread internationally. However, there appear to be differences in terms of technology use across various geographical regions according to the International Telecommunication Union (ITU). Recently, ITU Facts and Figures 2017 [1] demonstrated that mobile phone use has experienced the largest growth compared with other technologies over the last two decades. More specifically, worldwide mobile phone subscriptions per 100 inhabitants were 15.5 in 2001, 76.6 in 2010, and 103.5 in 2017. At the same time, subscriptions for landline telephones were 16.6 in 2001, 17.8 in 2010, and 13 in 2017. According to a study by ProQuest [2], the number of scientific papers and reports published on this topic has grown markedly. The study examined 26 scientific databases simultaneously (e.g., PsycINFO) using the search terms "mobile phone" or "cell* phone" and "smartphone". It was reported that 490 academic outputs were published in 2001, 3225 in 2010, and 8224 in 2017 (these results referred to scholarly peer-reviewed journal articles, as well as trade journals, magazines, conference proceedings, and other reports).

Negative aspects related to mobile phone use are often conceptualised within the umbrella term of Problematic Mobile Phone Use (PMPU; [3,4]). According to Billieux and colleagues [4–7], PMPU can be understood as a heterogeneous and multidimensional construct involving the potential negative effects of mobile phone use. Accordingly, these authors formulated an integrative pathway model to account for the various types of problematic mobile phone use (i.e., dangerous, prohibited/antisocial, and dependent). Based on this model, each pathway to mobile phone overuse (i.e., extraversion pathway, reassurance-seeking pathway, impulsive pathway) is underlain by specific psychosocial factors and individual differences. Although maladaptive mobile phone use was initially considered a public health issue in child and adolescent populations [8–11], over the past decade, mobile phone use has been considered to involve potential risks for all populations across the different dimensions of problematic use, namely dangerous, prohibited, or dependent use [4].

Regarding general health issues traditionally associated with mobile phone use, several studies have shown significant associations between mobile phone use and users' lifestyles and wellbeing. For example, Ezoe and colleagues [11] found that PMPU among Japanese female college students was associated with poor sleep, low physical activity, decreased work performance, and skipping breakfast. Similarly, Gallimberti and colleagues [12] observed that reading books, higher school marks, and longer hours of sleep were associated with low PMPU in Italian adolescents. Conversely, and in line with previous studies, other authors have reported PMPU to be positively associated with stress, depression, sleep disturbances, extraversion, female gender, young age, and poor academic or professional competence or performance [13–22]. Furthermore, Yang and colleagues [13] investigated the health and psychological problems associated with mobile phone use in adolescent Southern Taiwanese students and found that PMPU was associated with aggression, insomnia, smoking, suicidal tendencies, and low self-esteem.

For instance, two studies analysing young Swedish adults' perceptions of the need of being available at all times via their mobile phones [14,15] reported that mobile phone use was positively associated with stress, depression, and sleep disorders. Similarly, a recent systematic review carried out by Elhai and colleagues [16] found that PMPU was usually related to depression, anxiety, chronic stress, and low self-esteem. However, only depression and anxiety were consistently related to this problematic use, with medium and small effect sizes, respectively. In another paper, the same authors even stated that while depression was inversely associated with social PMPU (e.g., social networking, messaging), anxiety was positively related to problematic use as a process or being consumption-based (e.g., news consumption, entertainment, relaxation) [17].

Associated behaviours, such as dependency and/or compulsiveness, have also been reported when individuals check their phone display, and even when not interacting with their mobile phone directly. This is because auditory and/or tactile notifications prompt thoughts that affect attention, and which negatively impact on performance [18] (a phenomenon coined as 'technoference'; such use of mobile phones results in conflicts in interpersonal relationships and decreased wellbeing [19]). In addition to this, physical reactions, such as headaches and heat sensations, have been reported. In the same vein, Bickham and colleagues [20] found associations between PMPU and depression in North American adolescents. In sum, the existing evidence on smartphone use suggests a clear association between PMPU and decreased wellbeing, especially in young populations worldwide.

In relation to dangerous mobile phone use, PMPU has initially been negatively associated with safety behaviours [1,2], such as using mobile phones when driving, cycling, or walking. The importance of this factor is supported by the development of specific policies and regulations related to mobile phone use (i.e., to prevent road accidents). A study conducted in China [21] assessed unintentional injuries (i.e., road traffic injuries, pedestrian collisions, and falls) due to mobile phone use and psychopathological symptoms in adolescence. The most prevalent injury was collisions (followed by falls and other injuries), where adolescents experienced PMPU, as well as negative emotional, behavioural, and social adaptation symptoms. Another study from the United States (US) [22] reviewed the associations between motor vehicle crashes and PMPU in adolescents because drivers between 16 and 19 years in the US are the most likely to die as a consequence of distractions caused by mobile phones. The review evidenced that half of all adolescents texted on their mobile phone while driving.

Prohibition of mobile phone use (or its regulation) is another specific aspect of PMPU, and is usually associated with legal or public regulations. However, some individuals do not abstain from using phones in such circumstances (i.e., public spaces, such as libraries, cinemas, or theatres). According to Takao and colleagues [23], personality traits may be associated with these types of behaviours, such as self-monitoring (i.e., traits related to the tendency to control and regulate the public self) and approval motivations (i.e., the need for favourable evaluations from others). Both are associated with an extraverted personality, as indicated by previous research [14] because individuals with the extraversion trait are sensitive to social cues and peer pressure, which involves being prone to risk behaviours when using mobile phones constantly, even when their use is banned. This aspect of problematic mobile phone use can also be related to the fact that individuals use mobile phones in a way that interferes with social situations. A prototypical example is the act of snubbing someone in a social setting by using one's mobile phone instead of interacting, a phenomenon referred to as "phubbing" [24,25].

The most studied type of negative outcome associated with mobile phone use is dependence, also conceptualised as a genuine addictive behaviour by some researchers [9,26]. The introduction of the internet and instant messaging (IM) on mobile phones (i.e., smartphones) has been associated with mobile phone dependence [21]. Moreover, it has also been associated with sociability levels of mobile phone users [27–29] and peer pressure [28]. However, studies examining peer pressure have reported slightly contradictory findings [29], where PMPU has not necessarily been associated with peer support or social acceptance. Therefore, it appears there is a potential association between mobile phone dependence (especially texting) and levels of sociability in adolescent and young adult populations [27,28,30]. Other factors usually associated with this type of problematic use include emotional symptoms (e.g., stress, anxiety, and depression [31–33]), reward seeking [26], and heightened impulsivity [2,26]. Moreover, specific mobile phone use patterns have also been associated with dependent use, except for some entertainment uses, such as downloading or playing mobile games [26,34,35], or using the mobile phone for travel bookings, online payments, and online shopping [34].

In sum, on the one hand, a few authors have claimed that the negative nature of dependent mobile phone use is not always severe, such as Chung [36], who argued that levels of dependence in South Korean female adolescent mobile phone users (i.e., withdrawal, maladjustment, tolerance, obsession, and flashiness) are associated with high levels of interpersonal solidarity (i.e., shared sentiments, intimacy, and similarities). Similarly, other scholars [37] have alerted researchers concerning the risk of overpathologizing everyday life behaviours in the context of behavioural addictions research, such as PMPU. On the other hand, Chóliz [38] has claimed that mobile phone addiction is a clinically relevant condition. Therefore, further research is warranted to assess the underlying motivations behind dependent use.

In relation to the cross-cultural assessment of PMPU, only a few studies have been conducted [39,40]. A number of different scales have been used [5,22,41,42], and according to a literature review by Pedrero and colleagues [42], the 'gold standard' scale is the Mobile Phone Problem Use Scale (MPPUS [3]). Unfortunately, the MPPUS is a unidimensional scale, which is problematic given the hypothesized multi-dimensional nature of PMPU. Moreover, the structural validity of the MPPUS was only tested with exploratory factor analysis (EFA), and needs to be confirmed in further studies using confirmatory factor analysis (CFA) and measurement invariance (MI). Another contemporary instrument to assess PMPU is the Problematic Mobile Phone Use Questionnaire (PMPUQ; [4]), which allows the measurement of the multi-dimensional nature of PMPU and was validated through the conjoint use of EFAs and CFAs. The scale assesses the three aforementioned specific types of PMPU. It was initially developed with a four-factor solution, but was recently reduced to a shorter version with three factors (dangerous use, prohibited use, and dependence) and updated to contemporary smartphone use (PMPUQ-SV; [33,35,43]). The fourth factor, related to the occurrence of financial problems, was removed due to the evolution of smartphones (i.e., smartphones being relatively cheap to use compared to when they were first introduced).

Subsequent studies—including some cross-cultural ones [33,35]—have evaluated the factor structure of the PMPUQ in its long or short versions via exploratory [35,43] and confirmatory [33,43,44] approaches in different populations (e.g., young adults [33,43], adults [35,43,44]), and different European languages, especially English [33,35,43,44]. However, psychometric results have been contradictory because some studies have reported adequate properties [33,35], while others have not [43,44]. Finally, to the best of the authors' knowledge, no previous study has tested MI to establish the cross-validity of any of the PMPU scales (i.e., unidimensional or multidimensional) simultaneously across different languages using confirmatory approaches. This is a necessary step to move the field forward in order to establish cross-cultural MI of a scale to guarantee reliable and comparative findings across countries and languages.

The aim of the present study was to test the psychometric properties and measurement invariance of eight versions of the PMPUQ-SV. The languages selected were German, French, English, Finnish, Spanish, Italian, Polish, and Hungarian. A number of non-European countries using the same languages agreed to join the data collection in this first study. In addition to being able to perform future cross-cultural studies, there are a number of reasons for carrying out the present study to validate the PMPUQ-SV in several languages. Firstly, there is little empirical evidence regarding PMPU as a multidimensional construct, especially in adulthood. Secondly, PMPU has almost exclusively been investigated in relation to its addictive use rather than considering other potential problems (such as dangerous or prohibited use). Thirdly, the PMPUQ has been previously tested mostly using exploratory and confirmatory approaches, with no consistent results across different languages (e.g., English), but its MI across different languages remains to be investigated. Consequently, the present study investigated the multidimensional construct of PMPU across specific types of problematic mobile phone use described via the multi-group validation of the PMPUQ-SV across languages. Thus, the objectives were to (i) determine an optimal factor structure for the PMPUQ–SV among university populations using eight languages; and (ii) simultaneously examine the MI of the PMPUQ–SV across all languages in order to assess the linguistic comparability across the eight versions of the scale independently.

Therefore, the main purpose of the present study was to ascertain if the PMPUQ-SV is an appropriate psychometric tool for cross-cultural research. To the best of the authors' knowledge, this is the first study to investigate the three-factor model in a multinational sample and the first to conduct MI on a multidimensional model of the PMPU across multiple linguistic scale versions. Thus, the present study will help fill an important gap in the field of PMPU and make a contribution to the research area because it comprises robust cross-cultural research examining mobile phone use and its associated problems.

2. Materials and Methods

2.1. Participants and Procedure

A total of 5209 respondents participated in the study, which builds upon the Tech Use Disorders (TUD; [45]) project. The items examined in the present study were part of a longer online survey including other questions (e.g., other scales concerning use of technology or personality traits). Participants were not forced to answer questions (because the survey was completely voluntarily). After cleaning the dataset (e.g., removing missing values), a sample of 3038 participants remained. The sample included adults engaged in higher education environments in 2015. The ethics committee of the Psychological Science Research Institute of the Université Catholique de Louvain (Belgium) approved the study protocol in 2014. Participants provided informed consent and voluntarily participated following an assurance of confidentiality and anonymity. The invitation to participate in the online survey (hosted on Qualtrics) used two recruitment strategies: (i) the present authors inviting undergraduates to participate via their respective universities during their 2015 and 2016 lectures; and (ii) via electronic invitations in academic online environments (e.g., university emails, university research participant pools, university social networks, and university virtual learning environments). Missing data were treated with pairwise deletion to maximise the statistical power, and cases were considered to be missing at random (MAR). This left a total sample size of 3038 participants with some not included for several reasons (e.g., young participants were not yet drivers, etc.). The sample breakdown by each respective language is shown in Table 1, alongside key socio-demographic data and reliability estimations.

Consequently, a total of eight languages were included in the present study (see Table 1), which were provided by 14 countries participating in the present study via their respective academic environments: German (i.e., Germany: 12.61% of the sample), French (i.e., Belgium: 16.06%; France: 10.60%; Switzerland: 3.39%; Canada: 5.13%; others who filled in the French adaptation chose not to report their country: 0.23%), English (i.e., United Kingdom (UK): 1.81%, Norway: 1.71%; US: 0.13%; Indonesia: 0.20%), Finnish (i.e., Finland: 14.78%), Spanish (i.e., Spain: 5.13%), Italian (i.e., Italy: 9.48%), Polish (i.e., Poland: 8.49%), and Hungarian (Hungary: 10.24%).

2.2. Instrument

To assess potential PMPU, the 15-item PMPUQ-SV [33,35,43] was adapted from English into the other seven languages using a standard translation and back-translation method [46], except for French (as it was the original language [4]) (see Appendix A). Each subscale comprised five items, which were scored from 1 ('I strongly agree') to 4 ('I strongly disagree'), except for the items that were reverse scored [35] (see Table 1 for descriptive item scores). Overall scores ranged from 15 to 60, with higher scores indicating more potential problems due to mobile phone use. The Cronbach's alphas of the PMPUQ-SV across all languages ranged from 0.56 (English version; prohibited use) to 0.90 in the present study (German version: dependence; French version: dependence; English version: dangerous use).

Table 1. Demographic Information and item scores across all eight adaptations of the PMPUQ-SV.

	All	German	French	English	Finnish	Spanish	Italian	Polish	Hungarian
N	3038	383	1076	117	449	156	288	258	311
Women (N (%))	2193 (72%)	262 (68%)	829 (77%)	89 (76%)	308 (69%)	123 (79%)	190 (66%)	187 (72%)	205 (66%)
Age in (Yrs; mean (SD))	26.505 (9.395)	25.204 (6.602)	25.22 (10.034)	27.735 (11.319)	28.296 (9.06)	28.045 (11.642)	28.576 (9.555)	25.279 (6.965)	27.833 (9.032)
PMPUQ Score (mean (SD))	27.156 (6.869)	26.976 (6.547)	27.005 (7.177)	28.145 (5.564)	26.938 (6.584)	28.5 (6.696)	29.59 (6.533)	28.961 (6.399)	23.539 (6.159)
Cronbach's α									
Dangerous use	0.84	0.88	0.81	0.90	0.87	0.86	0.86	0.77	0.89
Prohibited use	0.69	0.65	0.74	0.56	0.62	0.66	0.68	0.66	0.75
Dependent use	0.88	0.90	0.90	0.83	0.85	0.85	0.84	0.82	0.89
Item Scores (mean (SD))									
1. Easy not to use mobile	2.359 (1.034)	2.460 (0.991)	2.352 (1.095)	2.462 (0.915)	2.341 (1.030)	2.455 (0.905)	2.581 (0.921)	2.391 (1.009)	1.971 (0.991)
2. Use mobile when driving R	1.569 (0.869)	1.525 (0.789)	1.402 (0.784)	1.393 (0.754)	1.933 (0.968)	1.549 (0.930)	1.874 (0.904)	1.721 (0.917)	1.354 (0.773)
3. Don't use when forbidden	1.737 (0.943)	1.593 (0.866)	1.830 (0.981)	1.632 (0.826)	1.506 (0.869)	1.821 (0.962)	1.839 (0.936)	2.128 (1.003)	1.508 (0.823)
4. Difficult not to use mobile R	2.179 (0.965)	2.285 (0.892)	2.214 (1.039)	2.308 (0.825)	2.049 (0.941)	2.393 (0.884)	2.345 (0.889)	2.236 (0.926)	1.772 (0.867)
5. Avoid using on motorway	1.417 (0.866)	1.324 (0.752)	1.467 (0.931)	1.308 (0.760)	1.379 (0.755)	1.319 (0.825)	1.360 (0.751)	1.721 (1.123)	1.296 (0.755)
6. Using mobile in library	2.354 (1.037)	2.590 (0.988)	2.423 (1.086)	2.624 (0.953)	2.336 (0.998)	2.757 (0.918)	2.205 (0.986)	2.031 (0.994)	1.965 (0.927)
7. Easy to live without mobile	2.473 (0.995)	2.527 (0.900)	2.377 (1.052)	2.778 (0.862)	2.715 (0.993)	2.653 (0.855)	2.784 (0.854)	2.442 (0.937)	1.929 (0.902)
8. Dangerous situations R	1.721 (0.965)	1.574 (0.782)	1.828 (1.102)	1.410 (0.697)	1.686 (0.846)	1.730 (0.996)	1.839 (0.929)	2.070 (1.011)	1.302 (0.636)
9. Use mobile when forbidden R	1.581 (0.806)	1.655 (0.753)	1.440 (0.754)	1.701 (0.757)	1.579 (0.804)	1.822 (0.900)	1.909 (0.954)	1.694 (0.829)	1.431 (0.701)
10. Lost without mobile R	2.205 (0.986)	2.016 (0.859)	2.213 (1.056)	2.607 (0.909)	2.245 (0.953)	2.160 (0.980)	2.345 (0.932)	2.395 (0.945)	1.939 (0.930)
11. Driving danger mobile R	1.379 (0.762)	1.295 (0.600)	1.437 (0.886)	1.248 (0.642)	1.425 (0.738)	1.299 (0.638)	1.529 (0.827)	1.434 (0.715)	1.125 (0.448)
12. Public transport	1.462 (0.711)	1.496 (0.647)	1.369 (0.709)	1.530 (0.566)	1.410 (0.751)	1.542 (0.668)	1.586 (0.684)	1.659 (0.869)	1.476 (0.621)
13. Hard to turn off mobile R	1.999 (0.980)	1.984 (0.880)	1.911 (1.023)	2.325 (0.936)	1.795 (0.920)	2.278 (0.978)	2.399 (0.948)	2.019 (0.906)	1.994 (0.987)
14. Driving concentration R	1.247 (0.597)	1.188 (0.459)	1.171 (0.505)	1.231 (0.578)	1.332 (0.703)	1.306 (0.651)	1.482 (0.787)	1.415 (0.755)	1.087 (0.353)
15. Use mobile in silent place	1.496 (0.749)	1.457 (0.620)	1.578 (0.851)	1.590 (0.697)	1.287 (0.594)	1.558 (0.769)	1.538 (0.672)	1.605 (0.813)	1.373 (0.659)

Note: R = reverse coded; PMPUQ-SV: Problematic mobile phone use questionnaire short version.

2.3. Analysis

2.3.1. Understanding Measurement Invariance

To investigate whether the PMPUQ-SV is psychometrically valid for use across different languages, an analysis of MI was conducted using multigroup confirmatory factor analysis (MGCFA). MI establishes whether various aspects of the latent structure of a model remain stable across multiple groups, being run in an iterative manner with a set of increasingly constrained confirmatory factor analyses (CFAs). Comparison tests are then undertaken to determine if reliable differences exist between these models [47], which would suggest groups have reliable variations at those specific levels. The first step in this procedure was to conduct individual CFAs in each language group and investigate model fit. Following this, a set of constrained and planned models were implemented as follows. Constraints are given in square brackets and are cumulative throughout:

- A test of configural (or 'pattern', (groups)) invariance that investigates whether the same number of factors and their respective items are the same across groups (i.e., does the specified CFA structure replicate across the groups tested?). Support for configural invariance would suggest that the three-factor solution of the PMPUQ-SV and respective items per factor are valid across groups.

- A test of metric (or 'weak', (loadings)) invariance that estimates whether the factor loading strengths are equivalent across groups. Metric invariance suggests that participants understand and respond to items in the same way across groups.

- A test of scalar invariance (or strong invariance, (thresholds)) investigates if group differences in factor means are unbiased [48], meaning latent scores can be compared across groups.

- A test of strict invariance (residuals) estimates whether observed items have the same residuals, meaning that items have the same measurement error terms across groups.

- An additional fifth model of strict invariance and equally constrained (means) tests if the entire mean structure is invariant. If supported, this suggests that the means of both the latent variables and observed variables are invariant across groups.

2.3.2. Ordinal Data Analysis

Given that all PMPUQ-SV items are assessed on ordinal scales, models that could support non-continuous item analyses were employed [49]. Therefore, multigroup analyses were run using the R program with RStudio [50] using the Lavaan [51], Psych [52], and SemTools [53] packages, all of which have options for assessing ordinal data in a CFA framework (see [54] for a tutorial). Accordingly, thresholds rather than intercepts were constrained. In all CFA models, correlation matrices used were polychoric and model fit statistics were estimated using diagonally weighted least squares scale-shifted (DWLSSS). DWLSSS has been found to be a more effective estimation method for ordinal data than maximum likelihood [55,56], the default estimation for most statistical software.

3. Results

3.1. Factor Structures

As the PMPUQ-SV is a relatively new scale and its first aim was to assess its psychometric properties to ascertain potential reasons concerning previous contradictory results [33,35,43,44], cut-off points for all indices were taken prudently. Firstly, individual CFAs were performed for the overall sample and individually in each language. The correlation matrix and factor loadings of PMPUQ-SV items across all linguistic versions can be found in Tables 2 and 3, respectively. Cut-off values for fit indices were applied as follows (although caution must be taken as these cut-off values appear to result in lower Type II error rates (with acceptable costs of Type-I error rates [57–61])): a Comparative Fit Index (CFI) between 0.90 and 0.95 is indicative of acceptable fit relative to the independent model, and from 0.95 is considered a good fit; Tucker Lewis Index (TLI) values greater than 0.90 have been used as acceptable fit models in the past, but since 2000, this has been increased to approximately 0.95 indicating good fit; Root Mean Square Error of Approximation (RMSEA) values less than or equal to 0.05 can be considered as good fit, values between 0.05 and 0.08 are acceptable, and greater than 0.08 could be considered a mediocre fit, but higher than 0.10 are considered a poor fit (ideally, if the RMSEA is greater than 0.05, the fit of the model is 'close' (i.e., such a model has a specification error, but this is not large; then sample size is a critical factor)); Standardised Root Mean Square Residual (SRMR) values must be less than 0.08 or close to 0.09 (or 0.10), as it is the most sensitive index to models with misspecified factor loadings, and a combination rule has been suggested (i.e., if the RMSEA is greater than 0.05 or close to 0.06, then the SRMR should be greater than 0.06, or close to 0.09–0.10, as it is usually acceptable for sample sizes that are equal to or less than 250 [59]). However, although reported here for the sake of transparency, χ^2 was not used to assess model fit, as it has been found to artificially inflate with an increasing sample size [62].

As can be seen in Table 4, the PMPUQ-SV in German, French, and English yielded good model fit statistics, whilst Hungarian and Finnish versions yielded adequate model fit statistics using less conservative cut-off scores. The Spanish version was almost acceptable, while the Italian and Polish versions had poor fit and were thus not carried forward for MI testing. Including the Italian and Polish versions would likely lead to the multigroup analysis immediately failing because the models already differ between the validated and non-validated languages in terms of factor numbers or structure. The English version was also removed because the highest response score for Item 12 (public transport) was not endorsed by any participants (with Lavaan requiring at least one response per level as a prerequisite).

Table 2. Correlation matrix of the 15 PMPUQ-SV items across all language adaptations.

							Item Number								
	1	2	3	4	5	6	7	8	9	10	11	12	13	14	15
1	-														
2	0.19 ***	-													
3	0.25 ***	0.22 ***	-												
4	0.58 ***	0.19 ***	0.30 ***	-											
5	0.09 ***	0.51 ***	0.33 ***	0.05 ***	-										
6	0.36 ***	0.07 ***	0.33 ***	0.33 ***	0.14 ***	-									
7	0.78 ***	0.22 ***	0.28 ***	0.56 ***	0.11 ***	0.39 ***	-								
8	0.19 ***	0.45 ***	0.31 ***	0.32 ***	0.35 ***	0.14 ***	0.20 ***	-							
9	0.23 ***	0.44 ***	0.51 ***	0.42 ***	0.31 ***	0.29 ***	0.29 ***	0.52 ***	-						
10	0.56 ***	0.13 ***	0.22 ***	0.56 ***	0.02	0.25 ***	0.63 ***	0.25 ***	0.32 ***	-					
11	0.12 ***	0.57 ***	0.24 ***	0.22 ***	0.41 ***	0.02	0.13 ***	0.53 ***	0.40 ***	0.19 ***	-				
12	0.08 ***	0.06 ***	0.18 ***	0.04 *	0.19 ***	0.12 ***	0.10 ***	0.08 ***	0.12 ***	0.01	0.08 ***	-			
13	0.53 ***	0.15 ***	0.27 ***	0.56 ***	0.05 *	0.23 ***	0.54 ***	0.25 ***	0.37 ***	0.62 ***	0.20 ***	0.09 ***	-		
14	0.15 ***	0.67 ***	0.32 ***	0.23 ***	0.49 ***	0.06 *	0.18 ***	0.56 ***	0.53 ***	0.20 ***	0.68 ***	0.20 ***	0.30 ***	-	
15	0.25 ***	0.08 ***	0.41 ***	0.25 ***	0.22 ***	0.41 ***	0.28 ***	0.22 ***	0.33 ***	0.20 ***	0.15 ***	0.38 ***	0.27 ***	0.21 ***	-

Note: All correlations are polychoric and p-values are FDR corrected for multiple comparisons, $* p < 0.05$, $*** p < 0.001$; PMPUQ-SV: Problematic mobile phone use questionnaire short version.

Table 3. Factor loadings of the PMPUQ-SV items across all languages.

	Factor Loadings		
	Dangerous Use	Prohibited Use	Dependent Use
14. Driving concentration	0.88		
11. Driving danger mobile	0.74		
2. Use mobile when driving	0.73		
8. Dangerous situations	0.73		
5. Avoid using on motorway	0.57		
9. Use mobile when forbidden		0.80	
3. Don't use when forbidden		0.63	
15. Use mobile in silent place		0.55	
6. Using mobile in library		0.52	
12. Public transport		0.26	
7. Easy to live without mobile			0.87
1. Easy not to use mobile			0.84
10. Lost without mobile			0.74
4. Difficult not to use mobile			0.73
13. Hard to turn off mobile			0.72

Note: PMPUQ-SV: Problematic mobile phone use questionnaire short version.

Table 4. Individual confirmatory factor analyses across all samples and for each language of the PMPUQ-SV 3.2. Measurement invariance.

Version	n	df	χ^2	p	CFI	TLI	RMSEA	RMSEA 90% CI	pClose	SRMR
All languages	3038	87	1858.371	<0.001	0.947	0.936	0.082	0.079–0.085	<0.000	0.074
German	383	87	231.642	<0.001	0.972	0.966	0.066	0.056–0.076	<0.000	0.069
French	1076	87	589.755	<0.001	0.973	0.968	0.073	0.068–0.079	<0.000	0.075
English	117	87	108.124	=0.062	0.976	0.972	0.046	0.000–0.072	<0.000	0.106
Finnish	449	87	383.929	<0.001	0.924	0.908	0.087	0.078–0.096	<0.000	0.092
Spanish	156	87	186.553	<0.001	0.940	0.928	0.086	0.069–0.103	=0.001	0.115
Italian	288	87	337.184	<0.001	0.915	0.897	0.100	0.089–0.111	<0.000	0.108
Polish	258	87	303.358	<0.001	0.880	0.856	0.098	0.086–0.111	<0.000	0.112
Hungarian	311	87	236.557	<0.001	0.954	0.945	0.074	0.063–0.086	<0.000	0.103

Note: PMPUQ-SV = Problematic mobile phone use questionnaire short version; χ^2 = Chi-square value, CFI = comparative fit index, TLI = Tucker–Lewis index, RMSEA = root mean squared error of approximation, pClose = provides a one-sided test of the null hypothesis that the RMSEA is equal to 0.05 in the population, SRMR = standardized root mean square residual.

To test for MI across languages, a series of MGCFAs with increasing constraints were conducted. The degree of difference (Δ) between the pairs of nested models was assessed using ΔCFI, ΔRMSEA, and ΔSRMR, as recommended by Chen [63], with respective cut-off values of ≤0.01, ≤0.015, and ≤0.03 for metric invariance and ≤0.01 for scalar invariance [64]. Satorra-Bentler χ^2 difference tests were also calculated between the nested models, although again, these have been found to produce unreliable estimates for large sample sizes, and therefore need to be interpreted with caution. Successive models were only calculated if the previous less constrained invariance in the hierarchy was at least partially supported.

Configural invariance was supported because the majority of fit indices were adequate, and so the next levels of constraint were investigated. Satorra-Bentler tests between all subsequent MI models were reliably different ($p < 0.001$; see Table 5), suggesting that each successive model had a poorer fit than the previous one (this provides evidence against invariance). At each stage, the changes in fit indices were inspected to assess whether this conclusion could be supported. Across all models, the changes in all fit indices were well below the pre-specified cut-off Δ-values, with the exception of ΔCFI for the scalar, strict, and mean models, which exceeded the ≤0.01 threshold at 0.012, 0.014, and 0.012, respectively. Considering the excellent values for the remaining fit indices at each stage, overall, the MI results provide evidence for metric invariance and partial evidence for scalar, strict, and mean invariance.

Table 5. Measurement invariance procedure conducted between German, French, Finnish, Spanish, and Hungarian for PMPUQ-SV.

Invariance	df	χ^2	p	CFI	TLI	RMSEA	RMSEA 90% CI	pClose	SRMR	$\Delta\chi^2$	Δdf	ΔRMSEA	ΔCFI	ΔSRMR
Configural	435	1567	<0.001	0.964	0.956	0.074	0.070–0.078	<0.001	0.084					
Config vs. metric ***										133	24	0.002	0.001	0.009
Metric	483	1654	<0.001	0.962	0.959	0.072	0.068–0.075	<0.001	0.093					
Metric vs. Scalar ***										165	54	0.003	0.012	0.006
Scalar	591	2154	<0.001	0.950	0.955	0.075	0.071–0.078	<0.001	0.087					
Scalar vs. Strict ***										272	30	0.005	0.014	0.008
Strict	651	2643	<0.001	0.936	0.948	0.080	0.077–0.084	<0.001	0.095					
Strict vs. Means ***										345	6	0.007	0.012	0.002
Means	663	3038	<0.001	0.924	0.939	0.087	0.084–0.090	<0.001	0.097					

Note: PMPUQ-SV: Problematic mobile phone use questionnaire short version; Satorra-Bentler $\Delta\chi^2$ Tests: Config vs. Metric: $X^2(5) = 23.930$, $p < 0.001$, Metric vs Scalar: $X^2(11) = 29.202$, $p < 0.001$, Scalar vs Strict: $X^2(7) = 69.105$, $p < 0.001$, Strict vs Means: $X^2(1) = 28.590$, *** $p < 0.001$.

3.2. Response Rates

Finally, in order to explore potential reasons for the violated ΔCFI for the fifth (means) model and if any items could be flagged up for refinement in future iterations, the response rates for each item were investigated across all different linguistic versions. As can be seen in Table 6, across all items for all languages, 75.2% of responses were in the 'disagree' or 'strongly disagree' categories. However, as items were reversed (i.e., 2, 4, 8, 9, 10, 11, 13, and 14), it should be interpreted that, for example, strongly agreeing on Item 14 (i.e., 'I use my mobile phone while driving, even in situations that require a lot of concentration') is more indicative of PMPU (i.e., dangerous use), but strongly agreeing on Item 12 (i.e., 'When using my mobile phone on public transport, I try not to talk too loud') is less indicative of PMPU (i.e., prohibited use). Moreover, a pair of items (i.e., Item 12 and Item 14) showed a particularly skewed response pattern with less than 7.6% and 4.9%, respectively, of respondents endorsing PMPU, to some degree, with both statements. Response patterns such as these may suggest that participants were not able to identify with these behaviours and that particular items that comprise the PMPUQ-SV may not be able to adequately discriminate respondents into distinct groups (i.e., as the vast majority of respondents reject these items). Taken together, the MI results illustrate that some of the items of the PMPUQ-SV with more skewed response patterns may prove consistently difficult to identify with across French, German, Hungarian, Finnish, and Spanish respondents.

Table 6. Item response rates per response category across all languages for PMPUQ-SV.

Factor	Item	All Languages			
		Strongly Agree (%)	Agree (%)	Disagree (%)	Strongly Disagree (%)
Dangerous	14. Driving concentration [R]	1.8	3.1	13.1	82.0
	11. Driving danger mobile [R]	4.2	4.5	16.1	75.1
	2. Use mobile when driving [R]	4.7	11.4	20.0	63.9
	8. Dangerous situations [R]	8.1	12.3	23.3	56.3
	5. Avoid using on motorway	77.3	10.2	6.1	6.4
Prohibited	9. Use mobile where forbidden [R]	3.4	10.2	27.7	58.8
	3. Don't use when forbidden	55.1	22.2	16.7	6.0
	15. Use mobile in silent place	63.0	27.2	6.9	2.9
	6. Using mobile in library	27.7	23.7	34.0	14.6
	12. Public transport	64.1	28.3	5.0	2.6
Dependent	7. Easy to live without mobile	21.4	25.6	37.5	15.6
	1. Easy not to use mobile	26.6	26.1	31.9	15.3
	10. Lost without mobile [R]	11.2	27.3	32.3	29.2
	4. Difficult not to use mobile [R]	9.7	28.0	32.8	29.5
	13. Hard to turn off mobile [R]	9.4	19.8	32.1	38.7
	Mean *	*51.2*	*24.0*	*17.0*	*7.7*

Note: PMPUQ-SV: Problematic mobile phone use questionnaire short version; [R] = reverse coded for questionnaire validations, but actual score given here. * = mean when items 14, 11, 2, 8, 9, 10, 4, and 13 are reversed.

4. Discussion

The objectives of the present study were to determine an optimal factor structure for the PMPUQ–SV among university populations using eight different language versions, and to examine the MI of the PMPUQ–SV across all linguistic versions and across the eight versions. Taken together, the findings suggest that the PMPUQ-SV is a potentially appropriate psychometric tool to screen for prohibited, dangerous, and dependent mobile phone use in adults from countries using these languages (e.g., Europe and America). However, its psychometric properties can be nuanced depending on the respective language. Despite this, there are several potential reasons for adopting this tool. First, it is a very good psychometric tool for French and German mobile phone users, as its fit indices showed good fit in comparison with the other languages (i.e., $CFI_{French and German} = 0.97$; $TLI_{French and German} = 0.97$; $RMSEA_{French and German} = 0.07$; $SRMR_{French} = 0.07$, $SRMR_{German} = 0.08$). Second, in psychometric terms, the English and Hungarian versions were considered robust and the Finnish and Spanish versions were considered acceptable. However, the Italian and Polish versions did not meet the psychometric requirements.

4.1. Main Findings

Using the overall sample, the PMPUQ-SV performed well across its three theoretical factors in terms of their internal consistency, factor loadings, and CFA results. Only two elements were close to the limit of being psychometrically acceptable [59]. More specifically, the Cronbach's alpha for prohibited use was low because it is a coefficient sensitive to the number of items (i.e., the subscale only had five items), and it demonstrated that there was no poor interrelatedness between items or heterogeneous constructs, except for Item 6 (i.e., 'I don't use my mobile phone in a library') relating to prohibited use. This item does not load strongly enough and could perhaps be dropped in future PMPUQ versions. Furthermore, as evidence for metric invariance demonstrated, factor loadings were similar across the MI groups, so Item 6 was poor across countries. In fact, reliabilities were quite poor for prohibited mobile phone use [65].

It was also demonstrated that the RMSEA value was not ideal [59,60]. The French and German versions were psychometrically excellent, although the latter had the same issue with an acceptable reliability for prohibited use. Consequently, more in-depth research is needed to explore the phenomenology of this specific aspect of PMPU. Similarly, the English and Hungarian versions fitted the model well, although the reliability of the English version using Cronbach's alpha was only acceptable [66]. In addition, the Finnish and Spanish versions can be argued to be acceptable with restrictions due to their mediocre TLI, RMSEA, and SRMS values.

In sum, half of the linguistic versions tested in the present study fitted the proposed model well (i.e., ordered by their respective goodness of fit: French, German, Hungarian, and English). However, two require future testing (i.e., Finnish and Spanish) and the other two (i.e., Polish and Italian) require further review in relation to potentially different mobile phone use patterns in some countries and/or to methodological aspects (e.g., the translation and back-translation method applied), because both had large enough sample sizes to test its factor structure using a confirmatory approach. Regarding the English version, previous studies using this tool have also shown other psychometric weaknesses in relation to its reliability (e.g., in other studies, the α for prohibited use was 0.59 [35], and the α for the dangerous subscale was 0.67 [35], or 0.42 [43]), which are in line with the present findings regarding the limited internal consistency for prohibited use. Consequently, this needs to be cautiously interpreted due to the short length of this particular subscale. However, in relation to previous studies using the full PMPUQ or its short version, its factor structure usually corroborated the underlying theoretical model, except for the English studies, which reported a two-factor solution [43,44].

The lower loadings achieved in the overall sample for one of the items on the dangerous use subscale (i.e., 'I try to avoid using my mobile phone when driving on the motorway'), and four items on the prohibited use subscale (e.g., 'When using my mobile phone on public transport, I try not to talk too loud'), could be due to two reasons. First, mobile phone users are probably in a more pre-contemplative stage (i.e., they may not consider their mobile phone behaviour as problematic when asked about it, possibly denying or resisting this possibility), which is in line with research on compulsive internet use and other addictive behaviours [67,68]. Second, some items may not have been appropriate in the present day and age. For instance, 'I don't use my mobile phone in a library', which appeared appropriate in the present study because university samples were used, but (i) not all respondents may use libraries given the ease in which reading materials can be accessed remotely; and (ii) those who are library users can access their mobile phones using silent option modes (e.g., for checking the time or *Facebook* notifications, using IM, navigating, or listening to music through headphones).

When looking at the descriptive findings, the study also demonstrated that there appeared to be common usage patterns and preferences in relation to mobile phones for dangerous and prohibited use in the respective language versions. Items related to dangerous and prohibited use were very extreme (either strongly agree or disagree on the Likert scales), whereas items related to dependent use were more evenly spread across the response categories (from strongly agree to strongly disagree on the Likert scales). This may explain why a lower internal consistency was found for prohibited use, as well as the fact that the subscale only had five items. Underlying cultural differences may also explain this (e.g., English-speaking participants may have the most diversity in response to Item 12 (the item with lowest loadings on the prohibited use factor); for example, some cultures do not appear to mind talking on a bus, whereas other cultures do not like it at all). The study also demonstrated, in reference to the response patterns in Table 6, that participants endorsed much fewer PMPU behaviors when responding to items on the dangerous ($M = 5.025$) and prohibited factors ($M = 5.9$), relative to the dependency factor ($M = 12.24$). Furthermore, in a previous study [43], Item 12 was excluded from the analysis, because it did not share variance in the body of items.

The results in the present study also demonstrated that cultural differences in self-reported mobile phone usage patterns and contextual factors must be investigated in greater depth (e.g., driving regulations in the countries where the study was conducted). The PMPUQ-SV may be a good tool to initially screen for potential PMPU among adult mobile phone users in some languages (French, German, Hungarian, English, Finnish, and Spanish) if tested independently per country. However, the scale is only useful for mobile phone users who drive vehicles. Consequently, dangerous use is only associated with driving behaviour, instead of other dangers when using mobile phones (e.g., crossing the road). In future developments of the PMPU, it is recommended that the construct should not only be assessed with items related to driving behaviour [3,4,25] because other dangerous behaviours also exist and have been reported in recent research regarding safety, which can be included in future iterations (e.g., collisions or injuries when cycling or walking [24], such as '*I use my mobile phone whilst crossing the road*' [43]), especially if new scales are going to be tested using children, adolescents, or adults that are not drivers. Conversely, in countries like the US where driving is permitted during mid-adolescence [25], items addressing driving behaviours when using mobile phones are recommended (e.g., PMPUQ-SV). In other words, while almost all European countries allow driving individuals to drive from the age of 17 or 18 years old, in other countries, the ages at which individuals can drive are lower, such as 14–16 years old.

Regarding the strongest MI results, only the French, German, Hungarian, Finnish, and Spanish results can be compared when using these versions in a cross-cultural study [68] because it was only in these countries that configural and metric invariances resulted in obtaining the expected value [63,64]. However, the other types of invariance (i.e., scalar, strict, and mean models) slightly exceeded the threshold, but the model can still be considered tenable. In sum, the present findings suggest that the factor structure, loadings and intercepts, and residuals of the PMPUQ-SV are invariant across the French, German, Hungarian, Finnish, and Spanish language versions. Therefore, the present study provides evidence for the equality of meaning of the problematic mobile phone use construct in five out of eight languages, further providing confidence in future use of the PMPUQ-SV in cross-cultural research on PMPU. For instance, among some of the countries where the TUD project [45] was developed (i.e., Belgium, France, Switzerland, Canada, Germany, Hungary, Finland, and Spain), it appears that cross-cultural data can be reliably compared.

4.2. Limitations

The main potential limitations of the present study are the sampling and characteristics of the participants (i.e., convenience community-based self-selected samples), who were adults studying or working in universities (or who were related to those who study or work in higher education institutions). Nevertheless, a large sample was collected during the same period (i.e., in 2015), using similar strategies, and the same online survey, in order to guarantee the standardization of the procedures for collecting reliable data from the three specific aspects of PMPU. The data were also self-reported and are therefore subject to well-known biases and limitations that are inherent within such a methodology. The purpose of the present study was to evaluate the cross-cultural robustness of the PMPUQ-SV to facilitate the development of future epidemiological studies across different cultures as these studies can help better ascertain the potential problems on the phenomenology of maladaptive mobile phone use from a psycho-sociological perspective. The PMPUQ-SV is appropriate for specific types of mobile phone users and has partially been cross-validated, but still presents some weaknesses which need to be studied in future research (i.e., reliability and language adaptability).

4.3. Future Research Directions

PMPU is still open to debate in relation to its potential health and educational harms in individuals' daily lives. For instance, it is not clear if PMPU results from a contemporary psychosocial problem (facilitated through this technology and the online behaviours associated with it in individuals' daily lives) or from other potentially addictive technological behaviours [37]). PMPU is situated somewhere on the continuum between the absence of problems to severe problems, ranging from a normal daily behaviour to potentially dysfunctional behaviours (or as the consequence of an existing disorder [38]). Furthermore, mobile phones are being increasingly used by adolescents and young adults worldwide [1], and given that they are usually utilized mainly for communicative purposes (i.e., information and maintenance of social relationships), some degree of constant use is expected in Eastern and Western societies.

In recent years, research on PMPU has bloomed in East Asian countries, where the condition is often viewed and classified as an addictive behaviour. Recent studies conducted in this region have indicated the moderating and mediating roles of several sociodemographic factors (e.g., gender), usage patterns (e.g., history of mobile phone use), and psychological variables (e.g., personality traits, emotion regulation skills) [69–73]. Most of this research focused on addictive usage patterns (with scales such as the Mobile Phone Addiction Index [74]), and it would thus be relevant to adapt the PMPUQ-SV to these contexts to provide a tool able to measure different types of PMPU. Such adaptation would also allow for interesting cross-cultural studies to be conducted between, for example, Asian and European countries.

One of the first literature reviews that examined both problematic internet and mobile phone use between 1991 and 2005 using five scientific databases determined, at that time, that mobile phone addiction symptoms were less consistently reported than internet addiction symptoms [75]. Sanchez-Carbonell and colleagues stated in 2008 that the use of synchronous apps (such as chatting apps and online games) might increase the likelihood of developing an addictive behaviour, due to the time lapse between engaging in the act and receiving a reward. A recent longitudinal study [30] partially confirmed this hypothesis (especially in relation to social networking apps and messaging services such as *WhatsApp* and *Facebook*). However, recent research on PMPU has not provided this evidence yet [35], in comparison with other internet-related problems, such as gaming, which appears to be the most prevalent because of the immediate rewards [76]. A recent review of cell-phone addiction [77] concluded (irrespective of whether or not it is a genuine addiction) that mobile phones give rise to problems that increasingly affect daily life. For instance, even with the risk of unlimited use (due to the affordability of contracts), the conceptualisation of this problematic mobile phone behaviour is still debated. In general, there is still an overlap in definitions of problematic behaviours related to online activities, including PMPU, Internet addiction, gaming disorder, social network use disorder, and others. Future studies are needed to gather evidence on how a nomenclature can progress and improve.

5. Conclusions

The present study is the first to ascertain that the PMPUQ-SV is an appropriate psychometric tool for cross-cultural comparisons to determine future prevalence estimates of multidimensional PMPU (i.e., dangerous, prohibited, and dependent mobile phone use). This is the first study that has investigated PMPU in an international sample, conducting MGCFAs and MI on a multidimensional model of the PMPUQ-SV across multiple language versions. An optimal factor structure (i.e., three-factor model) was found for the PMPUQ–SV among different university populations using six language versions (French, German, Hungarian, English, Finnish, and Spanish), and the MI of the PMPUQ–SV was examined across eight linguistic versions. The results indicate that five of the language variants (i.e., French, German, Finnish, Spanish, and Hungarian) are comparable for future cross-cultural studies. The PMPUQ-SV has been validated for almost all languages tested in order to be used independently in countries using these languages, and parts of these versions can be used for cross-cultural comparisons. The present study contributes to the behavioural addictions field by cross-validating results that can be used for future cross-cultural research on PMPU.

Author Contributions: Conceptualization: O.L.-F. Data curation: O.L.-F.; Formal analysis: C.D. and L.V.J. Funding acquisition: O.L.-F., J.B. Investigation: O.L.-F., D.J.K., H.M.P., M.F.G., N.M., M.K., H.-J.R., A.B., A.-K.G., L.R., L.K., Y.M., A.R., P.G., Z.D., O.K., A.S., A.P., B.L.-K., J.C., M.C., J.J.Z., E.S. (Emilia Serra), M.D., L.R., D.Z., S.A., N.I.L., E.S. (Eva Suryani), J.M.H., J.P.T., and J.B.; Methodology, O.L.-F.; Project administration: O.L.-F.. Resources: O.L.-F. Supervision: O.L.-F. and J.B. Writing—original draft: O.L.-F. Writing, review and editing: O.L.-F., D.J.K., H.M.P., M.D.G., C.D., L.V.J., N.M., M.K., H.-J.R., A.B., A.-K.G., L.R., L.K., Y.M., A.R., P.G., Z.D., O.K., A.S., A.P., B.L.-K., J.C., M.C., J.J.Z., E.S. (Emilia Serra), M.D., L.R., D.Z., S.A., N.I.L., E.S. (Eva Suryani), J.M.H., J.P.T., and J.B.

Acknowledgments: The present study was supported, first, by the European Commission ("Tech Use Disorders"; FP7-PEOPLE-2013- IEF-627999) through a Marie Curie postdoctoral grant awarded to O.L.-F. (supervisor: J.B.). Second, by the Psychology Department QR Funding at Nottingham Trent University, through a Kickstarter bid grant (2017) awarded to O.L.-F. to develop studies on 'Internet and mobile phone addiction: Cross-cultural epidemiological studies'. O.L.-F. also acknowledges the support of Kim Hoffman from the International Center for Advanced Research and Applied Science (INCAAS), Peru; Carmen Margarita Ilizarbe Pizarro, Universidad Antonio Ruiz de Montoya, Peru; and Katarzyna Gajewska from the Polish Foundation for Humanitarian Aid 'Res Humanae', Poland. The Hungarian part of the study was supported by the Hungarian Scientific Research Fund (grant number: K111938; KKP126835). O.K. acknowledges the support of the ÚNKP-17-4 New National Excellence Program of the Ministry of Human Capacities.

Appendix A

English

In relation with your mobile phone/smartphone, please answer these questions on a scale from 1 to 4, the numbers corresponding to: 1 "Strongly agree", 2 "Agree", 3 "Disagree", 4 "Strongly disagree" The statement suits you:

1. It is easy for me to spend all day not using my mobile phone.
2. I use my mobile phone while driving.
3. I don't use my mobile phone when it is completely forbidden to use it.
4. Is it hard for me not to use my mobile phone when I feel like it.
5. I try to avoid using my mobile phone when driving on the motorway.
6. I don't use my mobile phone in a library.
7. I can easily live without my mobile phone.
8. I use my mobile phone in situations that would qualify as dangerous.
9. I use my mobile phone where it is forbidden to do so.
10. I feel lost without my mobile phone.
11. While driving, I find myself in dangerous situations because of my mobile phone use.
12. When using my mobile phone on public transport, I try not to talk too loud.
13. It is hard for me to turn my mobile phone off.

14. I use my mobile phone while driving, even in situations that require a lot of concentration.
15. I try to avoid using mobile phone where people need silence.

French

Concernant votre téléphone portable/smartphone, veuillez répondre à ces questions selon une échelle allant de 1 à 4, ces chiffres correspondant à : 1 "Tout à fait ", 2 "Plutôt bien ", 3 "Plutôt mal", 4"Pas du tout "
L'énoncé vous correspond:

1. Il est facile pour moi de passer toute une journée sans utiliser mon téléphone portable.
2. Je téléphone en conduisant.
3. Je n'utilise pas mon téléphone portable dans des lieux où il est formellement interdit de le faire.
4. Il m'est difficile de ne pas utiliser mon téléphone portable lorsque j'en ai envie.
5. J'évite d'utiliser mon téléphone portable quand je conduis sur l'autoroute.
6. Je n'utilise pas mon téléphone portable quand je suis dans une bibliothèque.
7. Je peux facilement me passer de mon téléphone portable.
8. Je me sers de mon téléphone portable dans des situations que je peux qualifier de «dangereuses».
9. Je me sers de mon téléphone portable dans des lieux où la loi l'interdit.
10. Je me sens perdu quand je n'ai pas mon téléphone portable.
11. En conduisant, je me retrouve en situation délicate alors que j'utilise mon téléphone portable.
12. Quand je téléphone dans les transports publics, je fais attention à ne pas parler trop fort.
13. Il est pénible pour moi d'éteindre mon téléphone portable.
14. En conduisant, j'utilise mon téléphone portable dans des situations qui demandent une concentration importante.
15. J'évite d'utiliser mon téléphone portable dans des endroits où il faut être silencieux.

German

Bitte beantworten Sie die nächsten Fragen in Bezug auf Ihr Smartphone/Handy auf einer Skala von 1 bis 4, die Zahlen entsprechend: 1 "Stimme sehr zu", 2 "Stimme zu", 3 "Stimme nicht zu", 4 " Stimme überhaupt nicht zu"
Wählen Sie die Aussage, die am besten zu Ihnen passt:

1. Es fällt mir leicht, den Tag zu verbringen, ohne mein Handy zu benutzen.
2. Ich benutze mein Handy, während ich Auto fahre.
3. Ich gebrauche mein Handy nicht, wenn es absolut verboten ist es zu benutzen.
4. Es fällt mir schwer mein Handy nicht zu verwenden, wenn mir danach ist.
5. Ich versuche zu vermeiden, mein Handy während der Autobahnfahrt zu benutzen.
6. Ich benutze mein Handy nicht in einer Bibliothek.
7. Ohne mein Handy kann ich problemlos leben.
8. Ich benutze mein Handy in Situationen, die als gefährlich gelten würden.
9. Ich verwende mein Handy an Orten, an denen die Nutzung verboten ist.
10. Ohne mein Handy fühle ich mich verloren.
11. Während ich Auto fahre, bringe ich mich in gefährliche Situationen, weil ich gleichzeitig mein Handy benutze.
12. Bei der Verwendung meines Mobiltelefons in öffentlichen Verkehrsmitteln versuche ich nicht zu laut zu sprechen.
13. Es fällt mir schwer, mein Handy auszuschalten.
14. Ich benutze mein Handy während der Autofahrt, selbst in Situationen, die viel Aufmerksamkeit erfordern.

15.   Ich versuche meine Handynutzung in Situationen zu vermeiden, in denen Menschen Ruhe brauchen.

Hungarian

Kérjük, válaszold meg az alábbi kérdéseket a mobiltelefonod használatával kapcsolatban egy egytől négyig terjedő skálán, ahol: 1 "Teljesen egyetértek", 2 "Egyetértek", 3 "Nem értek egyet", 4 "Egyáltalán nem értek egyet"

Mennyire értesz egyet az alábbi állításokkal?

1.   Könnyű számomra egy egész napot eltölteni anélkül, hogy használnám a mobilomat.
2.   Használom a mobilomat vezetés közben.
3.   Nem használom a mobilomat olyankor, amikor ez egyértelműen tilos.
4.   Nehezemre esik, hogy ne használjam a mobilomat bármikor, amikor csak kedvem van hozzá.
5.   Igyekszem nem használni a mobilomat, amikor autópályán vezetek.
6.   Nem használom a mobilomat, ha könyvtárban vagyok.
7.   Jól elvagyok a mobilom nélkül.
8.   Olyan helyzetekben is használom a mobilomat, amikor az mások szerint veszélyes lehet.
9.   Olyan helyen is használom a mobilomat, ahol ez tilos.
10.   Elveszettnek érzem magam a mobilom nélkül.
11.   Sokszor veszélyes helyzetekben találom magam vezetés közben a mobilhasználatom miatt.
12.   Amikor tömegközlekedési eszközön használom a mobilomat, igyekszem nem túl hangosan beszélni.
13.   Nehezemre esik kikapcsolni a mobilomat.
14.   Még olyan helyzetekben is használom a mobilomat vezetés közben, amik nagy koncentrációt igényelnek.
15.   Igyekszem nem használni a mobilomat olyan helyeken, ahol másoknak csendre van szükségük.

Finnish

Alla väittämiä matka-/älypuhelimenne käytöstä. Vastatkaa seuraaviin väittämiin valitsemalla itseänne parhaiten kuvaava vaihtoehto asteikolla 1–4: 1 "Täysin samaa mieltä", 2 "Jokseenkin samaa mieltä", 3 "Jokseenkin eri mieltä", 4 "Täysin eri mieltä"

1.   Minulle on helppoa olla koko päivä käyttämättä matkapuhelintani.
2.   Käytän matkapuhelinta autolla ajaessani.
3.   En käytä matkapuhelintani silloin, kun sen käyttö on ehdottomasti kielletty.
4.   On vaikeaa olla käyttämättä matkapuhelinta silloin kun haluaisin käyttää sitä.
5.   Yritän välttää matkapuhelimen käyttöä moottoritiellä ajaessani.
6.   En käytä matkapuhelinta kirjastossa.
7.   Voin helposti elää ilman matkapuhelinta.
8.   Käytän matkapuhelintani tilanteissa, jotka voidaan luokitella vaarallisiksi.
9.   Käytän matkapuhelintani silloinkin, kun sen käyttö on kielletty.
10.   Tunnen olevani hukassa ilman matkapuhelintani.
11.   Ajaessani huomaan olevani vaarallisissa tilanteissa matkapuhelimen käyttöni seurauksena.
12.   Käyttäessäni matkapuhelinta joukkoliikennevälineissä yritän olla puhumatta kovalla äänellä.
13.   Minulle tuottaa vaikeuksia laittaa matkapuhelimeni pois päältä.
14.   Käytän matkapuhelinta ajaessani autolla myös tilanteissa, jotka vaativat erityistä tarkkaavaisuutta.
15.   Yritän välttää matkapuhelimen käyttöä tilanteissa, joissa tarvitaan hiljaisuutta.

Italian

Per favore, indica quanto ciascuna affermazione è adatta a descrivere l'uso che fai del tuo cellulare/ smartphone, su una scala da 1 a 4. I numeri corrispondono a: 1. "Fortemente d'accordo", 2. "D'accordo", 3. "In disaccordo", 4. "Fortemente in disaccordo"

1.   E' facile per me trascorrere tutto il giorno senza utilizzare il cellulare.
2.   Utilizzo il cellulare mentre guido.
3.   Non uso il cellulare quando è assolutamente proibito usarlo.
4.   E' difficile per me non utilizzare il cellulare quando mi sento di farlo.
5.   Cerco di evitare di utilizzare il cellulare quando guido in autostrada.
6.   Non uso il cellular in biblioteca.
7.   Posso vivere facilmente senza il cellulare.
8.   Uso il cellulare in situazioni che potrebbero essere considerate pericolose.
9.   Uso il cellulare dove è proibito farlo.
10. Mi sento perso senza il cellulare.
11. Quando guido mi ritrovo in situazioni pericolose perchè utilizzo il cellulare.
12. Quando uso il cellulare su un mezzo di traporto pubblico, cerco di non parlare troppo forte.
13. E' difficile per me spegnere il cellulare.
14. Uso il cellulare quando guido, anche in situazioni che richiedono molta concentrazione.
15. Cerco di evitare di usare il cellulare nei posti in cui la gente ha bisogno di silenzio.

Spanish

En relación con su móvil/smartphone, responda por favor a estas cuestiones en una escala de valoración del 1 al 4, los números corresponden a: 1 "Muy de acuerdo", 2 "De acuerdo", 3 "En desacuerdo", 4 "Muy en desacuerdo"
La declaración que más le convenga:

1.   Es fácil para mí pasar todo el día sin usar el móvil.
2.   Uso el móvil mientras conduzco.
3.   Yo no uso el móvil cuando está completamente prohibido.
4.   Es difícil para mí no usar el móvil cuando quiero usarlo.
5.· Trato de evitar el uso del móvil cuando conduzco por la autopista.
6.   No uso el móvil en una biblioteca.
7.   Puedo vivir fácilmente sin mi móvil.
8.   Uso el móvil en situaciones que podrían considerarse peligrosas.
9.   Uso el móvil donde está prohibido utilizarlo.
10. Me siento perdido sin el móvil.
11. Me he encontrado en situaciones peligrosas debido al uso del móvil mientras conducía.
12. Cuando uso el móvil en el transporte público, trato de no hablar demasiado alto.
13. Es difícil para mí apagar el móvil.
14. Uso el móvil durante la conducción, incluso en situaciones que requieren mucha concentración.
15. Trato de evitar el uso del móvil en lugares en que la gente necesita silencio (o se ruega silencio).

Polish

Proszę odpowiedzieć na pytania dotyczące Pana(i) telefonu/smartfona, posługując się skalą, w której kolejne cyfry od 1 do 4 znaczą: 1 "Całkowicie", 2 "Raczej tak", 3 "Raczej nie", 4 "Wcale"
Stwierdzenie odpowiadające Panu(i):

1.   Łatwo mi spędzić cały dzień bez używania mojego telefonu komórkowego.

2. Rozmawiam przez telefon prowadząc samochód.
3. Nie używam telefonu w miejscach, w których formalnie jest to zakazane.
4. Trudno mi się powstrzymać od używania mojego telefonu komórkowego, kiedy mam na to ochotę.
5. Staram się nie używać telefonu, kiedy prowadzę saochód na autostradzie.
6. Nie używam telefonu kiedy jestem w bibliotece.
7. Z łatwością mogę obejść się bez mojego telefonu.
8. Używam mojego telefonu w sytuacjach, które uważam za « niebezpieczne ».
9. Używam mojego telefonu w miejscach, w których prawo tego zakazuje.
10. Czuję się zagubiony, gdy nie mam ze sobą mojego telefonu.
11. Prowadząc, zdarza mi się znaleźć w trudnej sytuacji podczas gdy używam telefonu komórkowego.
12. Kiedy rozmawiam przez telefon w środkach komunikacji publicznej, zwracam uwagę by nie rozmawiać zbyt głośno.
13. Źle się czuję, kiedy wyłączam mój telefon, nie lubię tego.
14. Prowadząc samochód używam telefonu w sytuacjach, które wymagają szczególnej koncentracji.
15. Unikam używania telefonu w miejscach, w których należy zachować ciszę.

References

1. International Telecommunication Union (ITU). ITU Committed to Connecting the World: ICT Facts and Figures 2017—Global ICT Developments. Available online: https://www.itu.int/en/ITU-D/Statistics/Pages/stat/default.aspx (accessed on 7 March 2018).
2. ProQuest. Search—All Databases. Available online: https://search.proquest.com/results/3E9BFDEC5154401PQ/1?accountid=14693 (accessed on 26 January 2018).
3. Bianchi, A.; Phillips, J.G. Psychological predictors of problem mobile phone use. *Cyberpsychol. Behav.* **2005**, *8*, 39–51. [CrossRef] [PubMed]
4. Billieux, J.; Van der Linden, L.; Rochat, L. The role of impulsivity in actual and problematic use of the mobile phone. *Appl. Cogn. Psychol.* **2008**, *26*, 1195–1210. [CrossRef]
5. Billieux, J. Problematic use of the mobile phone: A literature review and a pathways model. *Curr. Psychiatry Rev.* **2012**, *8*, 299–307. [CrossRef]
6. Lopez-Fernandez, O.; Kuss, D.J.; Griffiths, M.D.; Billieux, J. The conceptualization and assessment of problematic mobile phone use. In *Encyclopedia of Mobile Phone Behavior (Volumes 1, 2, & 3)*; Yan, Z., Ed.; IGI Global: Hershey, PA, USA, 2015; pp. 591–606. ISBN 9781466682399.
7. Billieux, J.; Maurage, P.; Lopez- Fernandez, O.; Kuss, D.J.; Griffiths, M.D. Can disordered mobile phone use be considered a behavioral addiction? An update on current evidence and a comprehensive model for future research. *Curr. Addict. Rep.* **2015**, *2*, 156–162. [CrossRef]
8. Martinotti, G.; Villella, C.; Di Thiene, D.; Di Nicola, M.; Bria, P.; Conte, G.; Cassano, M.; Petruccelli, F.; Corvasce, N.; Janiri, L.; et al. Problematic mobile phone use in adolescence: A cross-sectional study. *J. Public Health* **2011**, *19*, 545–551. [CrossRef]
9. Chóliz, M. Mobile-phone addiction in adolescence: The test of mobile phone dependence (TMD). *Prog. Health Sci.* **2012**, *2*, 33–44. [CrossRef]
10. López-Fernandez, O.; Honrubia-Serrano, M.L.; Freixa-Blanxart, M. Spanish adaptation of the "mobile phone problem use scale" for adolescent population. *Adicciones* **2012**, *24*, 123–130. [CrossRef] [PubMed]
11. Ezoe, S.; Toda, M.; Yoshimura, K.; Naritomi, A.; Den, R.; Morimoto, K. Relationships of personality and lifestyle with mobile phone dependence among female nursing students. *Soc. Behav. Personal.* **2009**, *37*, 231–238. [CrossRef]
12. Gallimberti, L.; Buja, A.; Chindamo, S.; Terraneo, A.; Marini, E.; Rabensteiner, A.; Vinelli, A.; Gomez Perez, L.J.; Baldo, V. Problematic cell phone use for text messaging and substance abuse in early adolescence (11- to 13-year-olds). *Eur. J. Pediatr.* **2016**, *175*, 355–364. [CrossRef] [PubMed]

13. Yang, Y.; Yen, J.; Ko, C.; Cheng, C.; Yen, C. The association between problematic cellular phone use and risky behaviors and low self-esteem among Taiwanese adolescents. *BMC Public Health* **2010**, *10*. [CrossRef] [PubMed]

14. Thomée, S.; Dellve, L.; Härenstam, A.; Hagberg, M. Perceived connections between information and communication technology use and mental symptoms among young adults—A qualitative study. *BMC Public Health* **2010**, *10*, 66. [CrossRef] [PubMed]

15. Thomée, S.; Härenstam, A.; Hagberg, M. Mobile phone use and stress, sleep disturbances, and symptoms of depression among young adults—A prospective cohort study. *BMC Public Health* **2011**, *11*, 66. [CrossRef] [PubMed]

16. Elhai, J.D.; Dvorak, R.D.; Levine, J.C.; Hall, B.J. Problematic smartphone use: A conceptual overview and systematic review of relations with anxiety and depression psychopathology. *J. Affect. Disord.* **2017**, *207*, 251–259. [CrossRef] [PubMed]

17. Elhai, J.D.; Levine, J.C.; Dvorak, R.D.; Hall, B.J. Non-social features of smartphone use are most related to depression, anxiety and problematic smartphone use. *Comput. Hum. Behav.* **2017**, *69*, 75–82. [CrossRef]

18. Stothart, C.; Mitchum, A.; Yehnert, C. The attentional cost of receiving a cell phone notification. *J. Exp. Psychol. Hum. Percept. Perform.* **2015**, *41*, 893–897. [CrossRef] [PubMed]

19. McDaniel, B.T.; Coyne, S.M. "Technoference": The interference of technology in couple relationships and implications for women's personal and relational well-being. *Psychol. Pop. Media Cult.* **2016**, *5*, 85–98. [CrossRef]

20. Bickham, D.S.; Hswen, Y.; Rich, M. Media use and depression: Exposure, household rules, and symptoms among young adolescents in the USA. *Int. J. Public Health* **2015**, *60*, 147–155. [CrossRef] [PubMed]

21. Tao, S.; Wu, X.; Wan, Y.; Zhang, S.; Hao, J.; Tao, F. Interactions of problematic mobile phone use and psychopathological symptoms with unintentional injuries: A school-based sample of Chinese adolescents. *BMC Public Health* **2016**, *16*, 88. [CrossRef] [PubMed]

22. Delgado, M.K.; Wanner, K.J.; McDonald, C. Adolescent cellphone use while driving: An overview of the literature and promising future directions for prevention. *Media Commun.* **2016**, *4*, 79–89. [CrossRef] [PubMed]

23. Takao, M.; Takahashi, S.; Kitamura, M. Addictive personality and problematic mobile phone use. *Cyberpsychol. Behav.* **2009**, *12*, 501–507. [CrossRef] [PubMed]

24. Chotpitayasunondh, V.; Douglas, K.M. How "phubbing" becomes the norm: The antecedents and consequences of snubbing via smartphone. *Comput. Hum. Behav.* **2016**, *63*, 9–18. [CrossRef]

25. Roberts, J.A.; David, M.E. My life has become a major distraction from my cell phone: Partner phubbing and relationship satisfaction among romantic partners. *Comput. Hum. Behav.* **2016**, *54*, 134–141. [CrossRef]

26. Kim, Y.; Jeong, J.-E.; Cho, H.; Jung, D.-J.; Kwak, M.; Rho, M.J.; Yu, H.; Kim, D.-J.; Choi, I.Y. Personality factors predicting smartphone addiction predisposition: Behavioral inhibition and activation systems, impulsivity, and self-control. *PLoS ONE* **2016**, *11*, e0159788. [CrossRef] [PubMed]

27. Lin, T.T.C.; Chiang, Y.; Jiang, Q. Sociable people beware? Investigating smartphone versus nonsmartphone dependency symptoms among young Singaporeans. *Soc. Behav. Personal.* **2015**, *43*, 1209–1216. [CrossRef]

28. Foerster, M.; Roser, K.; Schoeni, A.; Röösli, M. Problematic mobile phone use in adolescents: Derivation of a short scale MPPUS-10. *Int. J. Public Health* **2015**, *60*, 277–286. [CrossRef] [PubMed]

29. Roser, K.; Schoeni, A.; Foerster, M.; Röösli, M. Problematic mobile phone use of Swiss adolescents: Is it linked with mental health or behaviour? *Int. J. Public Health* **2016**, *61*, 307–315. [CrossRef] [PubMed]

30. Carbonell, X.; Chamarro, A.; Oberst, U.; Rodrigo, B.; Prades, M. Problematic Use of the Internet and Smartphones in University Students: 2006–2017. *Int. J. Environ. Res. Public Health* **2018**, *15*, 475. [CrossRef] [PubMed]

31. Long, J.; Liu, T.Q.; Liao, Y.H.; Qi, C.; He, H.Y.; Chen, S.B.; Billieux, J. Prevalence and correlates of problematic smartphone use in a large random sample of Chinese undergraduates. *BMC Psychiatry* **2016**, *16*, 408. [CrossRef] [PubMed]

32. Andreassen, C.S.; Billieux, J.; Griffiths, M.D.; Kuss, D.J.; Demetrovics, Z.; Mazzoni, E.; Pallesen, S. The relationship between addictive use of social media and video games and symptoms of psychiatric disorders: A large-scale cross-sectional study. *Psychol. Addict. Behav.* **2016**, *30*, 252–262. [CrossRef] [PubMed]

33. Lopez-Fernandez, O.; Kuss, D.J.; Romo, L.; Morvan, Y.; Kern, L.; Graziani, P.; Rousseau, A.; Rumpf, H.J.; Bischof, A.; Gässler, A.K.; et al. Self-reported dependence on mobile phones in young adults: A European cross-cultural empirical survey. *J. Behav. Addict.* **2017**, *6*, 168–177. [CrossRef] [PubMed]

34. Jiang, Z.; Zhao, X. Self-control and problematic mobile phone use in Chinese college students: The mediating role of mobile phone use patterns. *BMC Psychiatry* **2016**, *16*, 416. [CrossRef] [PubMed]

35. Lopez-Fernandez, O.; Männikkö, N.; Kääriäinen, M.; Griffiths, M.D.; Kuss, D.J. Mobile gaming and problematic smartphone use: A comparative study between Belgium and Finland. *J. Behav. Addict.* **2018**, *9*, 1–12. [CrossRef] [PubMed]

36. Chung, N. Korean adolescent girls' addictive use of mobile phones to maintain interpersonal solidarity. *Soc. Behav. Personality* **2011**, *39*, 1349–1358. [CrossRef]

37. Billieux, J.; Schimmenti, A.; Khazaal, Y.; Maurage, P.; Heeren, A. Are we overpathologizing everyday life? A tenable blueprint for behavioral addiction research. *J. Behav. Addict.* **2015**, *4*, 119–123. [CrossRef] [PubMed]

38. Chóliz, M. Mobile phone addiction: A point of issue. *Addiction* **2010**, *105*, 373–374. [CrossRef] [PubMed]

39. Baron, N.S.; af Segerstad, Y.H. Cross-cultural patterns in mobile-phone use: Public space and reachability in Sweden, the USA and Japan. *New Media Soc.* **2010**, *12*, 13–34. [CrossRef]

40. Lopez-Fernandez, O. Short version of the Smartphone Addiction Scale adapted to Spanish and French: Towards a cross-cultural research in problematic mobile phone use. *Addict. Behav.* **2017**, *64*, 275–280. [CrossRef] [PubMed]

41. Lopez-Fernandez, O.; Honrubia-Serrano, M.L.; Freixa-Blanxart, M.; Gibson, W. Prevalence of problematic mobile phone use in British adolescents. *Cyberpsycho. Behav. Soc. Netw.* **2014**, *17*, 91–98. [CrossRef] [PubMed]

42. Pedrero, E.J.; Rodriguez Monje, M.T.; Ruiz Sanchez De León, J.M. Mobile phone abuse or addiction. A review of the literature. *Adicciones* **2012**, *24*, 139–152. [CrossRef]

43. Kuss, D.J.; Harkin, L.; Kanjo, E.; Billieux, J. Problematic Smartphone Use: Investigating Contemporary Experiences Using a Convergent Design. *Int. J. Environ. Res. Public Health* **2018**, *15*, 142. [CrossRef] [PubMed]

44. Kuss, D.J.; Kanjo, E.; Crook-Rumsey, M.; Kibowski, F.; Wang, Y.W.; Sumich, A. Problematic Mobile Phone Use and Addiction Across Generations: The Roles of Psychopathological Symptoms and Smartphone Use. *J. Technol. Behav. Sci.* **2018**. [CrossRef]

45. Tech Use Disorders. Technological Use Disorders: European Cross-Cultural Longitudinal and Experimental Studies for Internet and Smartphone Problem Uses, 12 July 2017. Available online: http://cordis.europa.eu/project/rcn/189961_en.html (accessed on 14 July 2017).

46. Beaton, D.E.; Bombardier, C.; Guillemin, F.; Ferraz, M.B. Guidelines for the process of cross-cultural adaptation of self-report measures. *Spine* **2000**, *25*, 3186–3191. [CrossRef] [PubMed]

47. Van de Schoot, R.; Lugtig, P.; Hox, J. A checklist for testing measurement invariance. *Eur. J. Dev. Psychol.* **2012**, *9*, 486–492. [CrossRef]

48. Gregorich, S.E. Do self-report instruments allow meaningful comparisons across diverse population groups? Testing measurement invariance using the confirmatory factor analysis framework. *Med. Care* **2006**, *44*, S78–S94. [CrossRef] [PubMed]

49. Kim, E.S.; Yoon, M. Testing measurement invariance: A comparison of multiple-group categorical CFA and IRT. *Struct. Equ. Model.* **2011**, *18*, 212–228. [CrossRef]

50. RStudio Team. *RStudio: Integrated Development for R*; RStudio, Inc.: Boston, MA, USA, 2015; Available online: http://www.rstudio.com/ (accessed on 7 March 2018).

51. Rosseel, Y. Lavaan: An R package for structural equation modeling and more. Version 0.5-12 (BETA). *J. Stat. Softw.* **2012**, *48*, 1–36. [CrossRef]

52. Revelle, W. *Procedures for Personality and Psychological Research*; Northwestern University: Evanston, IL, USA, 2016; Available online: http://www.personality-project.org/revelle.html and https://cran.r-project.org/web/packages/psych/index.html; (accessed on 7 March 2018).

53. SemTools Contributors. SemTools: Useful Tools for Structural Equation Modelling. R Package Version 0.4-14. 2016. Available online: https://cran.r-project.org/web/packages/semTools/index.html and https://cran.r-project.org/web/packages/semTools/semTools.pdf (accessed on 7 March 2018).

54. Hirschfeld, G.; Von Brachel, R. Multiple-Group confirmatory factor analysis in R—A tutorial in measurement invariance with continuous and ordinal. *Pract. Assess. Res. Eval.* **2014**, *19*, 1–11. Available online: http://pareonline.net/getvn.asp?v=19&n=7 (accessed on 7 March 2018).

55. Mîndrilă, D. Maximum Likelihood (ML) and Diagonally Weighted Least Squares (DWLS) Estimation Procedures: A Comparison of Estimation Bias with Ordinal and Multivariate Non-Normal Data. 2010. Available online: http://infonomics-society.org/wp-content/uploads/ijds/published-papers/volume-1-2010/Maximum-Likelihood-ML-and-Diagonally-Weighted-Least-Squares-DWLS-Estimation-Procedures-A-Comparison-of-Estimation-Bias-with-Ordinal-and-Multivariate-Non-Normal-Data.pdf (accessed on 7 March 2018).

56. Muthén, L.K.; Muthén, B.O. *Mplus User's Guide*; Authors: Los Angeles, CA, USA, 2001; Available online: http://research.socialwork.wayne.edu/pdf/mplus-users-guide.pdf (accessed on 7 March 2018).

57. Flora, D.B.; Curran, P.J. An empirical evaluation of alternative methods of estimation for confirmatory factor analysis with ordinal Data. *Psychol. Methods* **2004**, *9*, 466–491. [CrossRef] [PubMed]

58. Hooper, D.; Coughlan, J.; Mullen, M. Structural equation modelling: Guidelines for determining model fit. *Electron. J. Bus. Res. Methods* **2008**, *6*, 53–60. Available online: http://arrow.dit.ie/buschmanart (accessed on 7 March 2018).

59. Hu, L.; Bentler, P.M. Cutoff criteria for fit indexes in covariance structure analysis: Conventional criteria versus new alternatives. *Struct. Equ. Model.* **1999**, *6*, 1–55. [CrossRef]

60. Browne, M.; Cudeck, R. Alternative ways of assessing model fit. In *Testing Structural Equation Models*; Bollen, K.A., Long, J.S., Eds.; Sage Publications: Beverly Hills, CA, USA, 1993; pp. 111–136. ISBN 978-0803945074.

61. Van de Schoot, R.; Lugtig, P.; Hox, J. A checklist for testing measurement invariance, Eur. *J. Dev. Psychol.* **2012**, *9*, 486–492. [CrossRef]

62. Marsh, H.W.; Balla, J.R.; McDonald, R.P. Goodness-of-fit indexes in confirmatory factor analysis: The effect of sample size. *Psychol. Bull.* **1988**, *103*, 391–410. [CrossRef]

63. Chen, F.F. Sensitivity of goodness of fit indexes to lack of measurement invariance. *Struct. Equ. Model.* **2007**, *14*, 464–504. [CrossRef]

64. Cheung, G.W.; Rensvold, R.B. Evaluating goodness-of-fit indexes for testing measurement invariance. *Struct. Equ. Model.* **2002**, *9*, 233–255. [CrossRef]

65. Tavakol, M.; Dennick, R. Making sense of Cronbach's alpha. *Int. J. Med. Educ.* **2011**, *2*, 53–55. [CrossRef] [PubMed]

66. Schmitt, N. Uses and abuses of coefficient alpha. *Psychol. Assess.* **1996**, *8*, 350–353. [CrossRef]

67. Khazaal, Y.; Chatton, A.; Atwi, K.; Zullino, D.; Khan, R.; Billieux, J. Arabic validation of the Compulsive Internet Use Scale (CIUS). *Subst. Abuse Treat. Prev. Policy* **2011**, *6*, 32. [CrossRef] [PubMed]

68. Prochaska, J.O.; DiClemente, C.C.; Norcross, J.C. In search of how people change. Applications to addictive behaviors. *Am. Psychol.* **1992**, *47*, 1102–1114. [CrossRef] [PubMed]

69. Jiang, Z.; Zhao, X. Brain behavioral systems, self-control and problematic mobile phone use: The moderating role of gender and history of use. *Personal. Individ. Differ.* **2017**, *106*, 111–116. [CrossRef]

70. Liu, Q.; Zhou, Z.; Niu, G.; Fan, C. Mobile phone addiction and sleep quality in adolescents: Mediation and moderation analyses. *Acta Psychol. Sin.* **2017**, *49*, 1524–1536. [CrossRef]

71. Lian, L. Alienation as mediator and moderator of the relationship between virtues and smartphone addiction among Chinese university students. *Int. J. Ment. Health Addict.* **2017**, 1–11. [CrossRef]

72. Gao, T.; Li, J.; Zhang, H.; Gao, J.; Kong, Y.; Hu, Y.; Mei, S. The influence of alexithymia on mobile phone addiction: The role of depression, anxiety and stress. *J. Affect. Disord.* **2018**, *225*, 761–766. [CrossRef] [PubMed]

73. Zhang, Y.; Lu, G.; Liu, Y.; Zhou, Y. Mediating effect of self-identity on relationship between interpersonal adaptation and mobile phone addiction tendency in college students. *Chin. Ment. Health J.* **2017**, *31*, 568–572.

74. Leung, L. Linking psychological attributes to addiction and improper use of the mobile phone among adolescents in Hong Kong. *J. Child. Media* **2008**, *2*, 93–113. [CrossRef]

75. Sanchez-Carbonell, X.; Beranuy, M.; Castellana, M.; Chamarro, A.; Oberst, U. Internet and cell phone addiction: Passing fad or disorder? *Adicciones* **2008**, *20*, 149–159. [CrossRef] [PubMed]

76. Griffiths, M.D.; Nuyens, F. An overview of structural characteristics in problematic videogame playing. *Curr. Addict. Rep.* **2017**, *4*, 272–283. [CrossRef] [PubMed]

77. De-Sola Gutiérrez, J.; Rodríguez de Fonseca, F.; Rubio, G. Cell-Phone Addiction: A Review. *Front. Psychiatry* **2016**, *7*, 175. [CrossRef] [PubMed]

Permissions

All chapters in this book were first published by MDPI; hereby published with permission under the Creative Commons Attribution License or equivalent. Every chapter published in this book has been scrutinized by our experts. Their significance has been extensively debated. The topics covered herein carry significant findings which will fuel the growth of the discipline. They may even be implemented as practical applications or may be referred to as a beginning point for another development.

The contributors of this book come from diverse backgrounds, making this book a truly international effort. This book will bring forth new frontiers with its revolutionizing research information and detailed analysis of the nascent developments around the world.

We would like to thank all the contributing authors for lending their expertise to make the book truly unique. They have played a crucial role in the development of this book. Without their invaluable contributions this book wouldn't have been possible. They have made vital efforts to compile up to date information on the varied aspects of this subject to make this book a valuable addition to the collection of many professionals and students.

This book was conceptualized with the vision of imparting up-to-date information and advanced data in this field. To ensure the same, a matchless editorial board was set up. Every individual on the board went through rigorous rounds of assessment to prove their worth. After which they invested a large part of their time researching and compiling the most relevant data for our readers.

The editorial board has been involved in producing this book since its inception. They have spent rigorous hours researching and exploring the diverse topics which have resulted in the successful publishing of this book. They have passed on their knowledge of decades through this book. To expedite this challenging task, the publisher supported the team at every step. A small team of assistant editors was also appointed to further simplify the editing procedure and attain best results for the readers.

Apart from the editorial board, the designing team has also invested a significant amount of their time in understanding the subject and creating the most relevant covers. They scrutinized every image to scout for the most suitable representation of the subject and create an appropriate cover for the book.

The publishing team has been an ardent support to the editorial, designing and production team. Their endless efforts to recruit the best for this project, has resulted in the accomplishment of this book. They are a veteran in the field of academics and their pool of knowledge is as vast as their experience in printing. Their expertise and guidance has proved useful at every step. Their uncompromising quality standards have made this book an exceptional effort. Their encouragement from time to time has been an inspiration for everyone.

The publisher and the editorial board hope that this book will prove to be a valuable piece of knowledge for researchers, students, practitioners and scholars across the globe.

List of Contributors

So-Young Park
Ewha Institute for Age Integration Research, Ewha Womans University, 52, Ewhayeodae-gil, Seodaemun-gu, Seoul 03760, Korea

Sonam Yang, Hyunseok Jang and So-Youn Park
Kyonggi University, San 94-6, Iui-dong, Yeongtong-gu, Suwon, Kyonggi-do 16227, Korea

Chang-Sik Shin
Daejeon University, 62, Daehak-ro, Dong-gu, Daejeon 34520, Korea

Olatz Lopez-Fernandez
Turning Point, Eastern Health Clinical School, Monash University, 110 Church Street, Richmond VIC 2131, Australia
International Gaming Research Unit, Psychology Department, Nottingham Trent University, Nottingham NG1 4FQ, UK
Laboratory for Experimental Psychopathology, Psychological Sciences Research Institute, Catholic University of Louvain, 1348 Louvain-la-Neuve, Belgium
Monash Addiction Research Centre, Turning Point, Easter Health Clinical School, Monash University, Clayton, VIC 3800, Australia

Beifang Fan, Bo Xie, Huimin Zhang and Yuhua Liao
Department of Psychiatry, Shenzhen Nanshan Center for Chronic Disease Control, Shenzhen 518000, China

Wanxing Wang, Tian Wang, Ciyong Lu and Lan Guo
Department of Medical Statistics and Epidemiology, School of Public Health, Sun Yat-sen University, Guangzhou 510080, China
Guangdong Engineering Technology Research Center of Nutrition Translation, Guangzhou, 510080, China

Montserrat Peris
Department of Personality, Evaluation and Psychological Treatments, University of the Basque Country, 20018 San Sebastian, Spain

Usue de la Barrera and Inmaculada Montoya-Castilla
Department of Personality, Assessment and Psychological Treatment, Faculty of Psychology, University of Valencia, 46010 Valencia, Spain

Konstanze Schoeps
Department of Psychology, Faculty of Health Sciences, European University of Valencia, 46010 Valencia, Spain

Wei Hong, Ru-De Liu, Ronghuan Jiang and Xinchen Fu
Beijing Key Laboratory of Applied Experimental Psychology, National Demonstration Center for Experimental Psychology Education (Beijing Normal University), Faculty of Psychology, Beijing Normal University, Beijing 100875, China

Yi Ding
Graduate School of Education, Fordham University, New York, NY 10023, USA

Rui Zhen
Institute of Psychological Sciences, Hangzhou Normal University, Hangzhou 311121, China

Rafał P. Bartczuk, Michał Wiechetek and Iwona Niewiadomska
Institute of Psychology, The John Paul II Catholic University of Lublin, 20-950 Lublin, Poland

Joanna Chwaszcz
Department of Psychology, Katolicki Uniwersytet Lubelski Jana Pawła II, 20-950 Lublin, Poland
Institute of Psychology, The John Paul II Catholic University of Lublin, 20-950 Lublin, Poland

Lutz Wartberg
Department Psychology, Faculty of Life Sciences, MSH Medical School Hamburg, 20457 Hamburg, Germany

Rudolf Kammerl
Department of Education, Chair for Pedagogy with a Focus on Media Education, Friedrich-Alexander-University Erlangen-Nuremberg, 90478 Nuremberg, Germany

Seongho Min and Min-Hyuk Kim
Department of Psychiatry, Yonsei University Wonju College of Medicine, 20 Ilsan-ro, Gangwon-do, Wonju 26426, Korea

Jinhee Lee and Joung-Sook Ahn
Department of Psychiatry, Yonsei University Wonju College of Medicine, 20 Ilsan-ro, Gangwon-do, Wonju 26426, Korea
Division of Child and Adolescent Psychiatry, Yonsei University Wonju College of Medicine, 20 Ilsan-ro, Gangwon-do, Wonju 26426, Korea

Vega González-Bueso, Juan José Santamaría, Laura Merino, Elena Montero and Joan Ribas
Atención e Investigación en Socioadicciones (AIS), Mental Health and Addictions Network, Generalitat de Catalunya (XHUB), C/Forn-7-9 Local, 08014 Barcelona, Spain

Daniel Fernández
Research and Development Unit, Parc Sanitari Sant Joan de Déu, Fundació Sant Joan de Déu, CIBERSAM, Dr. Antoni Pujadas, 42, Sant Boi de Llobregat, 08830 Barcelona, Spain
School of Mathematics and Statistics, Victoria University of Wellington, Wellington 6140, New Zealand

Hyera Ryu, Ji-Yoon Lee, Aruem Choi and Sunyoung Park
Department of Psychiatry, SMG-SMU Boramae Medical Center, Seoul 07061, Korea

Jung-Seok Choi
Department of Psychiatry, SMG-SMU Boramae Medical Center, Seoul 07061, Korea
Department of Psychiatry and Behavioral Science, Seoul National University College of Medicine, Seoul 03080, Korea

Marta Beranuy and Joaquín González-Cabrera
Faculty of Education, Universidad Internacional de la Rioja (UNIR), Avenida de la Paz, 137, 26006 Logroño, Spain

Juan M. Machimbarrena
Faculty of Psychology, University of the Basque Country (UPV/EHU), Avenida de Tolosa, 70, 20018 Donostia, Spain

M. Asunción Vega-Osés
Faculty of Health Sciences, Universidad Pública de Navarra (UPNA), Calle Cataluña, s/n, 31006 Pamplona, Navarra, Spain

Xavier Carbonell
Faculty of Psychology, Education and Sport Blanquerna, Universitat Ramon Llull. Calle Císter, 34, 08022 Barcelona, Spain

Halley M. Pontes
University of Tasmania, School of Psychological Sciences, Newnham Campus, Building O, Launceston TAS 7250, Australia
The International Cyberpsychology and Addictions Research Laboratory (iCARL), University of Tasmania, Launceston TAS 7250, Australia
International Gaming Research Unit, Psychology Department, Nottingham Trent University, Nottingham NG1 4FQ, UK

Mi Jung Rho and In Young Choi
Department of Medical Informatics, College of Medicine, The Catholic University of Korea, Seoul 06591, Korea
Catholic Institute for Healthcare Management and Graduate School of Healthcare Management and Policy, The Catholic University of Korea, Seoul 06591, Korea

Hyeseon Lee and Taek-Ho Lee
Department of Industrial & Management Engineering, Pohang University of Science and Technology, Pohang 37673, Korea

Hyun Cho
Department of Psychology, Korea University, Seoul 02841, Korea
Addiction Research Institute, Department of Psychiatry, Seoul St. Mary's Hospital, College of Medicine, The Catholic University of Korea, Seoul 06591, Korea

DongJin Jung and Dai-Jin Kim
Addiction Research Institute, Department of Psychiatry, Seoul St. Mary's Hospital, College of Medicine, The Catholic University of Korea, Seoul 06591, Korea
Department of Psychiatry, Seoul St. Mary's Hospital, College of Medicine, The Catholic University of Korea, Seoul 06591, Korea

Mark D. Griffiths, Christopher Dawes and Lucy V. Justice
International Gaming Research Unit, Psychology Department, Nottingham Trent University, Nottingham NG1 4FQ, UK

Daria J. Kuss
International Gaming Research Unit, Cyberpsychology Research Group, Psychology Department, Nottingham Trent University, Nottingham NG1 4FQ, UK

Niko Männikkö
Department of Social Services and Rehabilitation, Oulu University of Applied Sciences, 90220 Oulu, Finland

Maria Kääriäinen
Research Unit of Nursing Science and Health Management, University of Oulu and Oulu University Hospital, 90014 Oulu, Finland

Hans-Jürgen Rumpf, Anja Bischof and Ann-Kathrin Gässler
Department for Psychiatry and Psychotherapy, University of Lübeck, 23538 Lübeck, Germany

Lucia Romo and Yannick Morvan
EA 4430 Clinique Psychanalyse Développement (CLIPSYD), Université Paris Nanterre, France; U894 Centre de Psychiatrie et Neurosciences, (CPN), Inserm, 92000 Paris, France

Laurence Kern
EA 2931, Centre de Recherches sur le Sport et le Mouvement (CESRM), Université Paris Nanterre, 92000 Nanterre, France

Amélie Rousseau
Psychology Department, PSITEC EA 4074, Université Lille Nord de France, 59650 Villeneuve d'Ascq, France

Pierluigi Graziani
LPS EA 849, Aix-Marseille University, 13007 Marseille, France
Psychologie, Langues, Lettres et Histoire Département, University of Nîmes, 30000 Nîmes, France

Zsolt Demetrovics and Orsolya Király
Institute of Psychology, ELTE Eötvös Loránd University, 1064 Budapest, Hungary

Adriano Schimmenti and Alessia Passanisi
Faculty of Human and Social Sciences, UKE—Kore University of Enna, Cittadella Universitaria, 94100 Enna, Italy

Bernadeta Lelonek-Kuleta
Department of Family Science and Social Work, Katolicki Uniwersytet Lubelski Jana Pawła II, 20-950 Lublin, Poland
Institute of Psychology, The John Paul II Catholic University of Lublin, 20-950 Lublin, Poland

Mariano Chóliz
Department of Basic Psychology, University of Valencia, 46010 Valencia, Spain

Juan José Zacarés and Emilia Serra
Department of Developmental and Educational Psychology, University of Valencia, 46010 Valencia, Spain

Magali Dufour
Service de Toxicomanie, Faculte de medicine Université de Sherbrooke, Longueuil, Qc, J4K 0A8, Canada

Lucien Rochat
Department of Psychology and Educational Sciences, University of Geneva, 1205 Geneva, Switzerland

Daniele Zullino and Sophia Achab
Department of Psychiatry—Research Unit Addictive Disorders, University of Geneva, 1205 Geneva, Switzerland
Department of Mental Health and Psychiatry—Addiction Division, University Hospitals of Geneva, 1205 Geneva, Switzerland

Nils Inge Landrø
Clinical Neuroscience Research Group, Department of Psychology, University of Oslo, 0317 Oslo, Norway

Eva Suryani
Department Psychiatry and Behavior, School of Medicine and Health Science, Atma Jaya Catholic University of Indonesia, Jakarta 14440, Indonesia

Julia M. Hormes
Department of Psychology, University at Albany State University of New York, Albany, NY, USA

Javier Ponce Terashima
University Hospitals Cleveland Medical Center/Case Western Reserve University, Cleveland, OH 44106, USA

Joël Billieux
Laboratory for Experimental Psychopathology, Psychological Sciences Research Institute, Université Catholique de Louvain, 1348 Louvain-la-Neuve, Belgium
Department of Mental Health and Psychiatry—Addiction Division, University Hospitals of Geneva, 1205 Geneva, Switzerland
Addictive and Compulsive Behaviours Lab (ACB-lab), Institute for Health and Behaviour, University of Luxembourg, 4366 Esch-sur-Alzette, Luxembourg

Index